THE HEALTHY HOUSE

How to Buy One, How to Build One, How to Cure a "Sick" One

by John Bower

A Lyle Stuart Book
Published by Carol Publishing Group

First Carol Publishing Group Edition 1991

Copyright © 1989 by John Bower

A Lyle Stuart Book
Published by Carol Publishing Group
Lyle Stuart is a registered trademark of Carol Communications, Inc.

Editorial Offices   Sales & Distribution Offices
600 Madison Avenue   120 Enterprise Avenue
New York, NY 10022   Secaucus, NJ 07094

In Canada: Musson Book Company
A division of General Publishing Co. Limited
Don Mills, Ontario

Queries regarding rights and permissions
should be addressed to: Carol Publishing Group,
600 Madison Avenue, New York, NY 10022

Manufactured in the United States of America
10 9 8 7 6 5 4 3 2 1

Carol Publishing Group books are available at special discounts
for bulk purchases, for sales promotions, fund raising, or
educational purposes. Special editions can also be created to
specifications. For details contact: Special Sales Department,
Carol Publishing Group, 120 Enterprise Ave., Secaucus, NJ 07094

Library of Congress Cataloging-in-Publication Data

Bower, John.
       The healthy house : How to buy one, how to build one, how to cure
    a "sick" one / by John Bower.
             p.   cm.
        Bibliography : p.
        Includes index.
        ISBN 0-8184-0550-3
        1. Housing and health. 2. Indoor pollution -- Health aspects.
    3. Consumer education. I. Title.
    RA770.5.B69   1989   88-35147
    613'.5--dc 19   CIP

To Lynn, who suggested that I write this book, who encouraged me to persevere, who offered many helpful suggestions, and who desperately needed a non-toxic house in order to regain her health

Contents

Disclaimer

No materials and techniques mentioned herein constitute medical advice. The listing of a particular manufacturer's product is not an endorsement of that product.

Since individual tolerances to pollutants vary considerably, and since manufacturing processes change periodically, personal testing of materials is recommended when sensitivities are severe. However, even careful testing of small samples cannot simulate the exposure found in a completed house where larger surface areas and synergistic effects can be encountered. For extremely sensitive people, this should be done under the supervision of a physician. Testing procedures are covered in Appendix II.

READER INPUT

The science of building healthy houses is still relatively new and this book represents the best knowledge currently available. However, manufacturers are continually introducing new products and materials into the marketplace. Some will be healthy and, unfortunately, some will not. If you, the reader, have found materials or construction methods that should be included in a future edition of *The Healthy House*, I would appreciate hearing from you. I am also interested in materials that you have found to be particularly offensive. Your input can be invaluable. Please send your suggestions to:

John Bower
Ecologically Safe Homes
7471 N. Shiloh Rd.
Unionville, IN 47468

Introduction

Your house is not simply a benign structure that you make mortgage payments on and enter or leave at will. It is an active, enclosed system, and when you are inside it you are an integral part of that system. If your house is like most of the others being built in the United States today, it is composed of numerous individual components, many of which contain highly toxic chemicals. The carpeting and floor tile are chemically treated to render them stain resistant. The wall covering is chemically treated with mold inhibitors. The windows are made with chemically treated wood. These materials can be harmful in their own right, but when they outgas into the living space of your house, they can interact to form new toxic compounds.

Enter you and your family. You have now linked into this system for better or worse. Probably worse. When the components of your home outgas or give off vapors, they are contaminating the indoor air. These chemicals are then inhaled by the occupants. Some may be absorbed through the skin. There is an old adage that states, "You are what you eat." A contemporary version could be just as accurately stated, "You are what you live in." When you consider the number of hours spent in your home, it only makes sense to build it so that its healthfulness benefits your own.

The federal government has not yet begun to promote this concept. Many products with known negative health effects are readily available and are being advertised and sold by manufacturers and lumberyards. Examples include particle board (formaldehyde) and salt-treated lumber (arsenic). More concerned nations like West Germany and Sweden emphasize the importance of more healthful building products and techniques. They are cognizant of the fact that the ill health of their citizens is often related to their houses.

What ill effects can you expect by becoming a part of your toxic house system? Actually, you may experience anything from such minor complaints as headaches, insomnia, and skin rashes to severe joint pain, anxiety, and depression. At the present time much of the medical community is aware of the true cause-and-effect relationship; however, there is a growing minority of health care professionals who are well informed about the devastating consequences of living inside modern houses. Architects are becoming aware as well and "sick building" articles are now appearing in the journals of both of these professional groups.

Safe alternatives to the readily available toxic materials and practices *are* available. It takes only a little more time, planning, and money (but not much) to build a safe house instead of one that will be hazardous to your health. When you consider the benefits to your well-being that such a house can provide, the added commitment will seem insignificant indeed.

Based on documentation from a variety of sources, this book will help you become familiar with problems created by traditional building practices. It will also present, in a thorough manner, healthier alternatives. Addresses of all organizations and suppliers shown in bold type are listed in Appendix III.

This not a step-by-step instruction book on how to build one particular home, but rather, a reference book that can aid you and your contractor in building the type of home you require.

Here's to your house and your health!

JOHN BOWER

THE HEALTHY HOUSE

Chapter 1

Indoor Air Quality

People in the United States spend between 80 and 90 percent of their time indoors. This time may be divided between home, school, and workplace, or in the case of a child, the sick, or the elderly, it may be almost entirely in one location—the home. Our homes may be our castles, yet they hardly protect us from the many contaminants in the air. Indoor levels of organic chemicals have been shown to be many times the level in the air outside.[1,2,3] While no two houses are alike, it is becoming apparent that, in general, the air in most of them is much more dangerous than was believed just a few years ago, and the trend is getting worse.

The **Environmental Protection Agency (EPA)** regulates the outdoor air quality. Some people criticize the **EPA** for not doing its job very well, but the outdoor air quality has improved, especially in major metropolitan areas. Yet, more work needs to be done. From the point of view of indoor air pollution, the **EPA** has no regulations whatsoever since, by law, it is required to regulate outdoor air quality only. The **Occupational Safety and Health Administration (OSHA)** is charged with regulating air quality in the workplace, where there have also been improvements. However, there is evidence to suggest that 15–20 percent of the population will react to chemical exposures below the established thresholds.[4]

In our homes, it seems as though we are left to our own defenses when it comes to indoor air quality. The **Consumer Products Safety Commission (CPSC)** has jurisdiction over a few sources of indoor air pollution, yet the air quality continues to deteriorate. Measurements of various pollutants within houses can be extremely high, often many times that allowed by regulation in the outside air or in the workplace. Since our houses are where we spend the most time, this could easily evolve into the greatest health threat of our time. Some of the health problems that are currently seen are somewhat minor, such as sinus congestion or joint pain, while others are major, ranging from severe depression to death.

Modern Construction Practices

Houses used to be built of native materials. If there were a lot of stones lying around, they were used in building construction. If trees were plentiful, houses were constructed of wood. Eskimos built igloos with what was available to them. Today, our building materials are very similar throughout the civilized world. Plywood, asphalt shingles, and 2×4s are a common sight at construction projects everywhere. These almost universally used materials can lead to indoor air pollution and hence ill health.

Building with 2×4s was invented early in the nineteenth century. At that time they were cut locally out of whatever wood was handy. It is not uncommon to find an old house framed out of oak or maple if that was what happened to be growing nearby. Today, hardwood lumber is used primarily for furniture or it is burned in wood stoves; it is rarely used for construction. Currently, softwood is the predominant construction material and some drawbacks from a health point of view have been noted. With the invention of modern adhesives, plywood and particle board are widely used in modern buildings. They emit toxic formaldehyde fumes. Simulated woodgrain plastic doors, synthetic paints, synthetic carpeting, caulking, and insulation all contribute to an indoor environment that has never existed before.

With the advent of interior plumbing and electricity, we have introduced additional potential pollutants into our living space. The water that is piped into our houses is often contaminated with various chemicals which can not only be ingested but can be absorbed through the skin. Some volatile chemicals are vaporized and we inhale them during a hot shower. Electricity has given us many conveniences, including such things as the continuous cleaning oven which emits various toxic fumes whenever it is turned on. The plastic insulation on electrical wiring has also been known to outgas bothersome fumes.

When people cooked over an open fire there was usually plenty of ventilation. Moving indoors created indoor air pollution. Soot on the ceilings of prehistoric cave dwellings attests to the fact that we have been polluting the indoor air for many thousands of years. Today we have totally integrated our fires into our houses, most of which are very poorly ventilated. Unfortunately, natural gas, fuel oil, kerosene, and burning wood are very much a part of modern houses. It is no wonder that the major indoor air pollutants are products of combustion. Attached garages allow more combustion products to enter the living space. Often the garage is located directly under a bedroom; thus, while we are asleep we breathe the various odors given off by the family car, the lawn mower, and miscellaneous insecticides and solvents stored there.

Mobile Homes

Mobile homes definitely fulfill a housing need but they are notorious for emitting various chemicals into the indoor air. The most prevalent is, of course, formaldehyde. It is emitted from the insulation, particle board, wall paneling, and carpeting, and since most newer mobile homes are built fairly tight and energy-efficient, it can't easily escape. Some people have become so affected by the formaldehyde that upon moving out of their mobile home, they have found that they are so sensitized to other chemicals that they have trouble finding *any* tolerable housing.

Our Surroundings

In the distant past everyone lived in rural areas. With the formation of cities, diseases began to become prevalent as people lived close together. Streets and streams became open sewers, hence the water supply became tainted. Since fire was needed by all to keep warm and for cooking, the air began to be fouled as well. Today, we have the addition of automobile exhaust, factory emissions, lawn chemicals, agricultural chemicals, and cleaning chemicals. With the larger populations in the cities, we often have to drive for many miles before we come across any clean air.

Post 1970s

Since the energy crisis of the 1970s, we have added more insulation to tighten up our houses. The result is that many pollutants can no longer leak out through the cracks. We have, in effect, sealed ourselves inside our homes with no fresh air, somewhat like placing plastic bags over our heads. Fortunately, there are energy-efficient ways to have fresh air and also low energy bills. There is nothing inherently wrong with an energy-efficient house as long as fresh air is considered. Space capsules and submarines are among the tightest "houses" ever constructed and the air quality in them is good. With the number of potential pollutants in existence today, **NASA** and the Navy have realized the importance of limiting the use of indoor pollution sources.

Solar designs have become popular, as have underground houses. If treated correctly, these can provide healthful environments; if, however, the designer is inexperienced, they can be quite unhealthy. Someone with mold sensitivity should be very cautious about having a greenhouse as part of the living space. Similarly, the rock heat storage systems sometimes used in solar designs can introduce radon or mold spores into the living space. Underground houses can also be havens for mold if improperly designed. However, if health is considered, virtually any style or type house can be nonpolluting.

Modern Furnishings

It is amazing how many of our modern furnishings could not have existed a century ago. Synthetic fabrics, polyester padding, urethane foam, plastic tables, plywood shelving, plastic television cabinets, and sophisticated electronic equipment of every description all have the potential to pollute the indoor air. Washing machines smell like synthetic detergent. Dryers smell like fabric softener. There is mold in the drip pan under the self-defrosting refrigerator. Our beds are treated with flame retardants and the sheets are treated with formaldehyde. The paint on the wall is not a paint but a potentially dangerous chemical soup. Many people are made ill by all of these modern furnishings, and only a relatively few are aware of the cause-and-effect relationship. They often live with the muscle aches, run-down feeling, depression, and anxiety without realizing that their home is the cause of their ills.

An even more insidious lists of pollutants is to be found under the kitchen sink, in the laundry room, and on the shelf in the garage. Detergents, spot cleaners, ammonia, scouring powder, dishwashing liquid, drain cleaners, insecticides, mouse poisons, hair spray, air fresheners, cosmetics, antiperspirants, soaps, shampoos, mouthwash, disinfectants, glass cleaners, mothballs, and fabric softeners all have the potential to poison our indoor air. Fortunately, many people are now using more natural products and are finding many safe alternatives to the hazardous, toxic chemicals. Often, the natural alternatives are not only more healthful, they may be less expensive and can work better.

Outgassing

Outgassing refers to the emission of gases during the aging and degradation of a material. These gases are often toxic and even in small doses can have grave consequences as far as our health is concerned. The new car smell and the film that forms on the inside of the windshield are a result of the plastic interior's outgassing. The plastic surface is in effect evaporating and various gases are released into the air that we breathe. Most of the modern materials created in the last 50 years outgas to some degree. This outgassing accounts for a tremendous amount of indoor air pollution which can easily result in sinus and lung irritation. Some of the chemicals being released are so powerful that they can damage the immune system. Formaldehyde is very often outgassed from modern buildings materials, but there are many other chemicals being outgassed that have hardly been studied at all. Most of the materials recommended in this book have been shown to have minimal outgassing characteristics.

Testing for outgassing is done in special chambers that allow scientists to accurately determine what chemicals are given off by different substances. There are a number of these chambers around the country and they are revealing frightening information about the modern materials that we have begun to take for granted. The leader in this research is **NASA**.

National Aeronautics and Space Administration

NASA has done extensive research into the safety of materials used in spacecraft. Its scientists are concerned not only with the health effects inside the closed atmosphere in which astronauts live and work, but also with the question of how these chemicals affect the sensitive electronic and optical equipment. Since astronauts must perform many varied and detailed operations while on a mission, an important aspect of concern is impairment of function. A less than optimum atmosphere inside a spacecraft can mean that they will not be able to perform at peak efficiency.

Virtually everything that goes into a spacecraft is tested for its particular outgassing characteristics. Everything from fabric, paint, and caulking to adhesives, plastics, and foams is included in their computerized database.

NASA's testing is done in a closed chamber in which the item to be tested is heated to 120°F for 72 hours. This causes the volatile materials to be outgassed at an accelerated rate. The gases are then analyzed and quantified. Vacuum testing involves placing materials in a similar chamber where a vacuum actually sucks out the various volatile chemicals that would normally outgas at a much slower rate. Actual air samples taken during spaceflights are also analyzed. A typical computer printout will list the material name, manufacturer, generic description, testing data, and the chemicals that were outgassed with amounts. As an example, one particular adhesive was found to give off the following gases:[5]

Carbon monoxide	C5 saturated and unsaturated
Formaldehyde	aliphatic hydrocarbons
Acetaldehyde	2-butanone
Methanol	Methyl propionate
Methyl formulate	Benzene
Ethanol	Methyl isobutenate
2-propanone	Methylbenzene
2-propanol	Hexamethylcyclotrisiloxane

Obviously, there is a lot of valuable information in NASA's database. However, much of it is useful only to the space program because the materials tested are usually not encountered by the general public. Many of the products making up homes cannot be used in a spacecraft because of excessive outgassing. Residential fiberglass insulation outgasses too much formaldehyde to be used by NASA, yet we continue to install it in our homes with little thought as to the consequences. As with much of the other information gained by the space program, these data will undoubtedly eventually lead to many applications in the private sector. In the meantime, the answer for the general public is to use products that have little or no outgassing characteristics. Unfortunately, there are many people already exhibiting sensitivities to various outgassed chemicals. For them, avoidance is of prime importance.

Environmental Protection Agency

The **EPA** has developed a computerized database for "Indoor Air Source Emissions."[6] This has been done to better transfer valuable data to researchers, policymakers, and consumers' groups. Although not responsible for *control* of indoor air, the **EPA** has been mandated to *study* indoor air quality. This research includes measurement and monitoring, health effects, and source information. Extensive bibliographies and literature reviews have been assembled and are available to researchers in the field.[7,8,9] These contain reports and data from all over the world.

Although not nearly as extensive as **NASA**'s database, the **EPA**'s contains information more pertinent to the indoor air pollution that we breathe every day. Emissions and outgassing characteristics from such things as kerosene heaters, vinyl floor tiles, gas ranges, wall paneling, ceiling tiles, and wood stoves have been studied.

The **EPA** has developed its own Environmental Test Chamber. The studies being done differ in methodology from the **NASA** testing, but the goal is the same—to determine the chemicals that are outgassed from various materials.

Major Pollutants

Pollutants can be divided into two major groups: gases and particulates. Gases can come from a variety of natural processes such as animal and human metabolism, or geographic phenomena such as volcanoes or swamps, etc. Gases are also being generated by man-made products and activities. Combustion fumes, pesticide applications, and outgassing from synthetic products account for a tremendous amount of gaseous pollution in our homes.

Particulates are simply small particles of various materials that are floating around in the air. Asbestos falls into this category, as do pollens, mold spores, infectious agents, and house dust. Depending on their size, particulates may be filtered out of the air by the nose and sinuses, or they may travel deeply into the lungs. Wood and tobacco smoke are major sources of particulates. Cigarette smoke can contain highly toxic heavy metals such as cadmium and radioactive polonium. About 40 pounds of particulate dust will settle in an average six-room house every year.[10]

Most books and articles on indoor air pollution deal with only a handful of the substances that can affect health. The major indoor air pollutants are usually listed as including: carbon monoxide, carbon dioxide, sulphur dioxide, nitrogen dioxide, asbestos, radon, particulates, ozone, and formaldehyde. These pollutants have been studied fairly extensively and their effects are pretty well agreed upon. They are in fact the major pollutants. But the list of actual pollutants inside typical homes and offices can number in the hundreds.

Various organic chemicals, hydrocarbons, and their derivatives are quite common in the indoor air. An organic chemical, by definition, is one that contains carbon in combination with other atoms. Formaldehyde is one of the most commonly encountered organic chemicals. It contains one carbon, two hydrogen, and one oxygen atom. A hydrocarbon is a type of organic chemical that contains only atoms of carbon and hydrogen. Benzene is a hydrocarbon containing 6 carbon atoms and 6 hydrogen atoms.

A complete list of all the possible indoor air pollutants would take many pages and would be meaningless to anyone but a chemist. The pollutants resemble alphabet soup more than chemicals that we breathe every day in our homes: aliphatics, alkylbenzenes, keytones, polycyclic aromatics, chlorinated hydrocarbons, terpenes, alkanes, xylene, butylacetate, ethoxyethylacetate, etc., etc. The effects of many of these chemical are poorly understood; yet there are countless people who have eliminated them from their lives and seen dramatic improvements in their health.

Combustion By-Products

Particulates are common pollutants associated with combustion. The soot and ash seen leaving a chimney are typical examples. Several gases are also products of combustion. Since so many homes have some type of combustion source in them, these by-products are very serious indoor air pollutants.

Carbon monoxide is produced by the incomplete combustion of such materials as natural gas, wood, coal, oil, kerosene, gasoline, and tobacco. It is colorless, odorless, and especially deadly. The hemoglobin in our blood will take up carbon monoxide much more readily than oxygen, so relatively small amounts in the air can translate into deadly amounts in the bloodstream. The resulting oxygen deficiency can result in impaired vision and brain function, irregular heartbeat, headaches, nausea, weakness, confusion, and death.

Carbon dioxide is also colorless and odorless. It is formed during the combustion of carbon containing fuels and is also produced as a

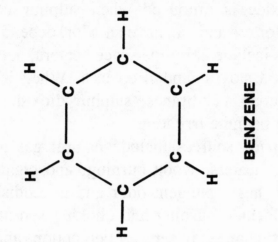

BENZENE

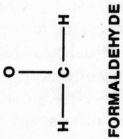

FORMALDEHYDE

Organic Chemicals

result of metabolism. Every time we exhale, we add more carbon dioxide to the air. Kerosene space heaters can introduce very high levels, causing symptoms such as: headaches, loss of judgment, dizziness, shortness of breath, or asphyxiation.

Sulphur dioxide is produced when sulphur containing fuels is burned. It is colorless and can have an odor, depending on the concentration. Sources include kerosene space heaters, natural gas or fuel oil appliances, wood stoves, and fireplaces. When it comes in contact with moist mucous membranes, sulphur dioxide forms sulphurous acid, which can be quite irritating.

Nitrogen dioxide sources include natural gas and fuel oil appliances, kerosene heaters, wood burning, and cigarettes. It is highly toxic, irritating, has a pungent odor and is reddish brown in color. Health effects include burning and choking sensations in the upper respiratory tract, changes in sensory perception, and irritation of eyes and skin.

Asbestos

Asbestos is a mineral that will separate into strong, thin fibers. It has been used in a wide variety of products because of its durability and heat-resistant qualities. Nearly 30 million tons have been used in the United States since the turn of the century. In some of its uses it is highly unlikely that it will cause any health problems. However, there are many applications where microscopic particles can be released into the air. Breathing these particles can result in asbestosis, a serious lung disease, or various forms of cancer. Unfortunately, lung disease may not be apparent until 15–20 years after exposure. In a number of cases, schools, libraries, offices, and hospitals have had to be closed due to asbestos in the air. Cleanup must be done with much care, since it often results in more asbestos being released than if nothing was done at all.

If an asbestos-containing product is solid and not disintegrating it is unlikely that it will release fibers. Sometimes a sealant can be sprayed on to hold the loose fibers in place. Various products such as "Crystal Aire II" by **Pace Industries** can be used for this purpose. Asbestos removal can be a very involved process, requiring great care.[11] If removal is necessary, the **Consumer Product Safety Commission (CPSC)** has a free booklet, *Asbestos in the Home*, that lists some general guidelines. Here it is stressed that anything containing asbestos fibers should be moistened before removal in order to prevent the very small particles from becoming airborne.[12] A more comprehensive booklet is available from the **EPA**.[13]

Various sources of asbestos in houses will be discussed in appropriate chapters in this book. In order to positively identify a material as containing asbestos, a sample should be submitted to a laboratory for analysis. The **CPSC** has a toll-free telephone number that can be used to locate a testing lab and to obtain information on sampling procedures. Other information can be obtained from the **Asbestos Information Center**.

Radon

Radon is a naturally occurring radioactive gas. It is odorless and colorless and is found in the soil in various parts of the country. When radon filters through the ground and enters a house, it goes through a radioactive decay process. It is when these decay products are breathed into the lungs that there is an increased risk of developing lung cancer. The **EPA** estimates that up to 20,000 lung cancer deaths each year are attributable to radon.

The primary methods of controlling radon involve ventilation and sealing entry points. Chapter 8 will discuss factors related to ventilation. Since radon enters a house primarily from the soil, the foundation system will have a major bearing on the amount of radon infiltration that takes place. Chapter 10 will cover this aspect more thoroughly. While radon can be emitted from some building materials, it is doubtful that they are major contributors,[14] although in a few instances they can certainly result in high levels. For example, if concrete is made with rock containing radium, it can release radon. If radon is found to be emanating from building materials, two coats of oil or emulsion paint can reduce emissions by about 15 times. However, several nails penetrating the paint can drop the reduction rate from 15 to 4.[15]

Radon is relatively easy to test for in the indoor air and if found, the risk can usually be minimized. For up-to-date information on testing devices, contact local or state Boards of Health.

Ozone

Ozone is a naturally occurring oxygen compound that exists in the upper atmosphere. It is a highly reactive gas with a pungent odor that can cause coughing, choking, headaches, and severe fatigue.[16] Other symptoms of exposure include eye, skin, and mucous membrane irritation. It can cause a breakdown of red blood cells which can contribute to breathing difficulties. Blurred vision and chromosomal aberrations have also been noted. Art galleries have reported that ozone can lead to deterioration of artwork.[17] Ozone can occur in the indoor air as a result of ultraviolet light or sparks from electric motors, electronic air cleaners, or negative ion generators. It is also a component of smog and can be given off by copying machines.

Formaldehyde

Formaldehyde is one of the most insidious of all the indoor air pollutants. It is a colorless gas that has a pungent odor only at very high concentrations. Symptoms of exposure can vary considerably, ranging from burning of eyes, tightness in chest, and headaches, to asthmatic attacks, depression, and death. Menstrual disorders of various types have been associated with formaldehyde exposure[18] and it has been shown to be a potent sensitizer. Exposure to formaldehyde can cause an individual to become sensitive to a wide variety of other chemicals that were previously not problematic. The effects of this can be devastating, and many people have been forced to move out of their homes into almost sterile environments in order to regain their health. According to an article in the *Journal of the American Medical Association*, "It has been suggested that between 4 percent and 8 percent of the population could become sensitized to formaldehyde and experience increasingly severe and prolonged reactions to diminishing levels of the substance."[19]

Formaldehyde has been shown to be carcinogenic and mutagenic in animals, and since animal studies can often be extrapolated to include human beings, the **National Institutes of Health and Safety** has recommended that "formaldehyde be handled as a potential occupational carcinogen."[20] However, in spite of long-term cancer concerns, it is becoming apparent that the chronic irritating symptoms associated with residential exposure and the sensitizing characteristics are a very real and more immediate public health problem.[21]

Formaldehyde is very cheap and can be used in a wide variety of applications. It is released from products such as permanent press fabrics, carpeting, particle board, plywood, insulation, paints, shampoos, and plastics. It is also found in tobacco smoke. With six billion pounds being produced annually,[22] it is a very difficult chemical to escape from.

While formaldehyde levels in homes will decrease considerably with time, if occupants have become sensitized to its effects, there may be no corresponding decrease in symptoms. Estimates of the half-life of formaldehyde outgassing range up to six years; however, this can vary substantially depending on the particular product and the geographic location.[23] As an example, the emissions of a formaldehyde source with a half-life of three years should be reduced to approximately 6 percent of the original level after a 12-year period.   If the half-life was six years it would take a total of 24 years to reach the 6 percent reduction level of emissions.

The best method of control involves actually removing the sources of formaldehyde from the house. This can be quite expensive if the source is insulation, particle-board subflooring, or kitchen cabinets. Since the outgassing rate is dependent on temperature and humidity, simply lowering the thermostat and not using a humidifier can significantly reduce emissions. Some of the sealants described in Chapter 19 can also be effective, as can air purifiers discussed in Chapter 22. Increased ventilation rates can also help.

There is an ammonia fumigation method of permanently reducing the high formaldehyde levels that are often found in mobile homes. This process uses a very strong, toxic ammonia solution (not household ammonia) and it has resulted in a 60 percent reduction in formaldehyde levels.[24] Since this procedure is potentially so toxic, it should only be done by a qualified person, wearing a respirator, and the house will need to remain unoccupied during the treatment. Ammonia fumigation will result in a fine dust of hexamethylene tetramine settling on interior surfaces. This is the end product of the reaction between the formaldehyde and the ammonia and should be thoroughly cleaned up after the treatment.

People as Pollution Sources
Besides occasionally smelling like goats, people and their activities can give off a wide variety of materials that can affect human health. It is widely known that viruses and bacteria can be passed from one person to another. Smallpox, measles, yeast infections, and AIDS are some obvious diseases that come to mind. Human activities such as using household cleaners and smoking are other clear sources of pollu-

tion; there are also a number of different chemicals that can be given off by human beings and animals as a part of metabolism that can contribute to indoor air pollution. A possible list could include:[25]

Acetone	Diethylketone
Acetaldehyde	Ethyl Acetate
Acetic Acid	Ethyl Alcohol
Allyl Alcohol	Hydrogen Sulfide
Amyl Alcohol	Lactic Acid
Ammonia	Methane
Butyric Acid	Methyl Alcohol
Carbon Dioxide	Phenol
Carbon Monoxide	Toluene

These are given off as normal by-products of living creatures. They are not necessarily associated with illness, but some people can react quickly to small amounts of these chemicals. It gives new meaning to the phrase, "You make me sick."

Synergism

Synergism refers to the joint action of two substances. With synergism, 2+2 may equal 8. In other words, the combined action may be greater than the sum of the individual actions. We have all heard about the danger of mixing alcohol and barbiturates. Together they can easily result in death, yet individually they are not nearly so potent. Chemicals are rarely studied together because the number of possible combinations would be astronomical. With hundreds of possible indoor air pollutants, many can and do act synergistically.

Tobacco smoke and radon gas are an example. When both are present in a room, the combined effect is considerably higher than the sum of the individual effects. The reason for this particular synergistic response is that radon tends to cling to the cigarette smoke particulates in the air and much more radon is then breathed into the lungs. When there is no smoke in a room, many of the radioactive particles attach to walls and furnishings where they decay harmlessly.

Summary

There are literally hundreds of other pollutants floating around in the air of our homes, both naturally occurring and man-made. Sometimes they are in relatively small concentrations and cause only subtle health effects. Most of these chemicals haven't been studied very thoroughly because they simply haven't been around long enough. Most have been invented since World War II and many more are being invented daily. "New and improved" actually means "new and improved, with unknown health effects." While the general population isn't immediately bothered by these lesser pollutants, there is an increasingly large segment of society that has been sensitized to them by such things as formaldehyde. These people actually react to so many different chemicals and in such small doses that they are often termed "allergic to the 20th century." The devastating effects on their lives should be a warning to the rest us about the dangers of these many substances that we have so readily accepted.

Chapter 2

Building-Related Illness

Building-related illness and sick-building syndrome refer to conditions that have only recently been discussed in the medical literature. Technically, a broken leg could be considered a building-related illness if it resulted from a fall down a flight of stairs. However, this condition usually refers to a disease that is caused by something in the air inside a building. The causes of building-related illness are both simple and complex. Obviously, the major indoor pollutants already discussed contribute to illness. They are certainly more prevalent today than at any other time in history and many more pollutants are being invented daily.

Symptoms

The symptoms of building-related illness can be many and varied. Legionnaires' disease results from exposure to a specific bacterium that has been found in damp locations, most notably commercial air conditioning systems. Typical symptoms include pneumonia, cough, fatigue, fever, muscle aches, nausea, etc.[1] It has also been known to result in death. Radon and asbestos exposure can be fatal as well. While death is certainly the ultimate symptom that anyone can experience, there is increasing concern over the many other "lesser" types of building-related maladies that are much more common.

The many modern chemicals in our home can cause symptoms such as uncoordination, dizziness, fatigue, nervousness, headaches, joint and muscle pain, abdominal pain, etc.[2] According to the **World Health Organization**, the following are common symptoms of the sick-building syndrome:[3]

Irritation of eye, nose, and throat
Dry mucous membranes and skin.
Erythema.
Mental fatigue, headache.
Airway infections, cough.
Hoarseness of voice, wheezing.
Unspecified hyperactivity.
Nausea, dizziness.

Allergies may be due to the various types of wood that houses are built of, as well as to house dust that is generated by different building materials. Some methods of construction can inadvertently promote mold growth, and incorrectly designed ventilation systems can bring pollen or mold spores indoors and distribute them throughout the house.

Building materials containing heavy metals such as lead paint or arsenic-treated lumber can poison the occupants. While small exposures may have no immediately apparent effect, these toxins can build up in our systems over the years, eventually resulting in illness. Many of the synthetic cleaning products that are used to maintain our homes are considered hazardous wastes. They are legally not allowed to be placed in sanitary landfills, yet we fill our homes with their odors.

Many people seem overly concerned about the carcinogens that are to be found in houses. It is sometimes assumed that if a material doesn't cause cancer, then it must be safe. Unfortunately, some indoor pollutants are teratogenic, meaning that they can result in birth defects such as deformities or serious malformations. Those that are fetotoxic can result in death to unborn children.[4] Others may cause chromosomal damage that will show up in future generations. Heart disease and damage to the immune system are other common negative effects of indoor air pollutants. People sensitized by such things as formaldehyde often report many types of reactions to the volatile chemicals in the air. Some are so sensitive to the modern materials in their environment that they must live in very restricted surroundings in order to remain free of symptoms.

Practically every material commonly used in modern building construction can result in some type of illness. Fortunately, there are many ways to minimize the risk by carefully selecting materials and building techniques.

Increased Sensitivity

People seem to be exhibiting more symptoms related to their environment than in the past. Allergies are more common today than just 50 years ago,[5] and sensitivities to outgassed chemicals are increasingly being recognized. It has been suggested that one reason for this apparent increased sensitivity is that the average citizen of today is genetically and biologically different from the average citizen of generations past.[6] This is because the food that we eat and the air that we breathe are totally different than that to which human beings have adapted over thousands of years. Our bodies are trying to adjust to a 20th-century environment that is radically different from any other environment in human history.

Two or three generations of eating prepared food, processed flour, and food additives have resulted in subtle changes in our bodies. Sugar is no longer an occasional treat, it is a daily staple. Manufactured foods abound, with less nutritional value than the whole, real foods that they have replaced. It is estimated that the average individual consumes at least one gallon of fungicides, bleaches, dyes, antibiotics, preservatives, moisturizers, and emulsifiers per year.[7] As a result of years of eating less nutritious foods and food additives, our systems no longer have the stamina to resist the assaults of environmental pollutants. The many negative health effects of our modern diet and life-style have been well documented by Charles T. McGee in *How to Survive Modern Technology*.[8]

The air that we breathe every day, both indoors and outdoors, is contaminated with chemicals that have never existed before. This means that our lungs are constantly required to deal with an unnatural pollutant burden. This stress is occurring every minute of every day and results in our bodies having less ability to handle an acute pollution emergency. This constant exposure has resulted in people having less resiliency than they had in the past, and more illness. Much of this illness is attributable to the toxic, allergenic, and carcinogenic materials that we have been using in our houses.

Subliminal Exposure

We are all exposed to a certain amount of air pollution that can be referred to as the background level, or subliminal exposure. Subliminal advertising relies on flashing a message on a television or movie screen so fast that the viewer doesn't consciously register what he is being told. Movie theater operators found that by flashing a picture of hot buttered popcorn on the screen for a fraction of a second during a movie, they could get viewers to go to the lobby and line up to buy popcorn without realizing why. This method of advertising is so effective in reaching the subconscious mind that its use has generally been banned. Subliminal exposure to pollutants can also affect people in a real but subtle way.

According to one scientist, "The greatest danger of pollution may well be that we shall tolerate levels of it so low as to have no acute nuisance value, but sufficiently high, nevertheless, to cause delayed pathological effects and spoil the quality of life."[9] We tend to become accustomed to the constant level of pollution around us because the effects are not suddenly devastating. In later life when the years of subtle exposure have contributed to chronic bronchitis, heart disease, or cancer, we have no idea why we are sick.

Pollutants can affect life in many ways, some of which are not immediately detrimental to health. If your tissues contain pollutants not needed for growth and development, this is known as your pollutant burden. It is often a result of subliminal exposure to chemicals. We all have multiple pollutant burdens to some degree, and large sectors of the population have enough pollution in their systems to cause various physiological changes. Sometimes these changes have no apparent significance, but at other times they can be seen as sentinels of disease. A certain percentage of us have high enough pollutant burdens to result in immediate sickness of some type, and for a few, the levels are fatal.[10]

The important thing for society at large to realize is the fact that we all are subliminally exposed to chemicals and that a high percentage of society is already being subtly affected. Unfortunately, for many people the results won't manifest themselves for decades. For others, the effect is immediately devastating.

Who Is at Risk?
People who spend a lot of time indoors are at risk of developing a building-related illness. That seems to include all of us, and in fact it does, but certain groups are especially at risk. Children, the elderly, and the infirm are more susceptible to any type of illness than the rest of the population. A newborn baby in a recently remodeled nursery can be at risk due to the variety of chemicals present in the new build-

ing materials. Children can have respiratory rates up to ten times faster than adults, hence they take in more indoor pollution per pound of body weight,[11] and a child's immune system is not fully formed until about age 10.[12] Conversely, the immune system of older people is on the decline, thus they are at an increased risk. Someone with an existing disease or someone living in an area of high outdoor pollution is more susceptible to indoor pollution because the immune system may already be overloaded.

Since we are all young, old, or sick at one time or another, we are all at risk at different times in our lives. Jet lag, shift work, hormonal changes, and everyday stress can also make someone more susceptible to indoor air pollutants.

Individuals who exhibit respiratory symptoms during a smog alert are likely to be susceptible to indoor pollutants. Someone whose eyes burn or water when entering a carpet store or newly remodeled room are probably reacting to formaldehyde and are in danger of developing more severe symptoms. Hyperactive children are also at risk.

Anyone with an immune system irregularity is in jeopardy of contracting a building-related illness because of the constant danger of having that system overwhelmed. Asthmatics and those with heart disease or respiratory disease are especially vulnerable. Smoking and drug abuse also contribute to risk. It has been estimated that the percentage of the population in a high-risk group at any one time may be as high as one-third.[13]

There are certainly many people exhibiting symptoms at much lower levels of pollution than the general population. This reinforces the point that the once considered safe level of exposure is not, in fact, safe enough. For the hundreds of outgassed pollutants that have been little studied, there are people who exhibit obvious symptoms. They act as early warning signs to the general population much as the canaries warned coal miners of unclean air in the mines. Canaries are more susceptible than most people to air pollution and they were taken into the mines to help predict when the air reached dangerously polluted levels. When the birds stopped singing and died, the miners knew it was time to seek fresh air.

Today's canaries are the people who are more susceptible than the population at large. Their lives have been radically affected by everyday exposures to air pollution. The rest of us should become aware of what bothers them because the odds are that it bothers us as well.

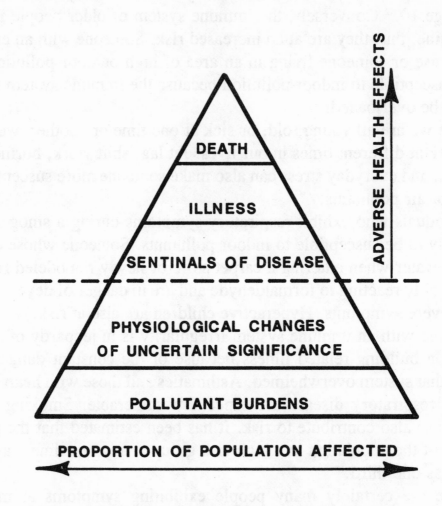

From *Archives of Environmental Health,* Volume 27, September
1973, pp. 151-154. Reprinted with permission of the Helen Dwight
Reid Educational Foundation. Published by Heldref Publications, 400
Albermarle St. N.W., Washington, D.C. 20016. Copyright © 1973.

Spectrum of Biological Responses to Pollutant Exposure

Their symptoms show up immediately while ours may not show up for years. This condition is known as chemical hypersensitivity syndrome.

Chemical Hypersensitivity Syndrome

Chemical hypersensitivity syndrome is known by a variety of names. Total allergy syndrome, 20th-century disease, environmental illness, ecological illness, and immune system disregulation are all names for the same condition. It involves an increased sensitivity to a wide variety of chemicals that are encountered daily. These substances are usually petrochemicals or their derivatives. The reactions and symptoms do not fall into the traditional allergist's definition, so they are usually not considered true allergies. Reactions can occur to exhaust fumes, synthetic fragrances, synthetic fabrics, plastics, food additives, printer's ink, etc. In short, practically everything in our modern environment can cause problems.

These reactions are often compared to addictions.[14] Since they involve exposure to chemicals encountered every day, addictions to them are possible. For some, getting their daily "fix" of exhaust fumes puts them on somewhat of an even keel. In the meantime their health gradually worsens as the daily exposure takes its toll. It isn't until total avoidance restores a healthy feeling of well-being that they realize to what depths their health had declined. A case study will help to illustrate this condition.

Chemical Hypersensitivity Syndrome Case Study

As a girl, LR grew up in a large metropolitan area and experienced symptoms of depression, insomnia, malaise, and nervousness. Many of these symptoms got worse as she grew older, yet were not nearly so severe when she was in the country. Whenever she went shopping with her family, she became weak and had to sit down often to catch her breath. She became increasingly uncomfortable around such things as cigarette smoke and exhaust fumes. In college, she found her health was markedly better in an older dormitory. When she moved into a newly constructed apartment, her health deteriorated rapidly. An art major, she found that her thinking got fuzzy in oil painting and water-color classes.

After marriage, living in a new duplex, the fumes emitted from the building materials caused burning and watery eyes as well as severe mood swings. Her health steadily deteriorated until after several moves, she and her husband moved into an older home in the country. Here she felt better than she had in years, although her health was still poor. They later purchased another house, again in the country, that needed some major rebuilding. After several years of construction work on the house, a part-time furniture refinishing business, and graphic design art work, LR's health collapsed.

She could hardly walk because of back and muscle pains. Her lungs ached. Her stomach was so irritated that she could barely eat anything. Her vision was blurred. Her sinuses were inflamed. Her gums were sore and bleeding. She hallucinated whenever she was able to sleep. She suffered chronic bladder and vaginal yeast infections. Practically every system in her body caused her problems.

She tracked down what she thought was the culprit: formaldehyde. It was emitted from the new carpeting, new bedroom furniture, new kitchen cabinets, new draperies, and new bed linens. When the bedroom was cleared of the suspected causes, her health seemed a little better. The house by now had been completely rebuilt and, as planned, it was time to sell it and hopefully make enough profit to build a new one and get out from under a mortgage payment. After the sale, they moved into a tract house that was old enough to have no new formaldehyde sources. During that summer, LR's health seemed much better; however, during the following winter it rapidly deteriorated. Whenever the natural gas furnace ran, she felt horrible. It was assumed that insecticides had been sprayed into the ductwork, causing the problem. The fresh paint was also suspected.

As they continued to search for land to build on, they moved into another rental that hopefully was healthier. This too, was old enough not to have any new formaldehyde sources. It seemed like a nice spot, with woods and a small stream on one side; however, her health steadily got worse. The house had natural gas heat, was next door to a gasoline station, and across from a doughnut stop where truckers let their diesel engines idle while they drank coffee. It was here that she saw chemical hypersensitivity syndrome mentioned on a television news program. Suddenly all of her symptoms fell into a pattern. It was now obvious that her current residence was probably one of the worst places that she could have chosen to live. She realized that she was reacting to not only formaldehyde, but to petrochemicals in general, and a wide variety of their derivatives. Every cleaning product under the sink was a problem, as were synthetic fabrics. Her wardrobe had to go. The upholstered furniture had to go. An unscented soap and detergent had to be found. Most importantly, a safe house had to be built because it was obvious that she was reacting to such things as carpeting, wall paneling, and the natural gas furnace.

Several years later, LR is slowly regaining her health. Her house is as pollution-free as possible, but she cannot tolerate a trip into town because of the many possible chemical exposures. She remains so sensitive that upon returning from town, her husband must shower and launder his clothes to remove any traces of exhaust fumes, cigarette smoke, or synthetic fragrances. Her artwork is now limited to using a metal mechanical pencil on 100 percent cotton rag paper inside a special vacuum reading box. One of her biggest regrets is that no one knew about chemical hypersensitivity syndrome when she was in grade school. She could then have avoided so many of the exposures that seemed so safe. Then she would not have lost so much of her tolerance.

There are doctors, known as clinical ecologists, who specialize in the treatment of chemical hypersensitivity syndrome. Members of the **American Academy of Environmental Medicine**, they have developed a variety of techniques for helping people cope with the condition, depending on their individual sensitivities. Special diets can help those sensitive to food additives. There are neutralization techniques to counteract the effects of some inhalants. Treatment techniques vary between both individuals and physicians. It is agreed, however, that the most important thing that can be done to improve one's health is avoidance of the chemicals that are causing the problem.

There are two national support groups for individuals with chemical hypersensitivity syndrome. The **Human Ecology Action League (HEAL)** and the **National Foundation for the Chemically Hypersensitive** are both nonprofit organizations that can direct people to local support groups. Membership in these groups is growing rapidly as more and more people become sensitive to their surroundings.

Implications of Chemical Hypersensitivity Syndrome

People with this condition exhibit symptoms to extremely small amounts of pollution, amounts that have long been assumed to be safe. They sometimes react to concentrations of pollutants so low that they cannot be measured by conventional instruments.[15] Therefore, it must be assumed that people are more sensitive to indoor pollution than was once commonly believed. Not only is it becoming apparent that sometimes devastating health effects can result from these low levels of contaminants, but that these are levels to which we are all exposed every day.

After removing many sources of indoor air pollution from the homes of sensitive individuals, improvement in health is often noted. For people with chemical hypersensitivity syndrome, this is often done as a matter of immediate survival. In many situations, as the indoor environment is cleaned up, other members of the family begin to see improvement in their health, as minor symptoms vanish. Suddenly, they realize that they too had been reacting to the poor indoor air quality. Their immediate symptoms were just not as severe. The implication of this for society at large is that we may all be affected by the small concentrations of pollutants that surround us. It is just that those with chemical hypersensitivity syndrome are reacting sooner and more severely.

Summary

The symptoms attributable to building-related illness run the gamut of everything from sinus congestion to death. Practically any symptom that can be listed can be caused by a building. People with chemical hypersensitivity syndrome may report symptoms mimicking almost every known disease.

Since we spend so much time indoors, it only seems logical that we should strive to make the indoor environment as unpolluted as possible. Unfortunately, many modern buildings have very poor indoor air quality, and as a result, they are a cause of much unnecessary illness. However, buildings can be designed and built to provide a healthful environment. Living in such a building can often reverse the negative side effects of living in a polluted building. It can also help to insure that a building-related illness or chemical hypersensitivity syndrome will not develop in the future.

Chapter 3

Finding a Safe House

Finding a safe place to live may be a difficult process, but as all prospective home buyers and apartment hunters know, finding any house or apartment that satisfies all of one's requirements is often difficult. Healthfulness is simply another requirement. Since all people are different, both in taste and genetic makeup, your healthful house may be quite different from your neighbor's. For example, one person may prefer hardwood floors while another may opt for ceramic tile. Both can result in nontoxic floors.

What to Look For
Since so many of the building materials in use today have the potential to pollute the indoor air, an existing house may need to be at least 30 years old not to have many outgassing sources. Of course, there are newer houses that can be just as pollution free, but they may be more difficult to find. Practically all houses being built today seem designed to foul the indoor air, yet it is possible to build a very safe house. All it takes is a little common sense and some planning.

Probably the three most important things to avoid when seeking safe housing are: carpeting, combustion appliances, and man-made wood products. This rules out most of the houses built during the last 30 years. Carpeting has been promoted as being plush and luxurious, but in fact, it is more important to recognize that it is often associated with indoor air pollution and building-related illness. Man-made wood products are notorious for emitting formaldehyde fumes. Formaldehyde is a fine product for embalming fluid, but it shouldn't be breathed by living people on a daily basis. Combustion appliances include anything fueled by natural gas, oil, coal, kerosene, or wood. We have already seen that they are responsible for the major indoor air pollutants.

There are many other possible sources of indoor air pollution, but these three seem to be the major contributors. If you do not have any severe health problems, eliminating these three groups of materials will be a big step toward clean air. If you already suffer from a chronic illness, or are otherwise at risk of developing a building-related illness, you should be even more selective. Plaster walls may need to be chosen instead of drywall or wallpaper. Hardwood lumber may need to be specified over softwoods such as pine. If your health is extremely poor, every item in the house's structure should be analyzed thoroughly.

How Safe Is Safe?

An *extremely* safe house is quite possible to build, but it would also be very expensive. It would involve the elimination of wood in favor of steel for the framing. Walls might need to be constructed of porcelain panels. Paints would probably need to be eliminated and special insulation would be required. A complicated air filtration system would then be necessary to keep the indoor air pristine. Fortunately, most people do not need a house that is built to these extreme standards.

A *reasonably* safe house can be built at only a modest increase in cost. Unfortunately, most builders are unaware of what goes into a healthy house, so when asked to work with new and unfamiliar materials, they may be unwilling to comply, or they may ask for a seemingly exorbitant price. This isn't necessarily price gouging; they just need to make sure that their estimate will cover all of the unknown factors. If a contractor knows exactly what is expected, and the plans exclude any unusual materials and techniques, then his price should be reasonable.

Older Houses

Older houses have a number of advantages over new houses. In the first place, any questionable materials will have had a number of years to outgas. New plywood might be a significant source of formaldehyde but 30-year-old plywood may be completely outgassed. It will even be difficult to find plywood in a house built before World War II. Older houses are more likely to have such things as hardwood floors and plaster walls. When the corner of carpeting is peeled back, it is not unusual to find a beautiful hardwood floor that has been hidden for years. If the cabinets are original, they could be made of solid wood. Most cabinets today are constructed with particle board that has a thin wood veneer. The veneer does practically nothing to seal in the formaldehyde fumes.

If an older house has had a lot of remodeling done to it over the years, it could easily have high indoor pollution levels so it might be better to look for a place "in the rough." One that needs some work can be remodeled using nontoxic materials. It can be an expensive proposition to have to remove recent remodeling and redo with different materials. In doing that, you end up paying for a room twice.

On the negative side, existing houses can have a long and unknown history. You can never be sure what kinds of insecticides or termiticides have been applied by previous owners. Chemicals that were once considered safe are now banned. You can no longer buy them, but their residues will linger for years. A former owner may have been very fond of perfume, leaving the closets saturated with the artificial fragrance. This can be an obvious source of irritation for a future resident who happens to be allergic to perfume. Materials such as asbestos or lead paint can be a problem in older houses as well.

A major source of trouble in some older houses is mold. Roof leaks and damp basements abound. Mold spores can be transported around the house by an old leaky furnace system. Since many older houses have oil or natural gas heating systems, an old, outdated system may actually be an advantage. It certainly won't add any value to the house, and can be replaced with a more healthful system.

The best thing about looking for an existing house is that is is already built and you can easily evaluate the neighborhood. There is no need to guess whether or not an oil refinery will be built across the street. Sensitive individuals can walk inside and see if the house has an adverse effect on them. It may even be possible to spend a couple of nights in the house to test one's tolerance for an extended period.

After reading this book, you should complete a list of the important health features that you want to consider for your particular needs. The odds are that you won't find the perfect house, but with some effort you should be able to find one with possibilities. A little remodeling could be in order, and that you might be able to have done before you move in. If you have severe sensitivities, there will be many aspects that will need to be considered. They will be covered in more depth in later chapters. But first we briefly discuss some particular types of housing.

Lustron Houses

There is one type of existing house that might well be very suitable for many sensitive people: a Lustron house. These houses were mass produced by a firm in Columbus, Ohio. Carl Strandlund's Lustron Corporation, in 1948, began producing houses whose unique feature was that they were built almost entirely out of steel, about ten tons in all. Most of the press coverage at the time was favorable, but the enterprise eventually failed due to lack of planning. About 3000 were produced and many still can be found in the Midwest.

These houses had an all-steel frame. The studs and rafters were all steel. All of the wall panels, both interior and exterior, were porcelainized steel. The roof shingles were porcelainized steel. The exterior panels were two feet square and are reminiscent of those used on some gasoline stations. Several pastel colors were available, and with a little polish, they still look good today. The doors and windows were also constructed of steel. They were all built on concrete slabs, which had to be placed very accurately because these houses were built to very close tolerances on an assembly line.

For someone concerned with outgassing, one of these houses might be worth considering. They are not, however, perfect. Generally they are located in cities, where outdoor air pollution could reach high levels. They are usually heated with oil, and they are not very energy efficient. Yet, all of these things could be remedied. Since they are bolted together, they can simply be unbolted and moved to a pleasant hilltop location in the country. The meager insulation can then be upgraded. Several have had their heating systems already changed. Baseboard heaters are fairly easy to add and the asphalt floor tile can be replaced with ceramic tile.

One disadvantage of these houses is that what you see is what you get. Since all the pieces fit together in a precise way, remodeling is difficult. The basic model was a 1025-square-foot two-bedroom unit, although a few three-bedroom units were built. If that isn't large enough, adding on could be difficult although two houses could be put together. Another drawback is the difficulty of hanging pictures on the steel walls. However, with a few magnets, they make great bulletin boards.

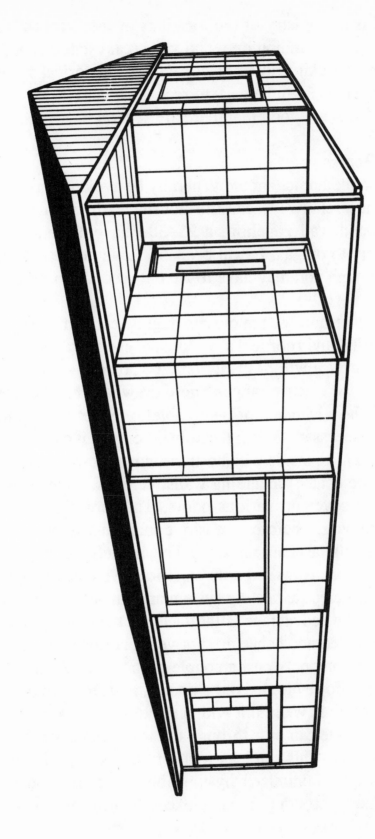

Lustron House

There is no registry of the locations of the Lustron houses. If you are interested in finding one, and your real estate agent doesn't know what you are talking about, check with the historical society or a local architect. They are quite easy to recognize, and if there is one in your area, the odds are good that there are several.

Mobile Homes

Newer mobile homes should generally be avoided, but an older model can provide relatively healthful housing. Although constructed with plywood and wall paneling, a 25–30-year-old model will have had many years to outgas. It will probably have an outgassed asphalt tile floor, although you may have to rip out recently installed carpeting to find it.

As in older houses, the closets may be contaminated with perfume or mothballs, and roof leaks could have created a mold problem. The electrical service will probably only be 50 amp—not enough for electric heat or an electric range. These drawback can be overcome, and you have the advantage of being able to move it to a more healthful location if necessary. When the home is empty, it can be relatively easy to coat the entire inside with an environmental sealant or paint. Everything can be coated, including walls, ceilings, cupboards, and closets in order to cover up various odors. The roof should be coated and allowed to outgas before a sensitive individual moves in. Roof coatings are usually asphalt-based, so they are definitely a potential source of air pollution. New 200 amp electric service can be added so that a nonpolluting electric heating system and range can be installed.

A general disadvantage is the fact that the older mobile homes are poorly insulated and hence are not very energy efficient. But since an older model may only cost a couple of thousand dollars, a high utility bill may be affordable. In cold climates, moisture can be a major problem. If the unit is well built with a tight exterior skin, moisture that is generated inside can pass through the walls and condense on the skin, inside the wall. This can lead to a serious mold problem; however, it can usually be minimized by the liberal use of exhaust fans in the kitchen and bathroom to remove excess moisture.

Apartments

Older apartment buildings are much more preferable than newer mass-produced units. Like older houses, they will likely have hardwood floors and plaster walls. Steam heat is often used in older apartments. Although the boiler may be gas or oil fired, it will usually be in the basement and if your apartment is on an upper floor, there may be no combustion products reaching there, unless the chimney is right outside your window. Even in small buildings, upper floors are preferable in order to get away from traffic fumes, and side streets are preferable to busy thoroughfares.

In major cities, large multi-story apartment buildings may have indoor parking garages on the lower floors which help to pollute the lower apartments. Sometimes these fumes can travel up elevator shafts or stairwells and reach the upper floors. Life on the upper floors can often, however, be quite tolerable. In fact, the best place to be in a city is as high up as possible, away from the pollution and smog.

The big danger in apartments is being contaminated by the smells, fumes, and odors from adjoining units. It is often possible to tell when the neighbors are smoking marijuana, spraying disinfectant, or painting, and odors from a neighbor's wood stove can seep through common walls.

Temporary Housing

Occasionally someone will suddenly find out that their devastating symptoms are being caused by their house and that the only solution is to move and move quickly. Yet, it may not be possible to find a new house or apartment immediately. This can be a frightening situation and the choices can be limited, but there are choices.

Some people have been able to live in a tent or camper in the back yard while remodeling is being done. Others have found refuge in a relative's or friend's house. However, new tents may be intolerable due to waterproofing chemicals and new campers may be constructed with potentially dangerous man-made materials. Similarly, a friend's house may be no more tolerable than the one that is being abandoned.

A clinical ecologist may be able to refer an individual to a safe place to stay. Local support groups for people with chemical hypersensitivity syndrome may be able to offer suggestions. Often, their members know of relatively safe places to stay. They may even have an empty bedroom that is available. **Ecological Ministries** maintains a national computerized list of nontoxic housing for both the short and the long term.

It may even be possible to find a relatively safe room already in your existing home, or such a room might be remodeled fairly quickly. This room can then become an oasis.

An Oasis

To make a room an oasis may be a reasonable alternative for a sensitive individual. In order to begin, the room must be emptied of all furnishings, including draperies, clothing, and carpeting. If this empty room continues to elicit symptoms, it may be necessary to seal some of the surfaces. A suitable paint or environmental sealant can be used to block any outgassing fumes, but may need to outgas itself for a time. If an immediate place to stay is required, the walls and floor can be covered with aluminum or stainless steel foil. The resulting "metallic look" can result in a very safe environment. If it is during the heating season, and the existing furnace elicits symptoms, then all of the registers in the oasis must be sealed and a tolerated auxiliary heater must be installed. If the bed is suspected of causing symptoms, it should be replaced with a metal box spring that has been covered with several cotton or wool blankets to provide padding. A room-size carbon air cleaner can also be helpful.

After an oasis has been created for the sensitive individual to retreat to, the rest of the house can be tackled on a room-by-room basis. The oasis can provide the safe environment needed for building up one's health. Often by spending eight hours of restful sleep in an oasis, an individual can cope with the rest of the house during the day, so that remodeling need not be rushed.

Remodeling or Building New

Whether you decide to build a new house or modify an existing house, you will probably require the services of a competent contractor. Unfortunately, many builders are unfamiliar with nontoxic construction materials and techniques. If you find that you must educate a contractor in the construction of a safe house, then you should familiarize yourself with the work to be done by reading the appropriate chapters of this book, and then let the contractor read those chapters as well. In that way you can both discuss intelligently the work to be performed. The **Environmental Construction Network** maintains a listing of builders familiar with non-toxic building techniques in the United States and Canada.

Since even many of the recommended materials require a period of outgassing, temporary housing may need to be secured, depending on the degree of an individual's sensitivity. It may be possible to have work done in one room, with an exhaust fan in the window, and the door shut. This may be enough to keep the rest of the house from being contaminated during the construction process. If you are an asthmatic, it may be very difficult to keep the dust to tolerable levels during any heavy construction.

If the remodeling required is very extensive, it may be more economically feasible to consider building a new house. One problem with a new house has to do with the fact that there are so many different materials used in its construction. Some may not be tolerable when tested individually, but may be OK when sealed inside a wall. So you may not know how safe a house is until it is actually completed. This will only be a consideration for extremely sensitive people, but should definitely be kept in mind. It can be an expensive proposition indeed to build a new house only to find that you can't live in it.

A healthful house may require the use of materials or techniques that increase the cost. Unfortunately, there is always a dollar sign involved, even when health is concerned. However, it is best to select the safest materials that you can afford. As nontoxic housing techniques become better known, these costs will inevitably drop. If expenses incurred are necessary to improve or maintain your health, they may be tax deductible. Deductible items include those things prescribed by a physician such as filters, and special transportation costs. Expenses that promote health, such as replacing a gas furnace with an electric furnace, may also be deductible if they are performed on the specific orders of your physician.

Since tax laws are constantly changing, it is important that competent advice be secured prior to taking deductions for remodeling a house. It may be necessary to obtain written statements from not only your physician, but also the contractor or real estate agent. All medical deductions must be proven, they are not simply allowed. The burden of proof is on the taxpayer, but as long as the Internal Revenue Service's guidelines are followed and a tax accountant's advice is adhered to, your listed deductions should be allowable.

Summary

Since everyone's housing requirements are different, it is important to determine your specific needs and make a list of the features that you want in a house. The various chapters of this book will help you form such a list. After analyzing your needs, you should be able to determine the feasibility of finding an existing house as compared to building a new one. Then you can proceed accordingly.

Chapter 4

Location, Location, Location

According to real estate agents, the three most important things determining the value of a house are: location, location, and location. For them, a location on a corner lot, near schools, shopping, and work may indicate the ideal place to live. Location is a very important thing to consider when searching for safe housing, but an entirely different set of criteria must be used. What a realtor considers remote for convenience reasons may be ideal for health.

Geographic Areas

People often wonder what part of the country is the most healthful place to live. Well-meaning friends are loaded with advice about the South being healthier, or the West, or the North, etc., etc. Unfortunately, there is probably no single geographic area that is the best place to live. All parts of the country have their unique types of hazards. The Southwest has been touted as having a dry climate that is perfect for asthmatics, but as Easterners have migrated there, they have brought pollen-bearing plants into the region. With irrigation, these plants have thrived and are spreading allergens into the wind.

Seashore locations have also been recommended. Here, there is the possibility of mold growth with an abundance of spores at certain times of the year. If there is any standing, stagnant water, it can be a breeding ground for many harmful organisms. Methane from swamp gas can also be a danger. Frontage on water is a desirable location for

41

many people, and as a result the area may be polluted by neighbors with wood smoke or lawn chemicals. With the prevelance of oil spills, it would not be uncommon to find an oily sludge on any ocean beach in the world.

The fresh country air in the Midwest is often fouled with agricultural chemicals, or with mold spores and pollen associated with farming. Even a tractor in need of a tune-up can pollute the air to a great degree.

Large cities are notorious for their air pollution, and this may extend for several miles beyond the limits of the city itself. Traffic and strip development along major highways can often extend the city's unhealthy air into the next town.

Even though there is no one perfect place to live, fortunately there are pockets everywhere that can provide the fresh air necessary for a healthful building site. The ideal site, however, can vary depending on your personal needs. The best spot for an asthmatic will be different from the site selected by someone with chemical hypersensitivity syndrome. The spot may very well be in the Southwest or at the seashore. Even though these places may not be perfect, if one knows what to look for, good sites can be found practically anywhere. The most important thing to do when analyzing any site is to look around thoroughly. Neighbors can often supply a wealth of information about a prospective property. For example, they can tell you how the people apply lawn chemicals, who burns wood, where the abandoned landfill is, the frequency of mosquito spraying, etc.

Maps

It is always helpful to have a good map when beginning the search for safe housing. With a map, you can easily see what surrounds a potential location. Unfortunately, the commonly available road maps will be of limited value. They will certainly supply you with the names of the roads and will enable you to find your way around unfamiliar parts of town or the country. They will not show the locations of houses. Nor will they show you any topographic information such as hills, drainage patterns, ravines, etc. For this information, 7½-minute quadrangle maps have been produced for the entire country by the **U.S. Geological Survey**. These maps are reasonably priced and are available either directly by mail through the **U.S. Geological Survey** or at selected locations in most states. These quadrangle maps cover approximately

$6^{1}/_{2} \times 8^{1}/_{2}$ miles at a scale of $1'' = 2000'$, and are color coded.

Besides showing the locations of roads, they will also show driveways and unpaved lanes. Rivers, ponds, and streams as well as intermittent creeks are also displayed. Houses and barns are easy to pick out, as are larger buildings such as factories. Real estate listings often list the township and section number. These too are to be found on these maps. The most comprehensive information, however, has to do with the topographic data that are available. Having been originally produced from stereoscopic aerial photography, they show elevations of a ground above sea level, so it is easy to pick out the top of a hill, where the valleys are, or how a ravine cuts through a particular piece of property. Other details that are incorporated include: boundaries of state or national parks, high voltage electric lines, gas wells, cemeteries, pipelines, some fence lines, and wooded areas.

It may be necessary to obtain several quadrangle maps to cover your entire county. Each one has a particular name and a key is available, so that you know which ones to request. With these maps, you can easily see just what is surrounding a particular house or building site. For instance, it may become apparent that there is a natural gas well just beyond the property line, or that there is a hidden farm field nearby, or that there are several houses in an upwind direction that will need to be investigated for burning wood. Names of property owners are not shown on these maps.

Another type of map that can be helpful is a plat map. Plat maps are usually available for the entire county and can be found in the local courthouse. These are usually contained in very large unwieldy books, but sometimes they have been reproduced into a smaller $8^{1}/_{2}'' \times 11''$ format by a local realtor or an abstract company for sale to the public. The type of information on a plat map includes the names of property owners and shapes of their property. If you find a location that looks promising, a plat map will supply you with the owner's name and owners of surrounding parcels. If a neighboring lot is owned by XYZ Nuclear Power Inc., a phone call may be in order to determine what they plan to build there. If a particular piece of property looks promising, even though it is not currently listed for sale, it might be worth a phone call. If you are told about a piece of property by a realtor, you can find it on a plat map and then look on a quadrangle map and see if there are any major drawbacks. This can save a tremendous amount of time driving around the countryside.

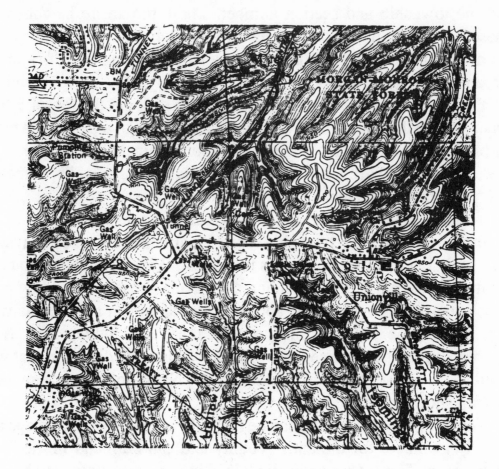

Portion of a 7¹/₂-Minute Quadrangle Map

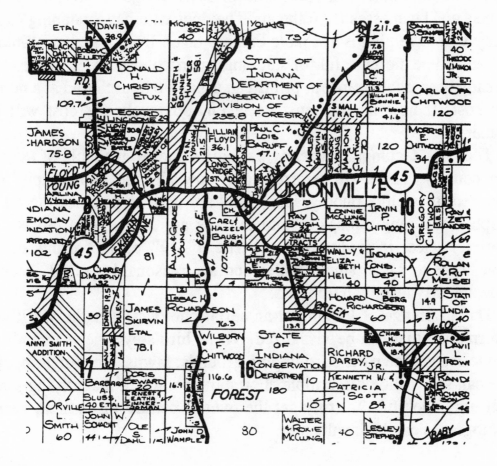

Portion of a Plat Map

Aerial Photography

Aerial photographs can also supply much information about the surrounding countryside when one is analyzing a piece of land. Most major cities have one or more aerial photographers listed in the telephone book. Some will specialize in such things as photographing homes and businesses from the air. The ones who have mapping capability will have photos available that are taken from a higher altitude. These will be more useful for studying a particular area. If an area has already been photographed, prints can usually be purchased at a nominal cost. If new photos must be taken, obviously the cost will be higher.

The **U.S. Geological Society** has aerial photos available of the entire country. These are referred to as low altitude photography (as opposed to satellite photography), and are used to produce the topographic quadrangle maps. Photo indexes are available, from which you can select individual photos. The 9″×9″ contact prints cover from three to seven square miles and are reasonably priced. Larger blowups may also be purchased.

The advantage of looking at an aerial photograph is the wealth of information that can be visualized. These bird's-eye views can allow you to see garden patches, dumping grounds, lawns, etc. Anything the eye can see will be discernible. For some photos, a magnifying glass will prove helpful. To truly get the overall picture of an area, aerial photographs can be invaluable.

Hills and Valleys

Some of the most polluted places in the world are in valleys. They can easily be more polluted than some of our major cities. A valley can fill up with smog and air pollution much like a bowl fills with water. The floor of a valley can, therefore, be much more unhealthy than a site on the rim. The winds through a valley often travel in the direction of a waterway, making the lower end more susceptible to air contamination. Farm fields can introduce pesticides and fertilizers as well as exhaust fumes into these geographic "bowls," filling them up with a variety of toxic smells.

On the other hand, hilltop locations can often be healthful sites. Breezes will tend to bring in a constant supply of fresh air. Like being on the top floor of an apartment building in a city, a hilltop location can put you above most of the surrounding air pollution; however, there is always the possibility of contamination. If an oil refinery is located upwind, the hilltop may not be very desirable.

In any case, the best test is to visit the site. Spending a day or two in the area will soon reveal if it is incompatible with your particular needs. Keep in mind that the air may be quite different on a weekend with people out for a Sunday drive than it will be during the week when the nearby factory is in operation. The purpose of this chapter is to list the possible sources of air pollution to watch out for, not to recommend a specific location. Practically every site will have both positive and negative points and, to repeat, the only true test for someone with extreme sensitivities is to actually visit the site and spend some time there. For someone with no apparent health problems but is interested in finding a place safer than the norm, these guidelines will not need to be adhered to quite as strictly.

Prevailing Winds

The climate patterns in the U.S. generally follow a path from west to east. Therefore, we usually consider the prevailing wind to be coming from the west. In general this is true, but is can vary tremendously in different areas of the country. It can also vary at different times of the year. Sometimes there may be an arctic blast coming out of the north, and at other times there may be a gentle southwestern breeze at the same location. The prevailing wind pattern can also be very site specific. Two areas a mile apart can have entirely different wind patterns.

The local topography is responsible for the variation of wind direction. A hill or mountain can cause the wind to blow around it rather than over, causing a predominantly southerly wind in a certain area, even though the wind is generally from the west. Lakes, fields, and woods can similarly have an effect on local wind direction.

The best way to determine from which direction the wind usually blows is to ask someone who lives in the neighborhood. Most people will know if the smoke from a factory tends to blow directly toward their house on a regular basis. Similarly, they will know if the dust from the gravel road is usually worse on one side, indicating the prevailing wind direction.

In some parts of the world, the action of the wind produces an abundance of positive ions in the air. Ions are simply electrically charged particles, and they occur everywhere. However, an excess of positive ions in the air result in an increase of serotonin in the body and symptoms such as irritability, insomnia, tension, or upset stomach. There are even reports of increased rates of suicides, accidents, and crime when these particular winds are blowing.[1,2] Physicians in these locales have been known to postpone elective surgery until the wind stops.

These dry winds are so well known that they have been given names. The Sharav in Israel has been shown to affect up to 25 percent of the population. Fortunately, these winds do not blow all the time. In the United States, the Chinook is known in the Pacific Northwest as is the Santa Ana in California. Local residents will know if the occurrence of these "devil winds" is common in a particular area.

Things to Avoid

The things to avoid can be quite numerous, and there are no iron-clad rules. The location to look for is the place with the cleanest air. This is often easier said than done. It will be impossible to list everything to avoid, because it could include practically every man-made object in existence as well as natural mold and pollen sources. Our purpose is to list the major problem areas.

Busy roads can be a source of polluting exhaust fumes, and on major highways and Interstates this will include both gasoline and diesel fumes. The air can also be contaminated through tire wear, spillage of freight materials, and littering. It has been shown that small animals living near high traffic areas have higher than normal concentrations of lead, cadmium, nickel, and zinc in their systems.[3] There may also be a proliferation of gasoline stations or restaurants, where fumes can build up. Gasoline stations can be especially polluting at night when the underground tanks are refilled and vent pipes spew a considerable amount of vapor into the air. Paved roads are often constructed of asphalt which can heat up in the bright sun and outgas. Asphalt patching compounds can also create problems for some people. Concrete road surfaces are much more inert, but they too are often patched with asphaltic compounds.

Gravel roads are notorious for being dusty. However, they will probably be less traveled than paved roads and will therefore have less exhaust fumes. Dust used to be controlled by highway departments by pouring used motor oil onto the gravel roads. This was discontinued when a commercially available road oil was developed specifically for the purpose. This product worked fine for controlling dust, but has since been banned because of its toxic potential. A water-based emulsion is currently being used in many areas that meets the newer environmental regulations. It still remains a problem for some people. If you live on a gravel road that is usually sprayed to control dust, you can talk to the local highway department and ask that they not spray in front of your house. They are usually happy to comply with such requests.

An even newer product for controlling dust has become available and is used by many road crews. It is the same chemical that northern crews use to melt snow and ice in the winter: calcium chloride. This is applied in a water solution, usually in late spring. It works by absorbing moisture from the air. This moisture then helps to keep the dust down, much like misting the road with a garden hose. Calcium chloride has a slight odor but seems fairly well tolerated by most people, although it has been known to cause automobiles to rust out prematurely.

Farm fields are usually worked several times each season and every time a tractor drives through a field more pollution is put into the air. Plowing can introduce a considerable amount of unhealthy dust into the air. This dust will not only contain soil, but also microorganisms that reside there. Chemicals that were applied in previous seasons can cling to soil particles and be transported by the wind. Planting can contaminate the air further with seed dusts as well as molds living on the seeds themselves. Fertilizing and spraying pesticides create their own obvious air pollution. Harvesting creates more dust from the crops themselves, and additional mold spores. While dust-related illness can be very devastating, as can be mold allergy, the greatest danger posed by a farm field is from the use of pesticides. Even the residues remaining on cotton after it has been processed into clothing can be intolerable to many people. In agricultural areas such as the Midwest, pesticides seem to be one of the major contributing factors in the development of chemical hypersensitivity syndrome. While many people consider exposure to agricultural pesticides to be acceptable, it must be remembered that pesticides are designed to kill living creatures, and human beings are living creatures just the same as insects. People exposed to toxic levels of organophosphate pesticides report altered brain functions such as understanding the speech of others, recognizing printed or written words, social withdrawal, anxiety, etc.[4]

Some obvious sources of pollution to avoid can include factories.

While the clean air standards are obviously tighter than they were in 1900, there are great strides still to be made. Accidental chemical spills or smokestack emissions are not uncommon even in a strictly run nuclear power plant. The average factory can release pollutants into the environment and never be caught violating the law because of the lax enforcement measures of the regulating agencies. Of course, all factories are not polluters. Many assembly plants, for example, are quite clean. The danger with them is that someone may be bothered by exhaust fumes because of the increased amount of traffic such as a business. Where there is more traffic, there is more air pollution due to exhaust fumes.

Smokestack industries have long been regarded as dirty. Many such factories were built years ago, before today's pollution control regulations came into effect and cleaning them up can be difficult. The tall smokestacks, which are often notorious air polluters, were developed to discharge pollutants high up in the atmosphere. This causes the contaminants to descend to earth in areas far from the plant. Therefore, living near such a smokestack may be healthier than living several miles away. The acid rain in the Eastern United States is attributed to the smokestack emissions in the Midwest. The pollutants have been successfully dumped in someone else's backyard.

While there is little direct evidence that acid rain has an immediate effect on human health, there is some indirect evidence. It is known that acidic water will leach metals such as cadmium, arsenic, zinc, and aluminum out of the soil. Drinking water from lakes and streams in these areas can result in a variety of diseases associated with ingestion of heavy metals. Acidic water may also result in less beneficial selenium being taken up, thus leading to selenium deficiencies. While there are apparently no serious effects resulting from acid rain contact with the skin, breathing trace quantities of sulfuric and nitric acid formed in the atmosphere can be injurious to human lungs. It has been suggested that high concentrations of acidic pollutants in the atmosphere were responsible for excess mortality in London in the 1950s, in the Meuse Valley in Belgium in 1930, and in Donora, Pennsylvania, in 1948.[5] Therefore, areas with high amounts of acid rain should be avoided.

Nearby houses can be sources of unhealthy wood smoke as can subdivisions that are served primarily by natural gas. Fumes from chimneys, dryer vents, and kitchen range hoods can send the by-products of natural gas combustion directly toward neighboring houses. Chemical lawn treatment companies have become quite numerous in recent years, as have the complaints of people bothered by chemicals. Some communities have been active in pushing stricter regulations for these firms because of the potential danger they pose for the population at large.

There have been studies reporting increased cancer rates in people living near high-voltage power lines.[6,7] Other symptoms such as disturbances in the cardiovascular system, the central nervous system, and lowered sexual capability have also been noted.[8] This could be due to either the electrical or magnetic fields surrounding the wires. Some people have reported increased sensitivities to these fields after a strong inciting event such as exposure to a strong unnatural field, dental work involving metallic fillings, etc. Symptoms can include experiencing leg cramps while passing an electrical transformer or slurred speech when near a computer terminal.[9] While electrical fields can be shielded by a properly grounded metal screen, panel, or conduit, magnetic fields cannot. Biological effects of magnetic fields include: irritability, fatigue, dizziness, altered appetite, headache, itching, burning, numbness, etc.[10] Both electrical and magnetic fields rapidly decrease in strength with distance, so it would be wise to live as far as possible from high-voltage lines. The strongest fields will be near lines carrying very high voltage such as 765,000 volts. Fortunately, most lines in residential areas carry considerably less voltage.

According to Soviet researchers, microwaves can induce dizziness, heart pains, irritability, diminished intellectual capacity, loss of hair, etc.[11] Cataracts have been noted in workers exposed to microwaves in radar installations.[12] In Vernon, New Jersey, parents in the vicinity of a high concentration of microwave satellite communications antennae found that the incidence of Down's syndrome (mongolism) was far higher than the national average.[13] Sources of microwave contamination to avoid would include radar installations, both commercial and military, and microwave communication towers.

It would also seem prudent to avoid living near television or radio broadcasting towers because of the powerful electromagnetic waves originating there.

Trees and plants have long been recognized as bothering allergy sufferers. Ragweed and goldenrod pollen are well known examples. For someone with conventional allergies, simply avoiding the most common pollen-bearing plants may be sufficient. However, for someone with severe sensitivities, a wider selection must be considered. Aromatic plants, such as mint, and many flowers have been known to elicit symptoms. For an individual sensitive to hydrocarbons, such things as creosote bushes and cedar trees should be considered. Most softwood trees contain various terpenes and other naturally occurring resins that can cause reactions. Some forests are routinely sprayed with chemicals.

Moldy conditions in places such as swamps and damp woods should be generally avoided, yet often, with a little planning, a swamp can be drained. This might then provide a healthful place to live. Similarly, a damp woods can be cleared out sufficiently to allow the sunlight and a breeze to penetrate, creating a suitable building site. Compost piles can generate tremendous amounts of mold spores and should definitely be avoided by a mold-sensitive individual.

Some areas are known for high radon concentrations. Such spots should be avoided. Local or state boards of health will be able to identify these high-risk locations. Volcanoes are obvious natural polluters that should be avoided because of their effects on the human system of breathing in toxic gases and ash.

Geophysical forces around earthquake fault zones result when there are changes in the stresses in the earth's crust. These tectonic stresses cause fields to develop that have both electromagnetic-like and gravity-like components. At least one researcher has theorized that these brief fields can cause unusual phenomena to take place.[14] Intense luminous displays, sometimes attributed to UFOs, could be a manifestation of this energy, as could some of the unusual movements of objects associated with poltergeists, so there may be reasons to avoid earthquake zones other than the obvious danger of severe tremors.

Landfills can pollute the air with dust, mold, and the smell of garbage. There will also be an increase in traffic flow and associated exhaust fumes. More importantly, they can pollute the groundwater as various contaminants seep deep into the ground. This can poison nearby water wells.

Utilities

All of the utilities serving a particular site should be considered. If the area is served by a municipal water system, the water should be analyzed. Besides the naturally occurring contaminants, drinking water can contain a wide variety of man-made pollutants. Some of these are intentionally introduced at the water treatment plant. Tests are run on such water supplies periodically and are available for public inspection. These tests may not be of much use to some sensitive individuals, because the measurement methods may not be able to record the low levels of contaminants to which they can react. Sometimes more sophisticated tests can be performed. Check with the local Board of Health for laboratories with these capabilities. Water from private wells is not required by law to be tested, but it too can be polluted because of the many chemicals that are continually seeping down into the aquifer. Since so much of our water supply has been contaminated, the best solution may be to filter the water. This is discussed more completely in Chapter 22.

Municipal sewage systems are convenient ways for cities to dispose of the thousands of gallons of waste produced every day. Today's treatment methods are tremendously better than simply dumping raw sewage into a river; however, there are still contaminants being discharged into the waterways from which drinking water supplies are taken. During heavy rains, sewage is often discharged directly to the receiving stream, bypassing the treatment process. This is deemed tolerable by regulatory agencies because the waste is diluted by the excess rainfall. For these reasons, the location of a house downstream from a municipal wastewater treatment plant is undesirable.

Manholes or wastewater pumping stations have been known to overflow causing sewers to back up into the houses. This can cause obvious health hazards. Usually, neighbors will know if these occurrences are commonplace.

Septic systems are typically used to treat the sewage from individual houses. If properly constructed and maintained, they will cause no health problems. If constructed in a swampy area or on a hillside, there is the possibility of the effluent leeching to the surface. Since shallow water wells can be contaminated by a septic system, Boards of Health generally recommend at least a 100-foot separation, and the well should be located on higher ground than the septic system.

Electricity and telephone poles are often treated with a toxic preservative which can outgas vapors for many months. If a new pole must be placed, it may be possible to request that a salt-treated pole be used instead of a creosote treated pole. Even though the salt treatment contains an arsenic compound, it will be considerably less odorous. In either case, poles should not be located near garden areas. Underground service is preferable, because no pole will need to be placed near the house.

Natural gas should generally be avoided in the healthy house. However, the country is crisscrossed with natural gas pipelines, so it may not be possible to avoid it completely. An all-electric subdivision will be preferable to one supplied with natural gas. The gas company will be able to tell you if there are any vent pipes, regulator stations, or underground storage areas nearby and neighbors will be able to tell you if these are known to leak gas fumes into the air.

Someone who has severe sensitivities may be somewhat isolated from the world due to intolerance of exhaust fumes, newsprint, etc. For them, television may be their primary means of information and entertainment. For this reason television reception should be considered. Traditional antennas have a limited range and may not function well in certain geographic areas. Cable TV is now available in a great deal of the country and may be a reasonable alternative. Home satellite dishes can open up a tremendous amount of stations to someone who is generally confined to home. A professional salesperson can evaluate the site for satellite reception.

Summary

In summary, everything can affect the healthfulness of a given location. For this reason, it is important to know as much about the site as possible. If you have walked around the property, spent a day or two there, looked at some maps or driven around the neighborhood and talked to people living nearby, you should have a good picture of its suitability. If you have learned enough to talk about a particular area for 30 minutes, then you probably will have learned if there are any obvious pollution sources that will be problematic. The important thing is to make an educated decision, one made with your eyes wide open, but if you are very sensitive your nose may tell you more than your eyes.

Chapter 5

Planning

During the planning stages of any project, many decisions need to be made. Designing a safe house is no exception. Some of the choices to be made will be similar in any house, such as the number of bedrooms, bathrooms, etc. Yet, in a safe house there are many additional things to consider, some of which will seem quite ridiculous and unnecessary to designers and builders of conventional houses. The health aspects of houses are just beginning to be understood, and as with any emerging technology, there will be a considerable lag until all houses are built in a healthful manner. This chapter will help you look at how the initial planning stages help to determine indoor air quality.

Since so many of the components of a house interact, it is important to plan any building project carefully. It can be very expensive to discover halfway into the construction process that a certain product is incompatible with the plan, or is unavailable in your geographic area. Since a few of the materials and techniques discussed in this book will be unfamiliar to some builders, a good set of plans is very important in order to minimize delays and misunderstandings.

Assessing Your Needs

All of your needs and requirements should be written down. As the list begins to grow, you will begin to notice that some things will conflict with others. For example, eliminating air pollution may be number one on your list, yet your spouse wants to be able to smoke. Compromises will be in order. Maybe your spouse would consider only smoking outdoors in exchange for a concession on your part.

The basic needs that should be addressed include: room number, size, and layout. Much of what we think we need in the way of rooms has been told to us by designers, builders, and real estate agents. For them, bigger is better because it means more profit. How often have you heard some people talk about never using their living room. All of their time is spent in the family room. Most people don't need a duplication of rooms. If a breakfast room is available, the dining room is rarely used. Does a family of three really need three bathrooms? Much of the high cost of today's housing is a result of buyers being sold more than they actually need. All houses should reflect the owner's true requirements.

Extra rooms not only cost money that increases the mortgage payment, they also must be furnished, heated, and cleaned regularly. This involves a lot of expense and effort for rooms that are only used a few times a year. Individuals with a chronic illness may not have the energy to clean a large house. Similarly, they may not have the energy to entertain a lot of guests on a regular basis, so a large house may be neither necessary nor desirable.

Other decisions, to be made early, are common to planning any house. Will it be a single or multistory, Colonial or Cape Cod, etc. The location, lot placement, and view will be considered. Every aspect of the house should be thought out. For someone with severe sensitivities, no detail will be too small to consider.

Special Needs

There will be many special needs that should be considered. If food allergies are a problem, it may be important to be able to close off the kitchen with a door, to keep cooking odors form permeating the rest of the house. A powerful exhaust fan should also be considered. It may be important to allow room for an extra refrigerator or freezer.

Someone sensitive to laundry odors from the washer and dryer, will want to consider a special room for those appliances. These can be placed in a room attached to the bathroom, so that the moisture from both rooms can be handled together.

Clothing and storage requirements will need to be addressed. It is important not to store clothing in an oasis because of possible contamination of the air by the clothes, dresser, shoes, etc. Dressers can be built into closets, and closets can be vented to the outdoors. This can be done with a small exhaust fan or in conjunction with a whole house ventilating system. Soiled clothing can contain mold as a result of dampness due to perspiration, or it can smell of perfume or cigarette smoke if the wearer has been around users of such things.

Books, magazines, and newspapers can be devastating to someone sensitive to printing ink. They should be stored in bookcases with glass doors. These too, can be vented to the outside. If these materials are too offensive for an individual to tolerate, they can be used inside a vacuum reading box such as those by **Living Source**. These units are similar in concept to laboratory ventilation devices. They allow a person to read with their hands and book inside a glass-topped box. A small fan then pulls fresh air into the box and exhausts contaminated air to the outdoors.

The garage often contains a number of toxic chemicals in the way of paints, solvents, fertilizers, insect repellents, etc. The largest polluter is, however, the family car. A hot automobile inside a closed garage will give off offensive smells that will easily seep into the house. An attached garage could have an exhaust fan installed to minimize any contamination of the air in the house. Such a fan could have a timer control so that when a hot automobile is pulled in, the fan could be turned on and allowed to run for an hour or so until most of the fumes have dissipated. Detached garages are highly recommended to keep these fumes from seeping into the living space.

If entertaining is important, it must be remembered that people's clothing and their hair act like sponges, absorbing a wide variety of chemical odors. They will bring these into your house along with the perfumes and other scented products that they are wearing. Unless a powerful ventilation system is installed, these smells will be absorbed by the walls and furnishings of the house. The smell of your guests can then linger for weeks after they have gone. This can result in the erosion of health for someone with sensitivities to artificial fragrances. A good alternative is to entertain only in warm weather outdoors, on a deck or patio. Garden parties can be quite enjoyable and it will be less expensive to construct and maintain a large covered patio than a large rarely used living room.

If you operate a business in your home, it may be necessary to isolate it from the living space if a family member is bothered by such things as printed materials, the plastic case on a computer, or the odors emitted from a photocopying machine.

Some sensitive people have decided to share their homes with others. This can be both a humanitarian gesture and a source of income.

Many people, on suddenly discovering that they are being made sick by their house, find that there is no place to turn for accommodations. It may be worth considering an extra bedroom and/or bath for such a situation. You may be surprised how much of a waiting list develops.

Ventilation

It should be decided early in the planning process how the house is to be ventilated. In temperate climates, opening windows will be adequate. In hot climates where air conditioning is necessary, or cold climates, it can be quite expensive to rely on open windows for fresh air.

Choices can include either spot ventilation or a whole house system. Spot ventilation is quite common, and includes kitchen and bathroom exhaust fans. This involves removing a pollutant at its source. Venting a closet can be a form of spot ventilation. With the advent of tightly built houses, it had been found necessary to provide a more general form of obtaining fresh air. Whole house fans and heat recovery ventilators are designed to fulfill this need.

These principles can be used in many different ways. For example, kitchen cupboards can be vented, as can appliances. If there is something that must be inside the house even though it bothers you, it can be vented. Use your imagination. If you are highly sensitive to your mother-in-law's perfume, in theory she could be placed in a glass booth and vented to the outside.

Reading boxes, central vacuum cleaners, and clothes dryer all have exhausts that must be considered when planning a ventilation system. If fresh, incoming air is to enter the house in one location, it may be possible to have the air pass through a particle or carbon filter. Ventilation will be discussed more fully in Chapters 6 and 8.

Materials

When selecting materials, it is important to decide what types of contaminants are to be minimized. Naturally occurring allergens such as molds and pollens can be handled as well as man-made chemicals. Pollens will generally be brought in from the outdoors, so filtering the incoming fresh air should help to eliminate them. They can also be given off by house plants, as can mold spores from the potting soil. Generally, if moisture is adequately controlled in the house, mold will be controlled as well. Eliminating man-made toxins is primarily a factor of choosing building materials carefully.

Building Codes
Most of the materials suggested in this book will comply with building codes. Occasionally, a residential inspector may be unfamiliar with some of the materials because they are not commonly available, or their use is primarily limited to commercial buildings. Showing the inspector some product literature will usually satisfy any questions. In some cases it may be necessary to obtain a variance from the code requirements. In such a situation it is important to present your case in a well thought-out and documented manner. As an example, the building code may require a bathroom exhaust fan, yet your design may rely on a whole-house ventilation system. The bathroom will still be ventilated even though there is no specific bathroom fan present. Technically this is a violation, but with an adequate explanation and readable drawings or plans, a variance should be allowed.

Solar Heating
Two types of solar heating have evolved over the years, active and passive. If designed correctly, both can result in a healthful way to obtain heat. Both will, however, require some form of auxiliary heat for those extended cloudy periods. For this reason, adequate insulation is stressed, no matter which method if chosen.

Active solar heating involves a mechanical system of some type. This will require considerable advance planning in order to insure that the heating system and the house interact and fit together properly. Often a complex distribution system is impossible to clean. Accumulated dust can be composed of a variety of natural and man-made contaminants. This will eventually reenter the living space, causing symptoms in sensitive people.

Many active systems use water or some other liquid to transfer the heat. If some form of antifreeze is used, a leak could soak into the structure and be difficult to sufficiently clean up if the homeowner is hypersensitive to such chemicals. All active systems use electrical motors in the form of fans or pumps. These can be a source of air pollution since they will emit fumes as they warm up during operation. The lubricating oil is often the culprit, but various electrical lacquers or insulations used have also been implicated.

Passive systems involve no extra equipment. The proper design of the house is all that is necessary. Window size and placement and amount of roof overhang control how much sunlight enters the house at different times of the year, This warm energy can, however, contribute to outgassing. Some people have noticed that their synthetic draperies are more odorous when warmed by the sun. Similarly, carpeting or other furnishings can outgas when heated. Of course, if these materials are not subject to outgassing, there should be no problem. One hundred percent cotton curtains and upholstery materials can minimize the problem.

Ceramic tile or concrete floors are often used in passive solar designs because they will store excess heat. This is then automatically released during the evening as the outside temperature drops. There are a few people who report that concrete, warmed by the sun, is subject to a small degree of outgassing, but fortunately this is not a common reaction. It is, however, worth testing for.

Superinsulated Houses

A variation on the passive solar concept has evolved in recent years, known as the superinsulated house. This involves combining passive solar heating with considerably more insulation than usual. It also requires that the house be built nearly airtight and fresh air be provided through a heat recovery ventilator. Superinsulated houses, if properly designed, can be excellent examples of construction for sensitive people.

A superinsulated house should not utilize any combustion appliances. The passive solar features will provide much of the heating, at virtually no cost. Since these houses are so well insulated, the back-up heat can usually be handled with small electric heaters, often at minimal cost. Annual heating bills in cold Canadian winters are usually below $200 for these designs. The necessary ventilation system can provide fresh filtered air on a continual basis, and a glazed ceramic tile floor can be both functional and relatively inert. Superinsulated houses are discussed more fully in Chapter 8.

Summary

As you read through this book, some of your initial requirements will undoubtedly change, but that is all part of the planning process. A designer's first idea is rarely the best. All good designs need to evolve.

Your list of needs will have many additions and revisions by the time construction begins. Don't be afraid to change your mind. In fact, you may change it several times. By the time the planning process is complete, you should have a thorough understanding of what goes into your safe house.

Chapter 6

Eliminate, Separate, Ventilate

The three most important rules to keep in mind when seeking healthful housing are: *eliminate, separate,* and *ventilate*. There are a number of things that can be done to improve the indoor air quality, but these are the most important principles to follow. As an example, if you had a strong poison in the house, the best thing to do would be to eliminate it, get it out of the house, or at least replace it with a less potent poison. If there was some particular reason that it needed to be in the house, the second best thing to do would be to separate it from the living environment. It could be placed in a jar. Thirdly, since the jar may not form a perfect seal, the area should be ventilated. Fresh air could be brought in or stale air could be exhausted. There are a number of ways that you can accomplish these three concepts. Usually they will need to be done in combination.

Eliminate

Eliminating potential pollutants is by far the most important consideration to insure clean indoor air. Some products emit such large quantities of pollutants that it would be virtually impossible to ventilate properly, and if it is the entire house that is outgassing, the only feasible way to separate the pollutants from the living environment would be to actually leave and not live in the house any longer. Unfortunately, this has been the only solution for a few individuals.

The best way to eliminate potential pollutants is not to use them in

63

the first place when building a house. There are alternatives to most of today's popular building materials that are either nonpolluting or considerably safer. When substituting a safer material, it may still not be perfect, but it will then be much easier to use the other two principles of *separate* and *ventilate* to clean up the air.

The most important things to eliminate have already been mentioned: carpeting, man-made wood products, and combustion appliances. There are substitutes for these items that will be discussed later.

If the problem materials are very old, they may have outgassed sufficiently for the pollutants to have eliminated themselves. This is why an older house may be very tolerable for a sensitive person, even though it may contain some questionable components. It should also be noted that the carpeting in an older house could be wool instead of a synthetic material and the paneling could be solid wood instead of plywood. The older materials were often not as polluting as our current "space age" versions. Yet, in other cases, older products may have had their own types of pollutants such as asbestos floor tile and lead-based paints.

Outgassing of new materials can often be hastened by heating them. A commercially baked-on enamel finish is often tolerable, while a conventional enamel paint could take many months to outgas by itself. Placing a material outdoors in the sun often hastens outgassing. You can also actually bake some problem materials in your own oven. This can be done outside the house in an electric range that is kept in the garage. It should never be done in the house or in a range that will be used for cooking, because of the danger of contaminating the inside of the house or the oven with the outgassed pollutants. If they are unhealthy to breathe, they will be unhealthy to eat.

Eliminating may also refer to something outside the house, as in the case of pollen-producing plants or even neighbors. If an individual is bothered by wood smoke, living next door to someone who heats with wood may be quite unhealthy. It may, in fact, be quite unhealthy for the neighbor as well. One may only feel the effects in 20 years when stricken with one of the "old-age" diseases such as arthritis. As the long-term effects of various pollutants are better studied and understood, it will be possible to know how many of our diseases could have been easily prevented. The fact that many individuals react to such things as burning wood and natural gas should be a warning to the rest of society to eliminate them as well. The symptoms of sensitive people, like dead canaries in coal mines, should be a message to us all.

If an existing house has some pollutants that must be removed, this must be done with care and must be well planned. Removing asbestos can sometimes cause a greater problem than if it is left in place. As a part of a solid material, such as asbestos-cement siding, it may be inert. Removal may result in much asbestos dust being generated and inhaled into the lungs. If removal involves carpeting and particle board subflooring, not only should the demolition be well planned to minimize such things as dust, but the new materials should be carefully selected prior to any work being done. Too often, someone has replaced an offending material with what was supposed to be a safer alternative, only to find out that it is just as bad. During the construction process, workmen can introduce offending odors into the house. Such things as cigarette smoke, fragrances, paint fumes, etc. can be absorbed by clothing and hair and as a result can pollute the air inside the house.

Eliminating can also refer to the wide variety of cleaning products and disinfectants under the kitchen sink. These items are often extremely toxic, and although inside sealed containers can leak poisonous gases into the kitchen.

Separate

There are several ways to separate a pollutant from the indoor living environment. The most effective is to encapsulate the material completely, to totally surround it and seal it entirely. It has been suggested that nuclear waste be encapsulated within glass to protect the environment. Encapsulating implies a 100 percent seal, yet this is rarely possible. Usually separating something means placing some type of barrier between it and the living space. While a 100 percent separation is rarely possible, a 90 percent separation is generally quite feasible.

As mentioned in the discussion of an oasis, metal foil can effectively separate an offending wall from the living space. The seams between sheets of foil can be taped to provide a better seal, but the adhesive tape has been known to bother some people. With care, the edges of the foil can be folded to provide an effective seal. An environmental sealant such as Crystal Aire I (**Pace Industries**) can seal in 94 percent of the pollutants if four coats are applied, or 97 percent with five coats. It may, however, take several weeks of outgassing before some individuals can tolerate the sealant. Kitchen cabinets constructed of particle board can be coated inside and out with either foil or an appropriate sealant, but it might be simpler to replace them with metal cabinets because of the limitations of the sealant methods. Insulation and the plastic sheathing on electrical wiring can often be effectively separated from the living space by using foil-backed drywall. While there are methods of totally sealing the drywall, as in the airtight drywall approach, it may not be necessary if a less polluting insulation or wiring are used. The paper surface of the drywall can pose a problem for some people. A tolerable paint can seal in the offending pollutants, but it must be chosen with care. Paint on the ceiling and walls constitutes a major source of indoor air pollution, simply because of the large surface area involved.

Separation can also involve the use of more cupboards, cabinets, and closets. Simply placing an offending object inside a closet will separate it from the actual living space. However, the object will continue to outgas whether it is in the bedroom or in the closet. This can cause pollutants to build up inside closets and cupboards. Opening the door can then release a cloud of polluted air. For this reason it is again best to eliminate as many polluting belongings as possible. For the remaining items, closets and cabinets can be ventilated.

Ventilation

After eliminating and separating, ventilation can remove the few pollutant sources that remain in the healthy house. If there are a lot of pollutants, they can be handled by ventilation, but the cost can be prohibitive. To adequately remove the toxics generated in a modern chemically laden house might require a huge exhaust fan with all of the windows open. The resulting heating bill for the month of January in Minnesota would be steep indeed. With only a modest number of contaminants, there may be only a modest increase in the heating bill. A superinsulated design with a properly designed ventilation system can not only provide a pollution-free indoor environment but also a low heating bill.

There are different ways of ventilating a house. An exhaust fan can be used to blow stale and polluted air outdoors. A window fan can introduce fresh air into a room. Heat recovery ventilators can provide fresh air in an energy-efficient manner. With ventilation, it is important to remember that when you blow air out of a house, somewhere there is going to be replacement air coming into the house. If a window is opened, that is probably where most of the replacement air will come from. If the house is constructed fairly tight, as many energy efficient houses are today, it may actually be necessary to open the windows to provide fresh replacement air. Without a properly designed ventilation system, replacement air will seep into the house through small cracks around window frames, doors, or electrical outlets. This is known as infiltration and a certain amount occurs in all houses no matter how they are built. Obviously, a tightly built modern house will have less infiltration than a 100-year-old farm house. Therefore, a tight house should have the windows open more often to provide fresh air.

The big drawback to infiltration is that it is uncontrolled. The amount of air blowing through the walls in the form of infiltration is a function of not only how the house is built, but also such factors as the weather and type of heating system. Infiltration can allow pollutants from inside the wall cavities to reach the living space. Bits of insulation or chemicals from its outgassing can be carried into the house. You never know how much infiltration is taking place. One day it may be providing sufficient fresh air and the next day very little. Similarly, opening a window is hardly an efficient way to obtain fresh air in the winter, and in warmer weather, pollen and dust particles can easily be brought indoors. If you own a house, you will need to consider your specific circumstances and arrive at the most efficient method of ventilation to achieve healthful fresh air.

Heat recovery ventilators were developed to provide fresh air inside superinsulated houses in an energy efficient manner. When installed properly, they can provide a constant supply of fresh air, which can be filtered if necessary. While they can easily be adapted to older houses, they have a fairly high initial cost which may not make them cost-effective. It may cost less money in the long run to simply install an inexpensive exhaust fan in a problem area. Heat recovery ventilators will be discussed in more detail in Chapter 8.

Kitchen range hoods and bathroom exhaust fans are methods of ventilating specific rooms. After eliminating most of the problem belongings in a house, the few remaining ones could be stored in one particular closet that has a small exhaust fan to remove the pollutants before they reach very high levels. It could be placed on a timer, so it would not be necessary to run the fan 24 hours a day. Ventilating a closet can also help to prevent the musty, moldy smells from accumu-

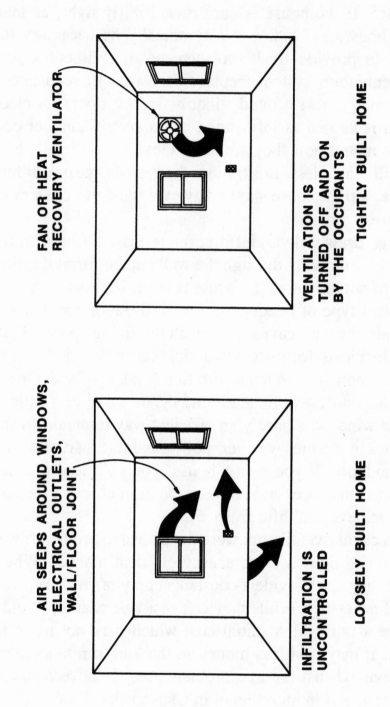

Infiltration vs. Ventilation

lating there. There are many things that can be ventilated locally in this manner. If you are bothered by the smell of a plastic television cabinet or the compressor on the refrigerator, they can be exhausted to the outside.

In a new house, it should be fairly easy for a professional to design a general ventilation system, perhaps using a heat recovery ventilator. This system could pull stale air from all the closets and exhaust it outdoors, while at the same time providing fresh, filtered air to a central location. In this way, the air in the house would constantly be circulating and changing. In an extremely tight superinsulated house, this method gives the occupants complete control over the air in the house. Since infiltration will be at a minimum in a tightly constructed house, the only air entering will be through the ventilation system. If there is a major pollution alert outside, or a neighbor is burning leaves, the fan can simply be shut off until the outside air is more tolerable. If a house relies on infiltration for fresh air, no such control is possible. It must be remembered, however, there is only so much air in a tight house and the ventilation system should not be shut off for extended periods. Sooner or later, the occupants will begin to use up the available supply of oxygen and the by-products of metabolism will start to build up.

Other Factors

There are other factors besides elimination, separation, and ventilation that affect indoor air quality. Adsorption is the process through which gaseous contaminants adhere to large surfaces such as walls. Cigarette smoke and mercury vapor will cling to walls and ceilings in this manner. These pollutants are, however, still in the room, they are just not floating around freely any more. It would be foolish to rely on this method of removing pollutants from the air, because there is a limited amount of wall space to which they can adhere. With a major source of toxic gas, the wall and ceiling surfaces would be filled rather quickly.

Absorption refers to the fact that porous surfaces such as brick and unfinished wood or drywall will actually allow air pollutants to soak into them much like a sponge absorbs water. Porous materials act as scavengers in this way, absorbing pollutants from the air. Again, with a large source of air pollution, it would not take long for these materials to absorb their limit, and then further contaminants would remain in the air.

It is also possible for particles to become electrically charged and become attracted to other oppositely charged particles. This can occur in an electrostatic air cleaner, or as a result of an ion generator. Plastic surfaces often have a static charge and as a result can attract dusts and other particle pollutants.

Summary
By keeping the three principles of *eliminate, separate,* and *ventilate* in mind during the planning and construction of a house, indoor air pollution can be minimized. Elimination of pollutant sources is by far the most important. If all of the problematic materials are successfully eliminated, then there may not need to be very much separation; however, ventilation should always be considered.

Chapter 7

Mold and Moisture

Mold and moisture will be discussed together because they usually are found together. If there is a mold problem in a house, there is invariably a moisture problem that contributed to it. The moisture can take the form of visible liquid water or invisible excess humidity in the air.

Mold

Mold is something that bothers many allergy sufferers. Molds, mildews, yeasts, rusts, smuts, mushrooms, etc., are all fungi, types of small primitive plants. They do not contain chlorophyll, so they must steal nourishment from other living plants or animals. They can also obtain their food from decaying matter or from a variety of building materials such as wood, paint, and wallpaper paste. In fact, there are so many food sources available for mold, that it would be impossible to remove them all. Since molds also require water for survival, the easiest way to control mold is to control excess moisture. While there are some molds that can survive on very limited amounts of water, most of the common allergenic molds can be controlled by keeping humidity levels in check.

Even though there are literally thousands of different types of fungi, only a few dozen are commonly found in our homes. These often result in mold allergy because of inhaled mold spores. The spores are the seeds by which the fungus reproduces. Most are extremely small in size, sometimes on the order of one micron (1 micron = 0.000039″). The larger spores can be removed with an ordinary air filter, but the smaller ones are quite difficult to remove because they simply pass through most standard filters. See Chapter 22 for a discussion of air filters.

Mold Allergy

Allergic reactions usually are a result of inhaling the spores and not the mold itself, because spores can become airborne due to their small size, while the larger "parent" mold cannot. If the larger organisms die and become broken up into smaller pieces, then they too can be blown through the air and elicit symptoms as they are inhaled by a sensitive person. Some people with mold allergies will react to such foods as mushrooms, cheese, dried fruits, vinegar, etc., because of their mold content.

The common symptoms of mold allergy include allergic rhinitis, bronchitis, sneezing, runny nose, congestion, eustachian tube obstruction, itching of the nose or eyes, fatigue, and weakness. Mold spores can enter the lungs causing asthma, a buildup of mucus, wheezing, and breathing difficulties. These symptoms are often quite uncomfortable, and in the case of a full-blown asthma attack they can be devastating. Dermatological and intestinal symptoms are also well documented. Cerebral symptoms can include: catatonic state, depression, crying, anger, confusion, fear, dizziness, anxiety, irritability, hostility, inability to concentrate, headaches, and hyperactivity.[1]

There are a number of fungi-related diseases that can be very serious. Some kinds of the mold *Aspergillus* can infect the entire body in an individual who has lung damage or a serious underlying illness. Spores from molds or fungus-like bacteria can result in a lung disease known as hypersensitivity pneumonitis. This condition usually resembles a generalized viral infection. Chills, fever, weakness, muscle pains, cough, and shortness of breath are typical symptoms, but if allowed to progress, it can result in lung and heart problems. Hypersensitivity pneumonitis is usually associated with certain occupations where there is considerable contact with mold. "Farmer's lung disease," "mushroom picker's lung," and "maple bark stripper's lung" are typical examples. It is also being diagnosed more and more in office buildings that have moisture/mold problems in their ventilation systems.[2]

For someone suffering from mold allergy, the best form of treatment is avoidance. This can be accomplished by eliminating the source of the moisture problem, and therefore the mold. As the mold is removed, symptoms will usually gradually disappear. Proper vacuuming, cleaning, ventilation, and dehumidifying will also help considerably. In the workplace, personal respirators can help, but in some cases a change of jobs is necessary.

Where Does Mold Grow?

Molds can grow practically anywhere there is moisture, oxygen, and something to eat. They are found in the soil and as high up as 10,000 feet in the air. Different varieties can be found in a dry desert, wet seashore, in a cold or hot climate. Since oxygen surrounds the planet, and there are so many possibiliities for food, curbing moisture and humidity is the primary method of control. In general, as the temperature and humidity fall in winter months, mold problems outdoors will decrease.

Mold can grow on rotting logs, in shady areas that are damp, on compost piles, etc. On farms, grains are subject to mold growth, so grain bins and silos are often problem areas for the individual with mold allergy. Workplaces such as bakeries, breweries, dairies, greenhouses, paper mills, upholstery shops, and woodworking industries all have the potential to irritate a mold allergic person.

If windows are kept open, the types of mold spores indoors and outdoors are similar. In buildings that are usually closed up, there can be entirely different species inhabiting the indoor environment than are found outdoors. The indoor and outdoor climates are different, therefore they support different types of organisms. Air conditioning often helps someone with a mold allergy for two reasons: 1. by removing humidity from the air it helps to create a drier environment that is less hospitable to mold growth, and 2. it requires that the windows be closed, resulting in the outdoor mold remaining outdoors.

In looking at molds in the house, we will be concerned with three basic areas: 1. outside the house, 2. inside the house, and 3. within the structure of the house.

Molds Outside the House

Mold can not only grow on the ground and on trees and plants, but it can grow on the house itself. This will be a problem when the house is located in a damp area of limited sunlight and little ventilation. A house deep in a forest can, therefore, be subject to mold growth. The best solution is to clear out enough of the vegetation to allow sunlight to penetrate and wind to pass through. In this way, the house will tend to remain dry and not provide the moisture necessary for the molds to grow.

On the roof, small organic particles of leaves, twigs, insects, etc., can accumulate. This will provide the necessary food, and if the roof is perpetually shaded by large trees, and as a result is damp, mold can result. Occasionally there will be enough organic matter to not only support mold, but also various mosses. Wood roofs can be especially susceptible if they are allowed to remain damp, and fungicidal treatments are often recommended. These chemicals, however, can be problematic for some sensitive people. The concrete roof tiles found in warm climates are very susceptible to fungal growth. They are somewhat porous and must be cleaned and painted every few years as they become black with mold. Occasionally, the asphalt used in composition shingles can become a food source for mold, as can the paint on a metal roof. Gutters can be terrible havens for damp rotting leaves and resulting mold. This can form a rich organic medium that larger plants such as trees can take root in. Downspouts should direct water away from the house or the result can be a damp basement or crawl space, resulting in a mold problem there.

The walls on the north side of a house will be more susceptible than the walls on the south side, because of the tendency to be slightly more damp in the shade. Absorbent wood siding will be more likely to remain damp longer than metal siding. A good paint film will generally provide more protection than a stain which can dry out and allow moisture to penetrate. Poorly insulated, air conditioned buildings can be cool on the outside of the wall, resulting in condensation and mold growth.

Rain does not always fall straight down. A driving rain can force its way into small cracks that don't appear to be a potential area for dampness to accumulate. Capillary action can cause rain to be drawn between pieces of siding, resulting in wetting from the back as well as the front. Porches should be designed to shed water. Entryways should be covered to prevent rain from entering the house when the door is opened. An ample overhang over windows will allow them to be opened during a shower without danger of water entering. Damp window sills are good places for mold to grow. Electrical or telephone wires entering the house can divert some rainwater into the structure if improperly installed.

The southeastern portion of the country from the Carolinas to Texas, and the west coast of Oregon have been shown to be the most likely areas of the United States for decay to occur in above ground structures.[3] These parts of the country are often humid and damp. This leads to fungus growth or decay. Extra efforts should be taken in these locations to insure that moisture problems do not occur.

In the area surrounding the house, almost anything can result in mold growth. Trees, shrubs, grasses, gardens, etc., can all support different types of mold at different times of the year. Compost piles can be significant sources, with visible clouds of spores rising into the air. The outdoor factors that seem to have the greatest effect are high levels of shade, high levels of organic debris, and uncared-for or natural landscaping.[4] The best solution to all of the mold problems around or on the outside of the house involves plenty of sunlight and fresh air to keep the area reasonably dry. The sun will tend to warm the area and evaporate the excess moisture. The wind will then carry it away.

Mold Inside the House
Molds can find a variety of foods inside the house. They can eat petroleum products found in paints, gases in the air, oils in the air from certain types of filters, wallpaper, leftover food, potted house plants, dried flowers, and Christmas trees. Garbage pails and dirty refrigerators are prime food sources as are dirty clothes in a laundry hamper or shoes damp with perspiration. If tap water is allowed to stand for a few hours, mold will soon begin to grow there. Carpeting has been shown repeatedly to be a source of mold growth.[5] Both carpeting and the padding can remain damp for days after a water leak or urination by pets. Shampooing is often attempted to solve a mold problem in carpeting, with the result that the freshly shampooed carpet remains damp for several hours, compounding the problem. Children are usually more susceptible to moldy carpet than adults simply because, being shorter, they are closer to it, and adults are rarely on their hands and knees playing. Carpeting should be especially avoided in the kitchen and bathroom.

Other sources inside the house include old furniture or picture frames, mattresses, clothing, and stored books or magazines. Wicker, especially plant baskets, can be an unusually bad source of mold growth. Sometimes, the growth on furnishings is so excessive that they must be removed and disposed of. Certain grouts and caulking materials around bathtubs and showers are susceptible to mold growth because of the dampness present. Clothes dryers should always be vented to the outside. A dryer vent can add a considerable amount of excess moisture into the air of the house.

The moisture necessary for mold growth can be in the form of liquid water or water vapor. Liquid water can enter the house from the outside through roof leaks, around leaky chimney flashings or through open windows. Plumbing leaks are often a source, as well as simply spilled water that runs under furniture. These are not everyday events and they will usually be corrected immediately while other moisture sources can be continuing occurrences. Toilet tanks and cold water pipes are often sources of condensation or "sweating" and hence a moisture problem. Water vapor can be generated by washing dishes, cooking, washing and drying clothes, and bathing. During normal metabolism, people add moisture to the air. A typical family of three will produce about 20 pounds of water vapor per day, most of which is from respiration and perspiration.[6] Unvented combustion appliances add moisture to the air, as well as other undesirable pollutants. Moisture can also enter the house from a damp crawl space.

We often add moisture to the air deliberately with humidifiers or by setting pans of water out to evaporate. In winter months, some houses can become extremely dry and it may be necessary to add moisture to the air for health and comfort, but humidifiers can harbor a variety of harmful organisms. Fungi, bacteria, and amoebae have been known to grow in the warm, wet environment, and then be blown into the air along with the desirable moisture. The only method of control appears to be frequent cleaning, but when a humidifier has become thoroughly contaminated, routine cleaning and disinfecting may not be enough to inhibit the mold growth. Steam type humidifiers are not reported to be a problem compared to cool-mist atomizing humidifiers,[7] nor are ultrasonic humidifiers. Mold will grow in standing water, so any humidifier can be contaminated with mold if it is not run for awhile. On restarting, ultrasonic models have been shown to kill the mold in them. However, mold particles can be spewed into the air, causing allergic reactions.[8]

Electrostatic filters used in heating systems have been shown to significantly reduce mold levels in the air.[9] They are, however, associated with producing ozone. Mold has been found growing on charcoal granules found in some air filters, but studies done in submarines have not found this to be a significant problem.[10]

Relative Humidity and Mold

The concept of relative humidity must be understood in order to fully grasp how water vapor can result in mold growth. Warm air can hold much more water vapor than cold air. When a given quantity of air is at 100 percent relative humidity, it is said to be saturated. When the air is saturated, it cannot hold any more water vapor. If this particular quantity of air is heated, we can add some more moisture, because as it gets warmer, it can hold more. If the air is cooled, it cannot hold as much moisture. When the temperature drops outdoors on a very humid day, the result is rain. The cooler air cannot hold as much moisture, so it simply unloads it in the form of a shower.

When saturated air, with 100 percent relative humidity, is heated, and can now hold more moisture, its relative humidity drops. As an example, it may now have 80 percent relative humidity. In other words, it is now 80 percent saturated. If the air is, say 50 percent saturated (50 percent relative humidity), and the temperature is lowered, the relative humidity increases. If the temperature is lowered enough, the saturation level can reach 100 percent. Outdoors, this means rain.

A certain amount of humidity in the air is desirable for human health and comfort, but too much will result in not only unhealthy mold growth, but also a proliferation of dust mites.[11] Generally, a relative humidity level below 70 percent will not support excessive mold growth. A problem can develop in a house because relative humidity varies from one area to another. It may be 70 percent in the living room but 90 percent in the bathroom. For this reason, levels should be kept below 40 percent in winter months to minimize problems. A 40 percent level in most of the house can easily mean that certain areas will approach 70 percent.

Inside a house, it is unlikely that rain will occur, but moisture can condense on cold surfaces. We think of the air indoors as being all the same temperature, but, in fact, there are many micro climates within our homes. In a poorly insulated house, it is often possible to feel cooler air near an outside wall in the winter. Very often, the air is warmer near the ceiling than it is near the floor. If the relative humidity in a house in the winter averages 50 percent (50 percent saturated), it will be higher near outside walls because the temperature is lower there. Windows can have condensation form on them because of their even lower temperature. In effect, they are cold enough for the relative humidity to rise above 100 percent and for "rain" to form. Windows with multiple glazing will minimize this occurrence. Metal window frames are notorious for being sources of condensation, but with the "thermal breaks" used in modern window construction, this too, can be minimized.

Mold doesn't require liquid moisture to survive. An area of high relative humidity is sufficient in most cases. The relative humidity can be high in bathrooms, laundries and kitchens where there is a lot of liquid water present. Exhaust fans will help to remove this excess moisture to the outdoors.

A clothes closet or built-in cupboards located on an outside wall can have a slightly lower temperature in the winter and consequently a higher relative humidity. Similarly, a piece of heavy furniture located on an outside wall can allow the temperature to fall near the wall or floor. Sometimes, a room will have poor air circulation and a corner will be somewhat cooler than the rest of the room, resulting in a higher relative humidity and mold growth. These problems are more likely to occur in poorly insulated homes and can often be relieved by improving the air circulation. Closet doors can be louvered, and furniture can be rearranged. In some cases, it may be necessary to position a small fan in a room to keep the air circulating.

In cold weather, draperies should be kept open. If they are closed, they will insulate the air space between the window and the drapes, resulting in an area of lower temperature. This translates into an area of higher relative humidity and a potential mold problem.

A concrete slab is often cooler than the rest of the room, so it can be another location for mold growth. Rugs tend to aggravate this problem by insulating the floor from the living space and allowing it to be even cooler. If a slab does not have a moisture barrier beneath it, such as plastic sheeting, moisture from the soil can actually rise up through the somewhat porous concrete by capillary action, causing the surface to become damp. This is known as "rising damp." There are various concrete sealers available through paint and hardware stores that can minimize this, but they can be problematic for some sensitive people, so they should be tested prior to use. Rearranging furniture to improve air circulation will also help.

After recent remodeling or construction, humidity levels inside the house can be very high because of the drying out of various building materials. New wood, plaster, drywall compound, and paint all contain significant amounts of water that will gradually evaporate over several weeks. Sometimes it can take an entire heating season to rid a house of this excess moisture.

In summer, with air conditioning, the air conditioner coil itself is much cooler than the air passing over it. This results in the warm, humid air condensing and giving up its moisture as it reaches a lower temperature. Air conditioners are designed to catch this excess water and either direct it outdoors or down a drain. There is usually a drip pan inside the unit to catch the water, and it can become a good place for mold to grow. Similarly, self defrosting refrigerators have a drip pan under them to catch the water from the defrosting cycle. This simply evaporates into the air rather than being directed to a drain, but while it contains water, it can be a significant location for mold to grow. Many people do not realize that there is such a pan under their refrigerator and are quite shocked to discover a large mold colony living there.

Mold Within the Structure of a House

Crawl spaces and basements can be havens for mold for several reasons. These areas are usually cooler than the rest of the house, and consequently will have higher relative humidity. They are also subject to moisture migration from the ground (rising damp). Foundation walls can have cracks or improper waterproofing and, therefore, admit water. Since these areas are under our homes, they are the logical place for plumbing leaks and water spills to end up. Occasionally, a broken pipe can empty raw sewage directly into a crawl space, unnoticed for days. Unless a house is built extremely tight, as in a superinsulated house, any mold spores found in the basement or crawl space will eventually find their way upstairs into the living area. These spores are so minute that they can pass through the smallest opening with ease.

Crawl spaces and basements can be built to minimize dampness and consequently, mold growth. These methods will be discussed in Chapter 10. Basic points involved are waterproofing, moisture barriers, insulation, temperature control, and ventilation. Unless these types of measures are taken, it is foolish to store personal belongings in these areas, because of the danger of them becoming food for mold.

Calcium chloride can sometimes be used to dry out a damp area. It is often available in hardware stores in winter months to melt snow and ice. Placed in trays or pans, it acts like a sponge, absorbing moisture from the air. It can help a damp situation but it won't cure a continuing problem. As it becomes saturated, it must be periodically changed. Dehumidifiers can also be used to dry out an area. A large capacity, automatic model is usually recommended for a damp basement or crawl space. They must either be hooked up to a drain or have their reservoir pan emptied as the moisture is converted from humidity to liquid water. Because of the water present, they can actually support mold growth, but the potential is much less than having a very damp basement.

Moisture within the structure can not only be unhealthy, it can also cause structural damage. Mortar in masonry joints can deteriorate when damp, resulting in a weakened foundation. Roof leaks or other sources of moisture within walls result in fungus attacks more commonly known as rot. A rotting structure can collapse in a cloud of mold spores. The mold growing within the walls will release thousands of spores which will certainly find their way into the interior of the house.

Burning natural gas or damp "green" wood can generate moisture in a chimney. This often collects in the ash clean-out pit which can be a good place for the mold to grow. A stainless steel chimney liner can help to increase the velocity of the flue gases and reduce the potential for condensation. Chimneys without caps can allow rain to enter, resulting in a similar problem.

Moisture within wall and roof cavities has become a potential problem in recent years as a result of houses being insulated without taking into consideration moisture migration. Just as heat passes through a wall into the cold outdoors, the moisture will also pass through a wall or ceiling. As the water vapor goes through the insulation, it becomes cooler and cooler, until it begins to condense *inside the wall*. This will result in wet insulation and framing lumber. When insulation is wet it loses much of its ability to insulate and when lumber gets wet it is in danger of attack by mold. Insulation containing formaldehyde resins will release formaldehyde gas more readily when damp. Urea-formaldehyde foam insulation has been shown to support mold growth.[12] When wood rots, it is actually being eaten by a fungus. Exterior paint failure is often a sign of a moisture problem inside the wall. As the excess moisture tries to escape through the siding, it will cause paint to blister.

Older houses, with little or no insulation, allow both heat and moisture to pass through the walls rather quickly. This can happen so fast that the water vapor doesn't have a chance to condense. When one of these houses is insulated, the passage of heat and moisture is slowed. This slower movement of moisture means that it can now have a chance to condense inside the wall cavity, resulting in a potential mold problem. In some climates this can form frost just inside the exterior sheathing, which melts as soon as temperatures rise in the spring. One solution would be to use a moisture barrier paint on the inside of the house in order to slow the passage of moisture through the wall. One such commercial brand is "Insulaid" manufactured by **Glidden Paint**. In a new house, it is a common practice to install a moisture barrier before the drywall or plaster is put up. If done correctly, this can help to alleviate potential moisture problems.

Ceiling moisture barriers are also important. In a cold climate as moisture rises through the insulation into the cold attic space, it can condense on the underside of the roof in much the same way that moisture condenses on a cold window pane. A moisture barrier will help in this case as well, but in most situations it is still very important to allow the roof system to breathe. This can be accomplished by the use of ventilators. A combination of eave and ridge vents usually works well. Other choices include gable end vents, roof vents, mechanical ventilators or electric fans. There will always be a little moisture passing into the attic, because no moisture barrier is 100 percent effective, so ventilation of this space is imperative. Another problem in cold climates that can occur when roofs are improperly ventilated involves ice damming. This occurs when the portion of the roof directly above the house is warmer than that directly over the eave. In this case, snow begins to melt and run down the slope. When it reaches the colder eave, it refreezes. In doing so, it can back up under the shingles and eventually result in water dripping inside the structure. There must be an air space between the insulation and the roof deck, and this space must be ventilated, or ice damming will occur. This problem is often found in insulation retrofits and in unvented cathedral ceilings.

Moisture inside a wall cavity may not be due to moisture migrating from the interior of the house. It can easily be a result of rain penetration, a leaky roof or gutters, or plumbing leaks.[13] No source of moisture should be overlooked if a problem is suspected. In the case of a severe mold problem within the walls, simply drying out the walls may not solve the problem. The wall cavity can contain a tremendous reservoir of spores and could easily continue sending them into the living space for months after the mold has ceased producing. The solution for a severe problem can be as drastic as removing the interior walls and cleaning out all vestiges of both mold and spores.

Moisture Barriers

Technically, if something does not stop 100 percent of the moisture it should be called a moisture retarder, not a moisture barrier. However, the terms "moisture barrier" and "moisture retarder" are often used interchangeably. They work by slowing the speed at which moisture passes through the surface of the wall. Diffusion is the term used to describe this slow form of moisture migration. Moisture barriers are rated in perms (permeance). A perm rating of zero means that no moisture will pass through the material. This will be a true moisture barrier. The higher the number, the more moisture will pass. Some typical perm ratings are:

Drywall	20.0
¼″ exterior plywood	0.7
1″ concrete	3.2
8″ concrete block	2.4
Enamel paint on smooth plaster	1.0
"Insulaid" paint (**Glidden**)	0.6
Shellac	0.4
4 mil polyethylene	0.08
Metal foil	0.0
Glass	0.0

In an existing house, a moisture barrier paint or the use of a foil type wallpaper may be the only choices for retrofitting a moisture barrier. In new houses, polyethylene sheeting is often used. This can become an effective moisture barrier because of its low perm rating, but it has been found to exhibit some problems and it is not a very effective air barrier. Some people may react to outgassing from the polyethylene itself. If electric baseboard heaters are used, the heat can cause the material behind them to degrade inside the wall and fall apart as it is warmed. Ozone generated by electrostatic precipitators or other appliances will also contribute to deterioration. This will obviously lead to a defective moisture barrier. Most superinsulated houses rely on very tightly sealed moisture barriers. Special detailing is required around any openings such as windows and electrical outlets.

Aluminum foil or stainless steel foil can also be used as a vapor barrier but, generally, they are available only in three-foot-wide rolls. This means a lot of taping of seams in order to achieve a tight seal, but it can be done to avoid the pitfalls of using a plastic material. Foil-backed drywall forms an effective moisture barrier.

Air Barriers

The importance of a moisture barrier has been recognized for some time as an important way to control moisture diffusion in walls. However, only recently has the importance of air barriers been understood. As air passes through openings in a wall, it can carry moisture with it. These openings are typically such things as electrical outlets and switches, small cracks around doors and windows, and gaps between the floor and the wall finish. As it turns out, an air barrier is considerably more important than a moisture barrier, although both are necessary.

A moisture barrier is effective in slowing the diffusion of water vapor through the surface of the wall. It does not need to be a perfect barrier to do this. If the barrier has a few holes in it, yet 98 percent of the wall contains a barrier, then, overall, it will be 98 percent effective as a moisture barrier. An air barrier, however, must be as close to 100 percent effective as possible. If an air barrier has a few holes in it, the various air pressures acting on the house (wind, stack effect, ventilation) will cause much air to be drawn through those holes. If that air contains moisture, and it often does, it can condense inside the wall and result in structural problems and mold growth. It has been shown that a 1″ hole in an air barrier will allow 100 times more moisture to pass by air than a 1″ hole in a moisture barrier will allow to pass by diffusion.

A construction technique that is gaining in popularity is known as the airtight drywall approach (ADA). In this method, drywall is utilized to form an interior air barrier. During installation great care is taken to insure that the drywall joints are sealed thoroughly, so that a virtually airtight house results. Special care is taken around windows, doors, electrical outlets, etc. It has been shown that this method can be quite effective in controlling air flow through the structure of the house. It is also a relatively easy method of construction. The airtight drywall approach is discussed more fully in Chapter 8.

Location of the Moisture Barrier and Air Barrier

It is very important to correctly locate the moisture barrier within the wall, ceiling or floor in order to avoid condensation within the structure and resulting damage or mold growth. Most of the books dealing with moisture barriers say that it should be located on the warm side of the wall.[14,15] While the location will obviously vary with the seasons, it is generally agreed that in cold climates, where January temperatures average 35° F or below, the moisture barrier should be on the interior side of the wall, close to the living space. It is also desirable in moderate climates to position the moisture barrier near the inside surface of the wall. Polyethylene is commonly used just beneath the drywall. In hot, humid climates, the moisture barrier should be near the exterior of the wall, near the outdoors. It is also usually stated that a wall should only contain one moisture barrier, not two. Two moisture barriers in a wall mean that water vapor can become trapped between them and condense. Therefore the rules of thumb are said to be: (1) in cold climates the moisture barrier goes on the interior of the wall, (2) in hot climates it goes on the exterior of the wall, and (3) use only one moisture barrier in any wall.

Contrary to these theoretically correct rules, many houses have been built that violate them without experiencing moisture damage inside the walls. Older houses typically have no moisture barrier whatsoever, and the theorists suggest that when such a house is insulated, moisture migration is slowed inside the wall and condensation can result. This rarely happens because the house is still leaky enough so that moisture doesn't get a chance to build up within the wall. Other houses have been built according to these rules and have had problems. This is often because no air barrier was installed. In new construction, the moisture barrier can be positioned in a theoretically incorrect position and not result in problems if its surface temperature will never get low enough to allow the relative humidity within the wall to reach 100 percent.

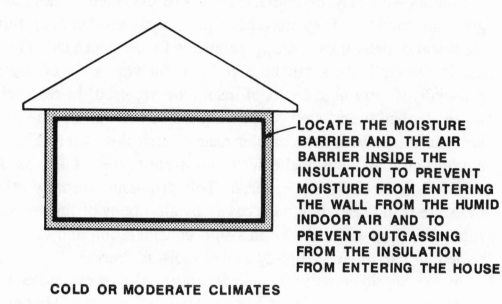

LOCATE THE MOISTURE
BARRIER AND THE AIR
BARRIER <u>INSIDE</u> THE
INSULATION TO PREVENT
MOISTURE FROM ENTERING
THE WALL FROM THE HUMID
INDOOR AIR AND TO
PREVENT OUTGASSING
FROM THE INSULATION
FROM ENTERING THE HOUSE

COLD OR MODERATE CLIMATES

LOCATE AN AIR BARRIER <u>INSIDE</u>
THE INSULATION TO PREVENT
OUTGASSING FROM THE INSULATION
FROM ENTERING THE HOUSE

LOCATE A MOISTURE BARRIER
<u>OUTSIDE</u> THE THE INSULATION
TO PREVENT MOISTURE FROM
ENTERING THE WALL FROM
THE HUMID OUTSIDE AIR

HOT, HUMID CLIMATES

Mositure and Air Barrier Locations

Houses with polyethylene moisture barriers often do not have very good air barriers. They may have poor seals around such things as electrical outlets, thus creating pathways for moisture laden air to get inside the wall. This can be a problem in very cold climates, and especially if very high levels of insulation are used. In research studies, water had been found condensing inside the wall in the vicinity of holes in the polyethylene barrier near electrical outlets.[16] This can be aggravated if an additional exterior moisture barrier is also used, such as a foil-faced sheathing material. This problem is usually related to moisture being carried into the cavity by air, not by diffusion. Superinsulated designs usually take this into consideration and use a tightly sealed air barrier and a tightly sealed moisture barrier.

In hot, humid climates, an interior moisture barrier has been shown to result in condensation at certain times of the day. However, the problem was no longer apparent if two moisture barriers, on each side of the wall, were used.[17] While two moisture barriers may be desirable in some situations to control moisture migration from humid air into the wall cavity, their use can result in moisture problems from other sources. For example, if moisture enters the wall from a roof or plumbing leak or from rising damp, condensation within the wall cavity can easily occur, resulting in rot or mold growth. In new construction, lumber can contain a substantial amount of moisture. This can become trapped between two moisture barriers and result in problems.

It will be advantageous to have an interior air barrier in a healthy house, no matter what the climate, to separate such things as insulation from the living space. In cold climates, the same material can be used to function as both an air barrier and a moisture barrier. Tightly sealed foil-backed drywall will perform this dual function. In moderate climates, there generally have been no ill effects noted with the use of an interior moisture barrier. However, in very hot, humid climates, there can be condensation within a wall when an interior moisture barrier is used. As the moisture migrates into the wall from the outdoors, it travels through the insulation until it reaches the interior side of the wall. If the living space is air conditioned, this surface will be cool. A moisture barrier here can result in the humid air condensing on the cool surface, within the wall. As noted above, if two moisture barriers are used, condensation does not occur, but this can result in other problems. In hot climates, an interior air barrier can be created by using tightly sealed drywall and a separate moisture barrier can be used in the outer portion of the wall.

In summarizing, a moisture barrier and an air barrier should be used on the inside of the wall in most climates of the United States. This controls the moisture and prevents outgassing of the insulation from entering the living space. The use of two vapor barriers within a wall should generally be avoided. In hot, humid climates, an interior air barrier should be combined with an exterior moisture barrier. While rules of thumb such as these can be handy, moisture migration can be quite an involved and technical subject. Rather than relying on such rules, the designer is advised to carefully analyze a wall, ceiling or floor section in order to determine if condensation is likely within the structure. This can be done by calculating the surface temperature of each component at different times of the year. This information, combined with the indoor and outdoor humidity levels, can be used to predict the humidity levels within the wall cavity. A psychometric chart can be used to determine if the relative humidity will reach 100 percent at any surface within the structure. Humidity of 100 percent will mean condensation with resulting mold growth and structural damage. High levels of insulation mean a slower migration of moisture through a wall, so these walls should be analyzed carefully to predict condensation potential.

Ventilation

Since most modern houses, and especially superinsulated houses, are built fairly tight, ventilation has an importance that it never had in the past. Houses used to be built so loose that the wind literally blew right through them. Today, with modern materials and construction methods, there is hardly enough fresh air indoors to breathe. If there are many outgassing materials present, the indoor air can be quite toxic. Moisture must be removed through ventilation in order to eliminate mold problems and fresh air must be brought in. Exhaust fans have been commonly used to reduce interior moisture to acceptable levels. With the advent of superinsulated houses, a device known as a heat recovery ventilator has been developed. These units are designed to provide a constant supply of fresh air, as well as remove excess moisture. They will also remove various stale odors.

Heat recovery ventilators simply supply fresh air and remove stale air in a manner that is much more energy efficient than opening a window or living in a leaky 100-year-old house. They are discussed more fully in Chapter 8.

Cleaning Up a Mold Problem

When a mold problem is encountered, the first and most important thing to do is locate the source of the moisture and eliminate it. When this is done, the mold can no longer produce spores. It may not be dead, but without moisture it will be dormant and will not produce spores. People often assume that a good, strong disinfectant will kill the mold and there will no longer be a problem, but if the moisture is not eliminated, the mold will simply return again and again. Many sensitive people are bothered by commercial disinfectants. In some cases, "Zephiran" (**Winthrop Pharmaceuticals**) is recommended for these individuals. It is available through pharmacies.

After the moisture problem has been solved, the area should be cleaned with soapy water and thoroughly dried. A portable electric hair dryer can be used to dry out a place that is hard to get at. Washing will not only help to remove any unsightly stains, but more importantly, it will remove the allergenic spores without sending them flying into the air. A portable vacuum is not recommended for cleaning up the microscopic spores because they will tend to pass through the vacuum's filter and be blown around the room. A central system with an outdoor exhaust will work much better. After cleaning the area, it may still remain somewhat stained. A wall might require repainting, a floor refinishing, or tile regrouting.

Borax or vinegar are often recommended for killing mold. They are quite good as cleaning products, but if the moisture problem isn't solved, it does no good to think about killing the mold. Mold counts are often 1000 times as high as pollen counts, so even if you successfully kill one colony, there are many more spores waiting to start a new one. This is why it is so important to remove the moisture supply.

Summary

Mold, a common allergen, can grow in many locations inside or outside of a house. It can also be found within the structure of a house. In order to control its spread, moisture must be kept in check. Both visible water and invisible high humidity levels can help to create an ideal environment for mold to grow rapidly. Controlling this moisture involves several techniques, depending on each particular situation.

Chapter 8

Airtightness and Ventilation

Modern construction practices have resulted in houses being built with less ventilation than in the past. The way houses used to be built, it would have been very difficult to achieve today's degree of airtightness. Sheet materials such as drywall and plywood mean that there are fewer cracks and seams for air to pass through. Windows and doors are now made of different materials that are designed to admit less air infiltration. When we introduce many potentially toxic materials into a living space with minimal fresh air, the result is often ill health. According to one informed architect, "You can build tight buildings as long as you don't fill them full of poisons."[1] Fortunately there are ways to achieving energy efficiency without sacrificing health.

Should a House Breathe?

Many people condemn the current trend toward airtightness and energy efficiency because of the negative health implications. Clearly, something needs to be done. According to an editorial in the *Journal of the American Medical Association*, "There is no doubt that unless a reasonable and logical plan is developed, the deleterious health impacts of excessive home tightening will be enormous."[2] As an analogy, if we compare our bodies to our houses, we can see the need for a house to breathe.

Our bodies don't breathe through various cracks and openings the way our houses have traditionally breathed. Our bodies are very well designed machines with a specific mechanism for admitting oxygen. We breathe through our mouths and noses, not through our skin. Our skin has, as one of its functions, to control moisture migration out of the body through perspiration. If we introduce toxic materials into our bodies, it is no surprise that illness is the result. If we view a house as an extension of our body, we can see that three basic principles must be understood: 1. A house must have a flow of air through it. 2. A house's structure should be designed to perspire correctly. 3. A house shouldn't contain toxic materials.

Toxic materials are to be avoided at all costs when designing a safe house. With inert building materials, less fresh air is necessary; however, it will always be necessary to supply the oxygen essential for life. It is also required for moisture control and removal of stale odors, but if fresh air is needed to counteract the effects of poisonous materials, a very large volume may be needed. In an existing house, some remodeling may be necessary to remove pollutant sources in order to achieve healthfulness, simply because it won't be feasible to install a huge ventilating system.

The breathing done by a tightly built house can be accomplished by simply leaving the windows open, but this is hardly energy efficient. Tightly built houses in Canada, Scandinavia, and other colder climates rely on a device known as a heat recovery ventilator for fresh air. Such a unit will not only supply fresh air but it will also remove average amounts of stale air. This is all accomplished automatically, in an energy-efficient manner. It will also be important for a house to be designed to expel large amounts of stale or moisture-laden air at certain times. Kitchen range hoods, outside clothes dryer vents, and bathroom vents will perform this type of function.

We have already seen how moisture can travel through wall and condense, resulting in mold growth within a wall cavity. With proper construction techniques, this problem can be eliminated. The result will be a very tightly built house. This will mean that a ventilation system will be even more necessary. The capacity of it will depend on the size of the house, number of occupants, and number of toxic materials inside the house.

Controlled Indoor Air

The concepts of how a house should breathe are unfamiliar to many designers and builders. Today's modern technology has bypassed many professionals, with the result that their thinking no longer applies to the way houses are currently being built. Loosely built houses "automatically" supplied plenty of fresh air for other occupants. The energy crisis of the 1970s had the result of adding insulation, weatherstripping, wood stoves, and less expensive natural gas heat. It wasn't until people began getting ill in these supertight houses that a problem was suspected. Many designers began advocating a return to a looser type of construction. Unfortunately, this type of thinking is not progressive. The correct answer is to analyze the problem and continue moving forward. A healthful, energy-efficient, state-of-the-art house is the result.

For very sensitive people, the concept of controlled indoor air has several advantages. When air passes through a house in a random, uncontrolled way, it brings with it mold and pollen spores. As the air passes through the wall itself, it can pick up small particles or odors from the insulation. On a cold day, there may not be enough fresh air entering the house, yet on a windy day there may be more than is necessary. When air passes through a structure in this way it is called infiltration. Tightening up a house reduces infiltration to a minimum. As a result, controlled fresh air through ventilation is now necessary. Air entering through a ventilation system or a heat recovery ventilator can be filtered, thus providing a very clean supply of fresh air for the occupants. It will be very difficult to filter out all of the smaller mold and pollen particles, but the improvement over the outside air during the ragweed season can be significant. If the outdoor air is very polluted, a complicated and expensive filtration system may be required. This is why a location far from pollution sources is desirable.

If an air filter contains a sufficient amount of activated carbon, it can remove a variety of chemical contaminants that are bothersome to many people. If a neighbor is burning trash or tuning up his automobile and the fumes are too much for the carbon to handle, the unit can simply be shut off until the outdoor pollution passes. It is important to remember that if the house is very tightly built, there is only a limited supply of oxygen present for breathing. This should be no problem if the ventilation system is only shut down for a few hours or even an entire day. Many people operate them at high speed for 12 hours, and turn them off for the remainder of the day.

Ventilation and Radon

Anything that causes a lowered air pressure inside a house can cause an increase in the amount of radon filtering through openings in the foundation. Of course, if there are no pathways for radon to enter the house, or if there is no radon existing in the soil, lowered air pressure won't result in radon in the house.

If a ventilation fan is used to blow air out of a house, there will be air entering the house somewhere else. In a loosely built house it may be difficult to control this infiltration. It may pass through the house in a variety of places, such as around poorly weather-stripped doors and windows or through cracks in the foundation. If there is an excess of infiltration, the concentration of radon will tend to be diluted. In fact, this is an easy method of radon reduction: increase the air flow through the house. However, if ventilation is used for this purpose, it is important to allow for the fresh air to enter the house somewhere other than through the openings in the foundation. Otherwise, an increase in ventilation would also mean an increase in radon.

A combustion appliance will need a supply of fresh air in order to keep the fire burning. As air is pulled into the combustion chamber and the burned gases rise up the chimney, a lowered air pressure in the house often results. Clothes dryers and kitchen range hoods can also cause a depressurization of the house if there isn't an opening somewhere else for fresh air to enter and balance the amount of stale air being exhausted.

If a house has gaps between a chimney or vent pipe and the ceiling, or around attic stairs, recessed ceiling light fixtures, etc., there is the possibility of wind creating a suction on the house as a whole. This can cause air to be pulled through these gaps, leading to depressurization. Therefore, these types of openings need to be sealed when it is necessary to reduce radon levels in a house.

Heat recovery ventilators should have the fresh and stale air streams balanced to avoid lowering the air pressure in a house. It is sometimes recommended that such a system be adjusted so that the house has a slightly higher pressure than the outdoors. In this way, pollutants tend to be expelled rather than drawn into the house.

The best solution for controlling radon is, of course, to prevent it from entering the house in the first place by one of the methods discussed in Chapter 10.

Heat Recovery Ventilators

Heat recovery ventilators are also commonly known as air-to-air heat exchangers. They do not produce heat, they simply recover heat that would otherwise be lost in the ventilation process. There are a number of different types, but basically they consist of a cabinet, a core, two fans, and some ductwork. The fresh air from the outdoors passes through one part of the cabinet, through the core, and into the house. The stale air from the indoors passes through another part of the cabinet, through the core, and then outdoors. As the two airstreams pass inside the core, they do not touch, but they do exchange their heat. In the winter, the cold outdoor air is warmed by the indoor air, so that by the time it enters the living space it is no longer like an arctic blast. Since there are varying temperatures inside the unit, water will condense within the cabinet. Drains are provided, which must be plumbed to a house drain. Some units are designed to remove excess moisture from the air, while others allow the moisture to be transferred between the two airstreams.

In theory, heat recovery ventilators do not leak between the two airstreams. In actuality, there is usually some leakage. Cross-leakage rates have been reported as low as 0 percent and as high as 40 percent.[3] Obviously, it is desirable to obtain a model with minimal leakage between airstreams.

Efficiency also varies.[4,5] Some units are reportedly rated above 90 percent; however, actual test results are often lower than manufacturer claims. Efficiency depends on both the indoor and outdoor temperature, humidity, and the fan speed. Therefore, the efficiency ratings for the same unit can vary, depending on how the testing was done.

If an 80 percent efficient unit is used when the outdoor air temperature is 0 degrees F. and the indoor temperature is 70 degrees F., then the 0 degree air will be warmed up to 56 degrees as it passes through the core. The 70 degree air is releasing its heat and will drop in temperature to 14 degrees by the time it reaches the outdoors. The 56 degree air will still need to be warmed up by heating system, but the cost will be considerably less than if a window was opened and 0 degree air was used for ventiation.

Heat recovery ventilators also work in the summer to cool the incoming air, but their greatest economy is in the colder climates where there is a much greater differential between the indoor and outdoor temperatures. In mild climates, where the temperature differential is

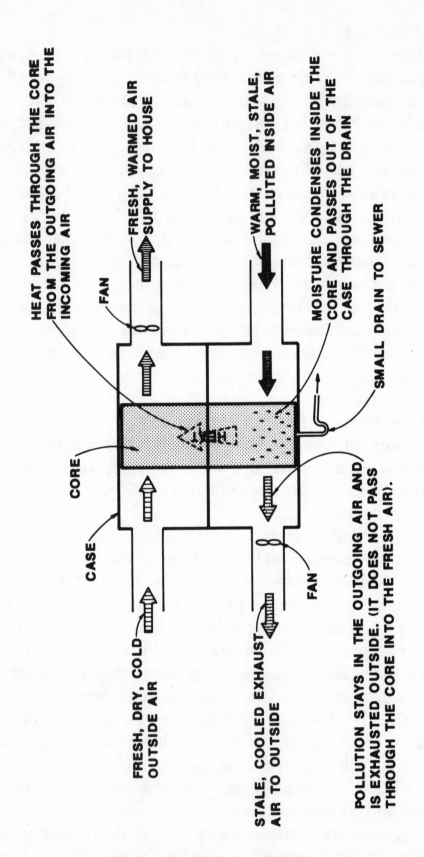

Heat Recovery Ventilator Schematic

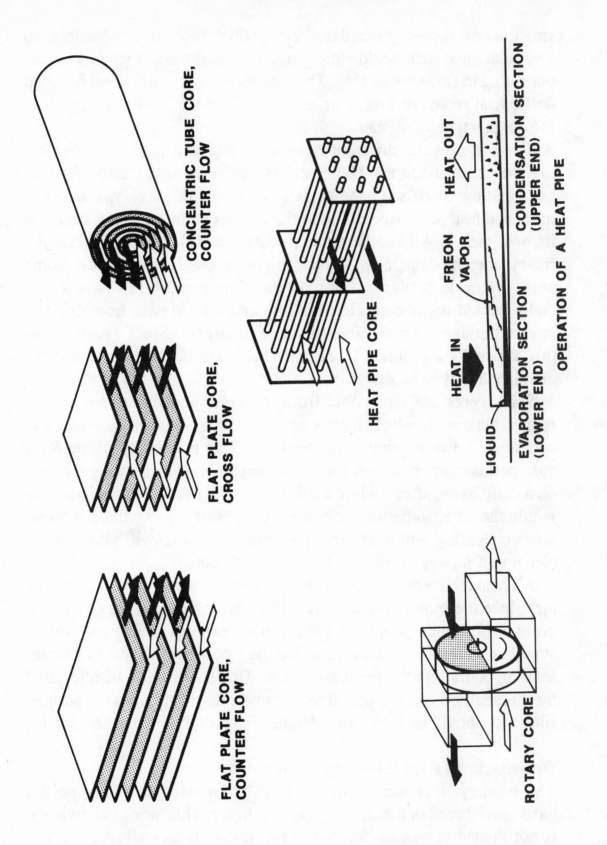

CONCENTRIC TUBE CORE, COUNTER FLOW

FLAT PLATE CORE, CROSS FLOW

FLAT PLATE CORE, COUNTER FLOW

HEAT PIPE CORE

HEAT OUT

CONDENSATION SECTION (UPPER END)

FREON VAPOR

EVAPORATION SECTION (LOWER END)

HEAT IN

LIQUID

OPERATION OF A HEAT PIPE

ROTARY CORE

Heat Recovery Ventilator Core Types

small, a heat recovery ventilator may not be economically feasible, so a ventilation system could simply use a fan and some ductwork, without trying to conserve energy. The amortized cost of a several hundred dollar heat recovery ventilator may not offset the modest energy savings in this type of climate.

There are several different types of cores, with flat plate cores being the most common. These are available in either cross-flow or counter-flow models. Other kinds of cores include rotary, concentric tube, and heat pipe. According to the various manufacturers, each has its own merits. All can be made to function well, but in general the rotary core models seem to have higher cross-leakage rates. Some cores are made of plastic, but most are aluminum. A few have a specially treated paper core. These allow moisture to pass from one airstream through the paper into the other airstream. Since excess moisture is usually a problem in a tightly built house, these units will not alleviate that type of situation.

Some cores are removable from the case, and others are not. A removable core is advantageous because it can be taken outdoors and occasionally washed with a garden hose. This is hardly feasible for a core permanently mounted inside the house. With air passing through on a daily basis, after a while a certain amount of dust will accumulate within the core, so periodic cleaning is necessary. Since there is moisture condensing within the case, a removable core will allow easier cleaning if mold growth ever becomes apparent.

All heat recovery ventilators have one or two small fans to move the air. Since the motors are usually within the airstream, they can be a problem for some people. As the motor heats up during use, oil or synthetic materials or lacquers inside the motor heat up and volatilize, sending odors into the fresh airstream. This can usually be alleviated by the addition of a carbon filter. Many units have a coarse particle filter that should be kept clean. High-efficiency filters can be added.

Drawbacks to Heat Recovery Ventilators

The primary drawbacks concern lack of knowledge. Many people have never heard of a heat recovery ventilator. This lack of knowledge is not limited to consumers, but to professionals as well. A good understanding of ventilation requirements, moisture problems, and system design is necessary in order to correctly specify and set up an installation. A lack of uniform testing standards make it difficult to compare the merits of different models. An excellent booklet, *Heat Recovery Ventilation for Houses*, is available from the **National Center for Appropriate Technology** to educate both builders and home-owners.[6]

Builders have resisted routine use because of the added expense, ignoring the fact that the hidden costs of ill health can be enormous. The size of some of the units is also a drawback because of the space required. Ductwork as well can take up room.

The primary consumer complaints concern the noise associated with a continually running system. A proper installation on rubber pads will minimize the vibration noise in the rest of the house. Register location also has an effect on noise. This can be minimized by careful positioning. Air silencers or "mufflers" are also available from some manufacturers, or they can be easily made in a sheet metal shop.

Sizing a Heat Recovery Ventilator

Small room-sized units are available, but these are of insufficient size to handle most situations; therefore, our discussion will be limited to whole house units or central systems.

Houses should be typically designed to provide one air change per hour (ACH). This should probably be considered a minimum. It may, in fact, be more than sufficient on most days, but there will always be times when it will be advantageous to turn the speed up to high and bring in plenty of fresh air. Human activities invariably produce undesirable odors, whether it is from cooking, or opening mail containing a scented advertisement. However, heat recovery ventilators are not usually designed to remove large amounts of indoor air pollution.[7] For example, an unvented gas range can require a tremendous amount of fresh air for combustion in order not to pollute this house. This type of pollution is best handled by a separate range hood. Combustion appliances should always have a separate source of air in order not to rob the occupants of necessary oxygen. Without proper combustion air, the occupants can succumb to carbon monoxide poisoning. Similarly, if the house contains a large amount of outgassing wall paneling, the best solution would be to either remove the paneling or seal it, for a very large heat recovery ventilator would probably not be economically feasible. They can certainly help a bad situation, but they may not provide enough air to be a cure. It may still be necessary to open

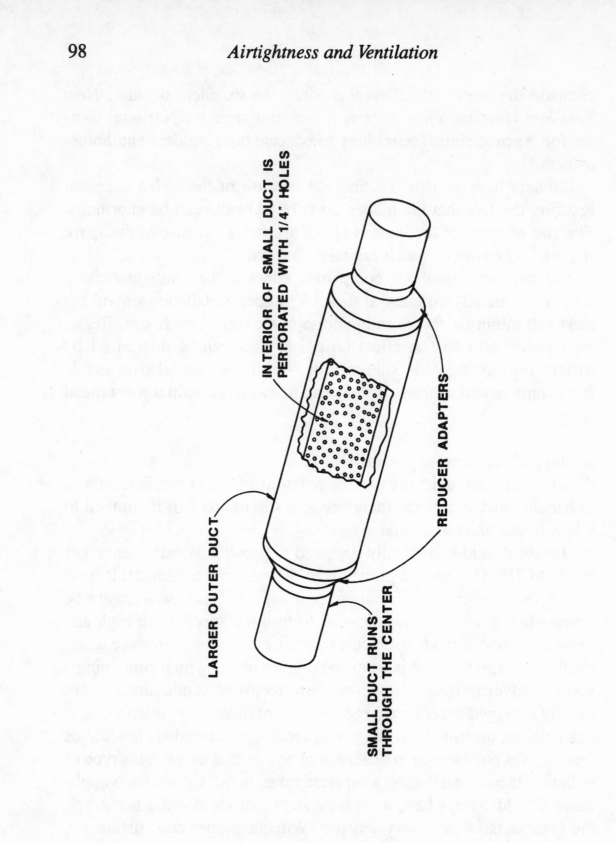

INTERIOR OF SMALL DUCT IS PERFORATED WITH 1/4" HOLES

REDUCER ADAPTERS

LARGER OUTER DUCT

SMALL DUCT RUNS THROUGH THE CENTER

Air Silencer

windows occasionally if, for example, burning toast fills the house with smoke.

In order to determine how large a unit will be necessary, the dimensions of the house must be known. As an example, we will consider a 30′×60′ two-story house with 8′ high ceilings. First, it is necessary to calculate the volume of the house by multiplying the width×length×height×the number of stories. In our example, 30′×60′×8′×2 = 28,800 cubic feet. If one air change per hour is desired, then 28,800 cubic feet will need to be exchange each hour. Since most units are rated in cubic feet per minute (CFM), this number should be divided by 60. 28,800/60 = 480 CFM. Therefore, a 480 CFM heat recovery ventilator will be required to provide a change of air each hour, or one ACH.

If a house has little or no toxic materials in its construction or furnishings, one ACH will usually be sufficient for most sensitive people. A house with a few toxic furnishings may require a slightly larger capacity. When in doubt, a larger unit should be selected over a smaller model. Even though the initial cost will be higher, in a tightly built house a ventilation system should not be considered a luxury; it is a requirement whose importance cannot be overemphasized. Fresh air is absolutely necessary for good health.

Sweden has made a 0.5 ACH a mandatory minimum if used continuously. In California, under winter design conditions, a 0.7 ACH minimum is required.[8]

Controlling a Ventilation System

The simplest method of controlling a ventilation system is to have no control, and this may be required in some building codes. Although it could be shut off at the main electrical panel, this method has some disadvantages. If all the windows are open on a nice day, there is no reason to have an additional ventilation system running. If there is a sudden source of outdoor pollution, as when a neighbor applies chemicals to his lawn, it will be desirable to shut the system off for a while.

Besides a simple on-off switch, three other types of controls should be considered: a variable speed control, a humidistat, and a timer. During normal everyday activities, it may not be necessary to provide one ACH. Most of the time, ½ ACH may be sufficient; therefore, a speed control will be an easy way to control the fan speed. Heat recovery ventilators are usually even more energy efficient at lower speeds. Since moisture can be a major problem in tightly built houses, a humidistat will be a helpful control. Many of the manufacturers provide them as a standard feature. The humidistat is usually mounted in the bathroom, so that as moisture levels rise during bathing, it will automatically turn on the ventilation system. A speed control in the living room can be wired together with a humidistat in the bathroom. In this way, the fan can be set to run at half speed during most of the day; yet when excessive humidity is generated by a hot shower, the humidistat will sense the excessive moisture and automatically turn the unit up to high speed. A time clock or a simple timer can be used to shut the unit off at a specific hour or turn it on in the morning. The control system can be quite simple, or as complex as one desires.

Where to Locate a Heat Recovery Ventilator

Some of the units are quite bulky, so an early planning consideration will be space. It is sometimes recommended that they be mounted in the attic or crawl space. These locations are hardly ideal because access is limited and regular cleaning may never take place. They may also be subject to freezing in these locations. There must be provisions for a drain to handle the water that will condense inside. A 3/4″ drain is usually sufficient.

A location in a utility room over the washer and dryer may be a good choice, or in a heated basement. In any case, it must be considered where the ductwork will be run. Generally, there will be four connections, each 6″ in diameter. Two will run to the outdoors and two will run to the indoors. The pairs of ducting should be separated at their ends. It will do no good to terminate the two outdoor ducts near each other, in which case the stale outgoing air will simply head back indoors by way of the fresh air intake. Similarly, if the ducts aren't separated indoors, the air will pass directly from one to another and the air in certain areas of the house will become stagnant.

The ducts running to the outdoors, and the unit itself, can become cold enough to allow moisture from the air to condense on the outside of them. These must be insulated in cold climates in order to prevent this occurrence. Some cabinets come with insulation already installed. Usually this is on the inside, where it can contaminate the airstream. It may be possible to remove the interior insulation and attach it to the outside of the cabinet. Without insulation, the cold cabinet could become wet with condensation. The problem can be alleviated by mounting the entire unit over a drip pan, to keep the surrounding area dry. Interior insulation can also be covered with metal foil to prevent the airstream from becoming contaminated. The supply duct outdoors should be located away from potential pollution sources such as automobiles, garages, plumbing vent stacks, dryer vents, etc.

Often, a single fresh air register and a single stale air register are recommended. This results in large areas of a house not being properly ventilated. If one fresh air register is used in the house, it can contain a single filter, depending on the design of the system. By using a single fresh air outlet in the center of the house, and several stale air registers around the perimeter of the house, a good circulation pattern can be developed.

"Creative" ventilation involves thinking about where the pollutants are generated and placing a stale air vent in that location.[9] Closets often can harbor stale odors. By placing a stale air vent in each closet, fresh air can travel from a central location, through a room, through the closet, and then outdoors. Cupboards can be vented in a similar manner. With proper thought, each room can have a constant supply of fresh air.

Clothes dryer vents, central vacuum exhausts, and kitchen range hoods should not be ducted through a heat recovery ventilator. Clothes dryers generate large amounts of lint that can rapidly clog the core. Central vacuum systems can do this as well, though not to the same degree because they contain a filter. Cooking odors contain particles of grease which can accumulate inside the core and become a fire hazard.

Sources

If one does not want to buy a heat recovery ventilator, plans are available for building one.[10,11] However, these models use plastic cores which should be avoided because of outgassing from the plastic. For the individual able to design a unit, flat plate aluminum cores without case or fans are available from **Automated Controls & Systems**. There are many different models being manufactured today and no single one is recommended in all situations. A suitable unit might be selected from the following partial list which does not include models that use either a treated paper core or a plastic core. Other more complete lists of manufacturers are available.[12,13] Since manufacturers are continually upgrading their products, it would be wise to review their literature for the following points:

1. Does the unit contain any plastic or treated paper components?
2. Is there any type of asphaltic or other coating applied?
3. If painted, is the finish baked on?
4. Can interior insulation be moved to the outside of the unit?
5. What controls are standard?
6. Is there an automatic defrost capability?
7. Can the core be removed for easy cleaning?
8. What is the published efficiency?
9. What is the published amount of cross-contamination?
10. Are auxiliary heaters or air-conditioning modules available?

Manufacturer	*Core Type*
Boss Aire	Flat plate, crossflow
Combustion Engineering, Inc.	Heat pipe
Des Champs Laboratories, Inc.	Flat plate, counterflow
May-Aire	Flat plate, counterflow
Mountain Energy & Resources, Inc.	Heat pipe
Nutech Energy Systems	Flat plate, crossflow
Xetex, Inc.	Flat plate, crossflow

Airtightness

Today, many houses are being built tighter with less ventilation, and the result is ill health. In the 1970s, a few houses began to appear that were being deliberately built as tight as possible.[14] They had mechanical systems to introduce fresh air. These houses were called "superinsulated" and their energy efficiency was phenomenal. In the midst of an energy crisis, they had heating bills of only $100 for the entire year. Some early mistakes lead to a very good understanding as to how a house can be both healthful and energy efficient. Moisture migration inside walls proved to be a very important consideration. Early superinsulated houses almost exclusively used a polyethylene air/vapor barrier, which can be bothersome to some individuals because of outgassing. Later designs incorporated what has become known as the airtight drywall approach (ADA).

Superinsulation

Superinsulated houses have four characteristics:

1. High levels of insulation.
2. An almost airtight and moisture-tight envelope.
3. Limited window area, with most facing south.
4. Fresh air is provided mechanically.

All of these factors combine to make a house truly energy efficient, but it may still not be healthful. If toxic building materials are used, the indoor air quality can remain poor. Yet with careful selection of materials, a state-of-the-art energy efficient *and* healthy house can be built.

Superinsulated houses can be built in any style from Cape Code to Colonial to Contemporary. The concept of superinsulation refers to a building system, not a specific design. Just as practically any house can have aluminum siding, practically any house can be superinsulated. It is relatively easy to design a new superinsulated house, but to upgrade an existing house can be difficult, primarily because of the problem of obtaining an unbroken air/vapor barrier. For a resourceful builder, this simply means some extra thought and care.[15,16]

In a superinsulated house, walls and ceilings are typically insulted to levels three or four times that of conventional houses. Floors are also highly insulated. Windows are generally triple-glazed and in some areas four panes of glass are being used. Every aspect of the house is very well insulated, but insulation alone does not make a house superinsulated. Special care is taken to insure that there are no shortcuts, known as thermal bridges, for heat to pass through the structure. There are several ways to achieve high insulation levels, but the most common seems to be by building the exterior walls 8″ to 12″ thick and filling the entire cavity with insulation. The easiest way of achieving this wall thickness is to actually build two walls and space them a few inches apart. This method of building has been practiced for many decades in ice house construction. It allowed ice to be stored throughout the year, before the introduction of mechanical refrigeration. Superinsulation construction techniques are not at all difficult, but are too involved to discuss totally here. The reader is directed instead to other sources on the subject.[17,18,19,20,21] Books and papers on the subject are available from libraries and bookstores.

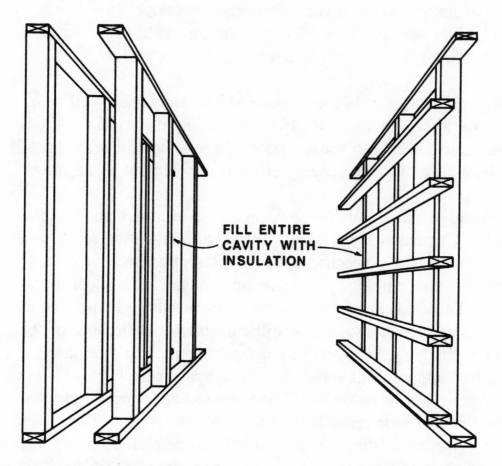

FILL ENTIRE
CAVITY WITH
INSULATION

DOUBLE WALL TECHNIQUE　　　　CROSSHATCH TECHNIQUE

Superinsulated Wall Framing

The airtight and moisture-tight envelope is of prime importance in a superinsulated house because of the potential for moisture damage inside the wall. Certainly, by making the house airtight, energy efficiency will be enhanced because it won't be necessary to heat the outside air that enters by way of infiltration. The barrier should be as moisture-tight as possible, because as insulation levels increase, the passage of moisture through the wall is slowed, and it can have a greater chance of condensing within the wall cavity.[22] As was discussed in Chapter 7, this can lead to mold growth and possible structural damage. If there are holes in the moisture barrier as are often found at electrical outlets, the water vapor will seek out those locations to pass into the wall cavity, much like a punctured inner tube will allow the air to escape from a tire.

A common method of achieving an air/moisture barrier has been the use of flexible polyethylene sheeting. This is applied directly to the studs, prior to the installation of the interior wall finish of drywall, plaster, or wood paneling. Various methods have been developed to seal this barrier around electrical outlets, plumbing penetrations, etc. One major disadvantage that has been noted with the use of a polyethylene barrier is that it can deteriorate inside the wall, unknown to the occupants, and become ineffective. This generally occurs behind electric baseboard heaters where the elevated temperatures cause the plastic to break down, become brittle, and fall apart. As noted in Chapter 7, polyethylene is a poor choice for an air barrier.

Window area is limited in superinsulated houses for two reasons. First of all, a lot of windows mean a lot of heat loss, and consequently, higher heating bills. Secondly, if there are a lot of south-facing windows, the house can be in danger of overheating in the winter. There has been an optimum percentage worked out for the number of windows for proper comfort and energy efficiency. The total window area should be between 10 percent and 15 percent of the total floor area. This will, of course, vary depending on the house's specific design and climate. For a 1000 square foot house, the window area should, therefore, be 100–150 sq. ft. Most of these should face south in order to obtain the maximum heat from the sun. Windows facing east will help the house warm up in the morning, after a night of cool temperatures. A correctly designed roof overhang will allow the windows to be shaded in the summer months when the solar heat is not desired.

Fresh air is provided mechanically because superinsulated houses are built so tight that there is not enough fresh air naturally blowing through the cracks to provide for the needs of the occupants. Heat recovery ventilators are the primary means of providing this needed air. These units can cost several hundred dollars, but this is often offset by the fact that superinsulated houses do not need furnaces. They are so energy efficient that small electric baseboard heaters are all that is required. Therefore, the money saved on a large heating system and complicated ductwork can be applied to the cost of obtaining fresh air in an energy efficient manner.

Airtight Drywall Approach

Because of the difficulties that can be encountered in installing a flexible polyethylene moisture barrier, a different method of construction has been developed. It also avoids the pitfall of having the vapor barrier deteriorate inside the wall cavity. The airtight drywall approach (ADA) was developed as an easy method of obtaining an air barrier. By utilizing foil-backed drywall, an effective moisture barrier is also obtained. This type of drywall is available from all of the major drywall manufacturers. It is not always kept in stock by local distributors, but it can usually be easily ordered. The actual construction techniques are not difficult, and can be applied to virtually any style of house.[23,24,25,26]

One method of using the ADA involves applying all of the drywall to the exterior walls before building any interior partitions. All of the joints and seams are then taped in the conventional manner. With special provisions around electrical outlets, windows, doors, etc., this provides a very tight air barrier. It is, however, an incomplete moisture barrier. Every seam between the sheets provides a potential path for moisture to diffuse into the wall cavity. Research has shown that this is not a problem because most of the moisture inside a wall cavity is carried there by the movement of air. With all of the joints and seams covered with drywall tape, a complete air barrier is the result. If the air is stopped by an air barrier, most of the moisture is stopped as well. Since the drywall is backed with aluminum foil, the majority of the wall does, in fact, have a very good moisture barrier. While the moisture barrier is of prime importance to keep water vapor from slowly diffusing through the wall, an air barrier is of greater importance. With a nearly perfect air barrier, the moisture barrier can be slightly imperfect.

Some of the methods utilized in the ADA will be unsuitable for very sensitive people. For example, intolerable foam rubber gaskets may be used in some locations to achieve a good seal. If it is not feasible to delay the erection of the interior partition walls, strips of plywood are used in some areas to achieve a seal. Aluminum foil tape can be used in many cases and it is generally well tolerated. It is available at some hardware stores and from heating/air conditioning suppliers.

Caulking is also used in ADA construction. It is often implicated in eliciting symptoms in susceptible individuals; however, it is very useful in this method of construction. If the ADA is being considered, it would be wise to test several caulkings early in the planning stages in order to find one that will outgas rapidly. See Chapter 19 for recommended caulkings.

From the standpoint of a very sensitive person, it will be advantageous to install and tape the drywall on all exterior walls prior to erecting any interior partitions. In this way, less potentially offensive materials will be needed to arrive at a good seal. Plumbing and electrical subcontractors generally do not like this method of scheduling because it means that they must be on the job site on two different occasions to do their rough-in work: once to work on the exterior walls, and once to work on the interior walls.

For information about the correct location of a moisture barrier in a wall and problems with moisture condensation within a wall cavity, see Chapter 7.

Summary

A state-of-the-art house must be viewed as a system. Insulation, moisture, ventilation, airtightness, healthfulness, and energy efficiency are all interrelated and should be considered together. Unfortunately, many builders and designers are not aware of the interdependency of the different concepts. The insulation contractor is unaware of the moisture problems caused by the drywall contractor. The heating contractor is unaware of the health effects caused by excessive home tightening by the other subcontractors. When considered together, the different aspects can combine to form an energy-efficient and healthy house. The best of all worlds is certainly a possible and achievable goal. Because of the interdependence of all of the components of a house, no chapter of this book will stand alone. Just as the leg bone is connected to the thigh bone, the drywall is connected to the ceiling joist. Our bodies are complicated machines whose different systems interact. Our houses are not quite as complicated, but the various components interact just the same. To ignore this fact can result in an unhealthy house.

Chapter 9

Concrete and Masonry

Concrete and masonry products can be used in a variety of locations in house construction. Concrete is often used in foundation and flooring systems, but can also be used for walls and roofs. Masonry is commonly used for walls, both above and below ground. In general, they are fairly well tolerated materials, but there are instances where they can and do cause health problems. Careful selection of products and components can, however, result in a safe installation.

Concrete

Concrete is a mixture of cement, aggregate, and water. When these ingredients are combined, the cement and water undergo a chemical reaction and solidify. If you place your hand on concrete as it hardens, it will feel warm, evidence of the chemical reaction taking place. Many people use the terms "concrete" and "cement" interchangeably. They are not the same thing, however. Cement is one of the ingredients of concrete, much like flour is one of the ingredients of bread.

There are several different cements that can be used in making concrete, although only one is commonly available. Similarly, there are different types of aggregates. Usually the aggregate used will depend on what is available in that particular geographic area. The water used will generally be tap water.

Concrete is usually finished to a smooth or brushed surface. There are, however, other attractive methods of finishing. Exposed aggregate can provide a more colorful and textured surface. Metal forms can be used to impress a brick or flagstone pattern in the surface before it solidifies. Concrete doesn't have to be plain and dull looking. With a little thought and planning, it can be used as a striking architectural accent.

Health Effects

Most sensitive people can tolerate concrete once it has cured; however, a few report various symptoms, which may be related to one or more of the ingredients. Reactions are more common to the wet mixture, before it hardens. At this stage, it is capable of causing a chemical burn.

Cement dermatitis is well known, though relatively uncommon, in the concrete industry. When water is added to dry cement, it produces calcium hydroxide, a very strong corrosive alkali. This acts like lye, with prolonged contact causing severe burns and skin tissue destruction.[1] This is usually the result of workmen walking in the wet concrete without proper protective clothing. The wet concrete can get inside loose-fitting boots and can splash up on unprotected legs. Burns can also develop when working with the dry mixture, before water is added. In this situation, the cement can react with perspiration on the skin, causing localized burning. Once the concrete cures and becomes hard, caustic burns are not a problem because the calcium hydroxide reacts with carbon dioxide from the air and becomes inactive.

This type of tissue damage can be so destructive as to cause third degree burns requiring skin grafting after a relatively short exposure of 20 minutes.[2] Various creams and lotions have been used as a preventive measure, but the best method is to avoid contact with wet cement or concrete. As with most reactions, there are some individuals who are more susceptible than others. Most concrete workers spend their entire lives without experiencing a single ill effect. Others may become burned on their initial exposure. Damage can be so severe as to cause injury to nerve endings with chronic pain being the result.[3]

Silicosis or white lung disease has been reported among workers in concrete plants. This is apparently due to dusts generated by the aggregate and not the cement. Symptoms can range from a slight cough to pneumonia.[4]

There are other, less devastating effects of working with concrete. A sandpaper effect from the cement particles or the aggregate can cause irritation. The perspiration-cement or water-cement solutions can remove protective oils from the skin, causing drying and cracking, or they can cause clogging of the pores.[5]

The home handyman should take proper precautions when working with concrete, but in general, these types of reactions are not a concern to the homeowner, because most people only come in contact with hard, cured concrete. Yet, there are a few people with various sensitivities who report adverse reactions to concrete after it has set. The surface of a concrete floor can wear from walking traffic, producing a dust that is very fine and can aggravate an asthmatic's condition, but there are other possible causes of symptoms. In order to locate the source of a hypersensitivity reaction, we will discuss the various components of concrete.

Cement

Cement acts like a glue to hold the concrete together. Type I Portland cement is the most commonly used today. Portland cement is the generic name for a type of cement, so named in 1824 because it resembled a type of building stone found in Portland, England. There are five different types of Portland cement available, with Type I being a general-purpose cement. Types II, III, IV, and V have been developed for specialized uses and are not normally encountered in general construction. For example, Type IV produces very little heat as it undergoes its chemical reaction with water and hardens. This quality is only important when large, massive structures are being built, such as Hoover Dam.

Type I Portland cement contains mostly calcium oxide, with lesser amounts of silica, alumina, and iron oxide. A small amount of gypsum may be also be added. The other types of Portland cement contain similar ingredients in different proportions. Other specialized types of Portland cement include: air-entrained cement (see discussion of admixtures), and various blended cements. These include Type IS (Portland blast furnace slag cement), Type IP (Portland-pozzolan cement), Type S (slag cement), and Type P (Portland-pozzolan cement).[6] These should generally be avoided by a sensitive person, because of their possible contamination with hydrocarbons.

Portland cement is made by heating the various ingredients to about 2800 degrees F. These materials melt to form clinkers which are ground into powder. When water is added to this powder to make concrete, it hardens. Aggregate is added to provide greater strength and bulk. Today, cement kilns are usually fueled by pulverized coal. As a result, there is a slight possibility that a small amount of hydrocarbon could contaminate the finished product. There are, however, other areas of more significant concern when analyzing why concrete could cause a reaction in a sensitive individual.

Before the development of Portland cement, natural cements were used. They consisted of varying ingredients that were excavated, heated, and ground into powder. These were used locally and their composition and properties were not consistent.

Another type of cement that is available today is aluminous cement, which is composed of bauxite with a high percentage of alumina. It is a rapid-hardening cement that gives a high early strength. This is an important consideration only in some specialized types of construction. Regular Type I Portland cement requires 30 days to reach 90 percent of its ultimate strength, although it is hard enough to walk on in a matter of hours. Aluminous cement hardens much more quickly. Aluminous cement is a specialized product that is not normally encountered in the residential construction industry.

Other materials can be considered cements, but they generally are not used to make concrete because of their relatively weak strength. They do have other purposes and will be discussed later. Materials such as hydraulic lime and quicklime are used in mortars. Plaster of Paris and Keene's cement are both gypsum cements.

Oxychloride cement, also known as Sorel cement, was popular in the past for use in flooring. Magnesite flooring is composed of oxychloride cement, magnesium chloride salts, and a filler such as sawdust, wood chips, sand, or asbestos. The liquid mixture was poured on a floor, leveled, and allowed to harden. Once hard, it needed to be sealed with something like tung oil. This type of flooring is no longer available and because of the sealing requirement, is not recommended for most sensitive individuals.

Type I Portland cement is by far the most widely used in concrete today. For someone with sensitivities that seem to be aggravated by concrete, a small quantity of Portland cement only should be mixed with a tolerated water, allowed to cure, and tested. The wet mixture should be avoided by the sensitive person and it should not be tested until a few days have elapsed. It may be advantageous to allow the sample to warm up in the sun after it has cured, in order to see if this hastens any possible outgassing.

Aggregate

Aggregate refers to the small stones added to the concrete mix. The strongest concrete consists of many different sizes of aggregate that are packed together in the cement/water mixture. A combination of sand and larger stones is usually used. The aggregate must be clean or the cement will not adhere.

The most common aggregates in use today are sand, gravel, and crushed stone. Sand and gravel are simply dug out of the earth. A variety of stones can be crushed to provide aggregate, including limestone and granite. These should pose no problem for someone with chemical intolerances. In the southeastern United States, seashells have been used for aggregate. There are some aggregates that can easily be problematic. Old concrete can be crushed and used for aggregate. If the old concrete was intolerable to a sensitive person, then if it is crushed and used as aggregate, the resulting new concrete may also be intolerable. In some parts of the country, slag from blast furnaces may be used, as well as fly ash, cinders, and volcanic material. These can contain hydrocarbon or sulphur compounds and should be avoided. Crushed sandstone, broken-up bricks, and other materials should not be used as aggregate if they are very porous. They could have absorbed a variety of odors prior to being mixed into concrete. Vermiculite, perlite, and expanded polystyrene can be used in light-weight or insulating concrete. If their use is anticipated, a sample of the concrete should be tested.

It is doubtful that any aggregate will elicit symptoms in most people because once the concrete is hard the aggregate will be encased in the cement. Most aggregates are basically rocks, and rocks are usually inert, but since there are no 100 percent safe building materials, various potential problem areas are mentioned here for the sake of completeness.

Radon can be given off by rocks in some parts of the country. This type of material should be avoided as a choice of aggregate, as should tailings or refuse material from uranium mines. Some of these materials have been used in the past. Today, most ready-mix concrete suppliers obtain their aggregate from only a few sources. Even though there are no radon testing requirements for concrete, enough houses are being tested today to determine if there are areas of large radon concentrations. If a supplier is producing concrete with excessive radon, it should be known fairly quickly if there are abnormally high numbers of houses in a given locality with radon problems.

Water

The water used in making concrete must be clean and relatively uncontaminated. If not, it can cause an adverse chemical reaction to take place when combining with the cement, resulting in a weakened concrete. Water stored in gasoline or oil cans should not be used. Nearly any water that is suitable for drinking can be used to make concrete. Usually the water comes from a municipal water supply or a private well.

Most water today has a variety of minor contaminants, some of which are naturally occurring, some of which are man-made contaminants, and some of which are added purposefully at water treatment plants. These contaminants are usually not found in sufficient concentrations to affect the strength of concrete. However, there are many sensitive people who have difficulty finding a water pure enough to drink. For a few of these individuals, the impurities in water may explain an intolerance to concrete. The pesticide residue, chlorine, or fluoride in the water may be released from the surface of the concrete, especially when it is warmed by the sun or a heating unit; however, it is doubtful if this is a significant factor.

While the three basic ingredients of concrete could each, theoretically, cause reactions in sensitive people, the most likely cause of intolerance to concrete involves a variety of chemicals that are incorporated into the concrete mixture called admixtures.

Admixtures

Admixtures are chemicals that are added to the basic concrete mix to give it different properties. Accelerators and retarders will affect the speed in which the concrete cures. Fungicides, germicides, and insecticides can be added. Colored aggregate can be considered an admixture. Other chemicals that can be added include: air-entraining agents, gas forming agents, pozzolans, expansion inhibitors, damp-proofing agents, permeability reducing agents, workability agents, grouting agents, expanding agents, and colorants.[7]

As a rule, admixtures will not be used unless they are specifically requested because of the increased cost. There are, however, exceptions. Air-entraining agents are often added to the powdered cement at the factory. They can be identified by the addition of the letter A to the cement's type number (eg. Type IA). They can also be added at the concrete plant as the concrete is being mixed. These admixtures are used in cold climates when concrete is to be placed outdoors. They are used routinely in sidewalks and patios that will be subjected to freezing winter temperatures. Air-entrained concrete has literally millions of microscopic air bubbles in it, up to 10 percent of the volume of the concrete. These bubbles help to absorb some of the pressure that concrete is subjected to in freezing weather. This reduces the likelihood of cracking. There are a variety of materials that are used as air-entraining agents, including: wood resins, fats and oils, wetting agents, soaps, sodium sulfate, hydrogen peroxide, and aluminum powder.[8] These are usually proprietary products whose precise composition is not relinquished by the manufacturers.

When ordering concrete from a supplier, the contractor is usually asked where it is to be used. If it will be used for a porch floor, air-entrained concrete may be automatically supplied. If it is to be used for a foundation footing or an interior concrete slab, it probably won't be supplied because these locations aren't subject to freezing temperatures. Some people do not realize that the air is added by the use of a chemical. It is sometimes assumed that it is incorporated with an air compressor of some type. Because of the chemical used, air-entrained concrete can be troublesome to some sensitive people, as can many of the other admixtures.

Another admixture that is often added to concrete without being specifically requested is a water-reducing agent. This may only be used in the amount of 20 oz. per cubic yard of concrete, but could possibly be bothersome to a sensitive person. Again, these are generally proprietary ingredients. As such, it will be difficult to determine their exact composition. A concrete supplier will, however, be able to tell whether or not such an admixture is used, and whether the concrete can be ordered without it.

Colorants are of several types. Aniline-based colors, common lampblack, or dyes should not be used. They may not be tolerable to sensitive individuals, they will not produce a high quality coloring job, and they can be subject to fading. Most Portland cement is gray in color, hence the concrete is also gray. The color will vary throughout the country, depending on the exact ingredients fed into the kiln. Type I Portland cement can usually be specially ordered in white, which is manufactured without iron compounds. This is often recommended when using various commercial colorants in order to obtain brighter colors in grouts and mortars.

As with all admixtures, colorants are generally not recommended for use with sensitive individuals. If they are used, it will be a good idea to test them prior to actually using them in a house. The colorants should be high-quality mineral pigments, such as those produced by **Davis Colors** or **Drakenfeld Colors**. Consult your local concrete supplier for the use of colorants, since they may keep a certain brand in stock that will prove suitable. Some colorants contain chromium or other heavy metal compounds that can be toxic, so they must be handled with care. While these materials may not affect someone immediately, heavy metals can build up in the body and cause effects later in life.

Pouring Concrete

There are several potential problem areas with concrete that do not involve the concrete itself. Concrete walls are usually poured into metal or wood forms. These are often treated with oil as a release agent, some of which will remain on the concrete and can produce symptoms in someone sensitive to petroleum products. They allow the forms to be removed easily and reused. A good coat of paint or wax can perform the same function but form oil is more popular. With care, uncoated forms can be used if required.

Reinforcing steel is often placed in concrete to give it added strength. This is desirable in most situations and should cause no tolerability problems.

Plastic moisture barriers are often placed under concrete slabs to prevent water from migrating up from the ground through the concrete. This too is very desirable, and although the plastic may not be tolerable on direct exposure, it will be separated from the exposed surface by a layer of concrete and should pose no problem.

Expansion joints are usually made of asphalt-impregnated insulation board. This will prove intolerable to many people. When needed in a long sidewalk or adjacent to a structure, expansion joints can be made out of redwood boards.

Muriatic acid is a good concrete cleaner that is available from hardware stores. It should, however, be thoroughly washed off before a sensitive person is allowed to be near the concrete. Muriatic acid is a powerful product that actually etches the surface of the concrete. It is primarily used to clean cement residues from finished surfaces such as ceramic tile. It should never be used near aluminum, as it will severely corrode it.

Curing compounds should be avoided. They help to retard the evaporation of moisture from the surface of the concrete. Curing can be accomplished by simply keeping the concrete damp with a garden hose. Dampening the concrete with water and then covering it with a sheet of plastic will help it to retain moisture. This may be left on for several days since the desired physical properties of concrete such as strength and durability will be enhanced by extended curing.

Concrete is somewhat porous and can stain easily. For this reason, sealants are often used. Most sealers are relatively toxic petrochemical derivatives. The exception is a product called sodium silicate. It is also known as water glass because even though it is available in liquid form, it is chemically similar to glass. It not only seals concrete, but it helps to cure and harden the concrete as well. A drawback is the fact that other paints or sealers will not adhere to the concrete once it has been coated with sodium silicate. When applied to concrete, it does not change its appearance, so if a color is desired, this is not the product to use. Sodium silicate is not always readily available. Chemical supply houses listed in the telephone book can often order it. Five-gallon quantities would probably be the minimum order. There are a number of manufacturers, including: **Ashland Chemical Co., Diamond Shamrock Corp.,** and **Du Pont Co.**

Masonry

Masonry refers to construction using such materials as concrete blocks, bricks, stone, tiles, etc. In general, the materials are fairly inert; however, there are possibilities for chemical contamination to occur. Mortar is used to bind the various materials together. Masonry walls are often strong enough to actually hold up a house, but they can be decorative as well. Masonry walls can be made much more attractive than a simple concrete block wall. Since masonry is usually well tolerated, we will discuss some of the more attractive materials as well as the functional ones.

Mortar

Mortar is a form of concrete. It too is a mixture of cement, aggregate, and water, but it has the addition of hydrated lime to increase its workability and improve its waterproofing qualities. What is known as masonry cement is simply a premixed product containing Portland cement and hydrated lime. To this are added sand and water to produce mortar. There are different types of mortars. All of the types have the same basic ingredients but in different proportions in order to obtain different properties. Type M, for instance, contains one part cement and 1/4 part hydrated lime, to which are added three parts sand. Masonry sand should be clean, angular, and of uniform size.

Hydrated lime is a product of limestone and should not affect most sensitive people any more than the other ingredients; however, if in doubt, testing should always be done prior to use.

Like concrete, the major problem area with mortar has to do with admixtures. One of the most common admixtures is antifreeze, which allows masons to work in temperatures below freezing. It is very important to make sure that the individual masons on the job understand that no admixtures are to be used in the house of a sensitive person without prior testing. These are often added to mortar mixes without knowledge of a sensitivity problem.

Mortar is colored more often than concrete. White Portland cement and white sand will yield a white mortar. This can be very attractive, yet hard to keep clean. If other colors are desired, use the same precautions as in coloring concrete.

Concrete Blocks

Concrete blocks are commonly available throughout the country. Being made of concrete, they are composed of cement, aggregate, and water. The aggregate is usually sand and slightly larger particles but in some cases can be another material. Concrete blocks are sometimes referred to as cinder blocks because cinders can be used as the aggregate to reduce weight. Expanded polystyrene beads can also be used to reduce weight and increase the insulative value. While standard concrete blocks with a sand aggregate are usually well tolerated, any unusual aggregate should be tested by a sensitive person.

Concrete blocks are somewhat porous and can absorb odors, depending on where they are stored. Blocks stored, for example, near a gasoline pump can absorb a certain amount of gasoline odor and bother a sensitive person. When new blocks are delivered to the construction site, they should be tested by a sensitive person prior to being used. This should be done after the fumes of the delivery truck have

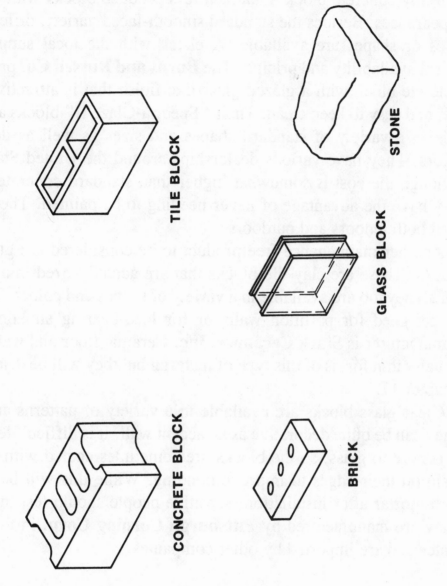

TILE BLOCK

STONE

GLASS BLOCK

CONCRETE BLOCK

BRICK

Masonry Materials

dissipated. Most reputable block companies will exchange blocks if a proper explanation is given.

Many concrete block manufacturers produce blocks with different appearances. Besides the standard smooth-faced variety, different textures or shapes are available. A check with the local supplier will reveal availability and pricing. The **Burns and Russell Co.** produces a concrete block with a glazed glass-like finish that is attractive, durable, and easy to keep clean. Their "Spectra-Glaze II" blocks are available in a variety of standard shapes and sizes as well as dozens of colors. They have various dealerships around the United States, and although the cost is somewhat higher than standard concrete blocks, they have the advantage of never needing to be painted. They can be used both indoors and outdoors.

Another maintenance-free product to be considered are glazed tile blocks. These are clay tile blocks that are actually fired in a ceramic kiln. They too are available in a variety of shapes and colors. They can be designed for partition walls or for load-bearing situations. One manufacturer is **Stark Ceramics, Inc.** Ceramic floor and wall tile are actually thin forms of this type of material but they will be discussed in Chapter 17.

Clear glass blocks are available in a variety of patterns and sizes. They can be quite decorative as an accent wall. It is difficult for mortar to adhere to glass, so the blocks are sometimes coated with a plastic resin on their edges to improve bonding. While this will be covered with mortar after installation, sensitive people should test them first. They are manufactured by **Pittsburgh Corning Corp.** in the United States and are imported by other companies.

Bricks

Bricks are made of clay or shale that has been fired and hardened in a kiln. They are usually not as hard as other ceramic materials that are fired at higher temperatures. Bricks are generally well tolerated. Harder bricks will be less likely to absorb moisture or odors. Bricks are available in many colors, sizes, shapes, and textures. Though usually confined to outdoor use, bricks can be used indoors as well, often resulting in a very decorative wall, but they may be difficult to clean because of their texture.

Building bricks are rather plain in appearance. Face bricks have better durability and appearance. Some brick is produced with a glazed, glass-like face that is highly durable, attractive, and easy to clean. Fire brick is made of a special type of clay that can withstand the high temperature inside fireplaces, boilers, etc.

Stone

Stone can be either cut into very uniform shapes or used in a natural rough state. Common varieties include: limestone, sandstone, granite, and marble. Stone provides a nice accent both indoors and outdoors. Softer stones are more absorbent of odors and can be easily stained. In general, the only danger in using stone masonry is the possibility of obtaining some material that emits radon. Outdoors this would not be a problem. Today, most quarries will know if there is radon in the area, so the danger in using stone should be minimal.

Summary

For the most part, concrete and masonry materials are well tolerated by sensitive individuals. With a few precautions, such as avoiding admixtures, and adequate testing, there should be no reason that an ecologically safe house shouldn't contain these materials. With proper design considerations, and selection of materials, concrete and masonry can yield a very warm and attractive house.

Chapter 10

Foundation Systems

The purpose of a foundation is to support the house and transmit its loads to the soil. The type of soil in the area will partially determine the design of the foundation in order to minimize uneven settlement which could result in cracking of the structure. The design of the foundation, as well as the choice of materials used, can have an effect on healthfulness. Since foundations act as bridges between the house and the ground, they can allow radon gas to pass from the soil into the house. Soils typically contain a certain amount of moisture and their temperature is often lower than that of the air. This combination of moisture and lower temperature can easily translate into a mold problem. Our discussion of foundations will, therefore, be concerned primarily with radon, mold, and material selection.

Material Selection

Concrete and masonry are popular choices for use in foundations. They are usually well tolerated by sensitive people, but there are a few cases where they can be the cause of reactions. Since they are made of raw materials that come from the ground, there is the possibility that they can contain radon; this possibility should not be overlooked, but the problem of radon in building materials themselves seems relatively rare in the United States. It is more prevalent in Europe.[1] Infiltration of radon from soil gas through the foundation into the house is by far the largest contributor to indoor radon levels.[2]

Radon, ground water, and termites can easily pass through very small cracks in a foundation; thus, where there is danger of uneven settlement, a reinforced concrete foundation may be a better choice than unreinforced masonry because of its ability to withstand greater loads. Most residential foundations are designed on a "rule-of-thumb" basis, but with weak or unusual soil conditions it may be wise to have an architect or engineer perform some soil testing or analysis in order to insure the integrity of the foundation. Cracking can not only be unsightly, it can be unhealthy as well.

Pressure-treated wood containing arsenic salts is beginning to be used for foundations.[3] It has advantages of being less costly, easier to insulate, and easier to finish; however, it can contaminate basements with arsenic. Children playing on these basement floors can easily get arsenic dust on their clothes and hands, and inadvertently into their mouths. These treated wood products are typically guaranteed for 25 years, considerably less than the expected life of a house. What happens in 50 or 75 years if much of the preservative has leached out into the soil and there isn't enough of it left to be totally effective, and a toxic termiticide is then required? A wood foundation does not appear to be a healthy choice for our families either for the short term or the long term.

Waterproofing materials in the past were composed primarily of Portland cement mixtures but they were not always effective. Today, a wide variety of plastic membranes, films, and bituminous mastics are very popular. They can be very bothersome to sensitive people, but once covered with soil they will be more tolerable. Since the upper portion of such materials is very near the level of the ground, there is the possibility of outgassing bothering someone sitting outdoors near a coated wall. There is also a small possibility of vapors passing through cracks in a foundation into a crawl space or basement, contaminating those areas. Very sensitive persons should select these materials carefully and insure that they are well separated from the living space.

Drainage and Moisture

For all types of foundations, good drainage is imperative. Soil that contains very much water and freezes in the winter can put tremendous pressure on a foundation and actually push the structure with enough force to cause structural damage. The resulting cracks will then allow moisture to pass through the foundation causing potential mold problems, and they will be pathways for termites.

Foundations depend on several techniques to remain dry. Of primary importance is positive surface drainage away from the house.

The ground should slope so that any rainfall or snowmelt flows away from, not toward, the structure. This can usually be done by building the house up high enough so that it can be graded correctly during backfilling. The amount of slope does not need to be great, but it does need to be sufficient to direct surface drainage away from the house. Six to eight inches of fall in ten feet is usually sufficient for grassy areas. Gutters and downspouts should help to direct water from the roof away as well. Without gutters, large quantities of rain water can be deposited on the ground near the foundation. In this case, the ground should have a steeper slope to move the water away from the structure.

Since there can be a certain amount of moisture in the soil itself, some type of system is required to keep it from finding its way through the foundation into the crawl space or basement. Various types of coatings and underground drains have been developed to do this. In areas where there is a high water table, the requirements are more severe in order to keep the foundation dry. Sump pumps may be needed to direct any such water to a storm sewer or ditch; however, during a power failure, the sump pump will not operate, and water can back up causing problems.

Moisture passing through a foundation generally involves mold growth and can result in deterioration of mortar joints and structural damage. If cracks can allow moisture to enter, then radon can enter as well. Crawl spaces with mold growth can create millions of mold spores that will seep through spaces in the floor or get into heating ductwork and be transported throughout the house. Basements used as living spaces can be uninhabitable for someone with mold sensitivities if there is a moisture problem.

Ground water is present in two basic ways. The level of the liquid water in the ground is referred to as the water table. It is at this level or below that water can be removed from the ground with a well. The depth varies considerably throughout the country and it can vary seasonally during periods of high precipitation. Water can also be present in the soil at higher levels than the water table due to capillary action. This is also called "rising damp."[4]

Capillary action can be responsible for water rising as much as 11 feet up through the soil from the water table. Clay and silt are especially vulnerable to this phenomenon. Less rise is found with sand and none with gravel. If you dip the end of a piece of paper towel into a glass of water, you will notice the towel becoming wet above the surface of the water. It is rising by capillary action. Some soils, concrete, and masonry act in this same way. The actual water table may be several feet below the ground surface, but capillary action can be responsible for liquid water and water vapor at much higher levels. This dampness can rise up through a concrete slab or masonry foundation, resulting in a moisture problem.

An easy way of controlling this is to excavate some of the soil having high capillarity and replace it with gravel. Another is to use a moisture barrier, usually 6 mil polyethylene, under the foundation system. This should be done under a concrete slab on grade and on the floor of a crawl space. A metal termite shield will prevent "rising damp" from reaching any wood framing, avoiding the possibility of rot from damp wood. A wooden plate in contact with masonry is required by most building codes to be chemically treated or be a naturally resistant species, like redwood, in order to be protected from such moisture.

In order to keep moisture from penetrating the walls of the crawl space, a Portland cement parging was originally used. It was simply troweled onto the outside of the wall as a barrier to ground moisture. A commercially prepared Portland cement-based product that will perform this same function is "Thoroseal Foundation Coating" by **Thoro System Products, Inc.** Although it contains some additives, it is often well tolerated by sensitive people when used as an exterior foundation coating. It is generally not intended to be used as a decorative finish coat. Since these types of products can develop cracks if the wall itself cracks, flexible (and odorous) plastic or asphalt coatings are more popular. If the wall develops a small crack, they can stretch and bridge the gap, maintaining a seal. They rely on being a barrier only, something like a swimming pool in reverse, with the wet ground on the outside and the dry basement on the inside. If there is a very high ground water level, the pressure against any coating can be enough to cause leaks to form in very minute openings. The traditional method of lowering the pressure of the ground water has been to place one or two underground perforated plastic drain tiles around the perimeter of the house and to backfill with stone. Any groundwater then seeps down through the stone and into the drain tile and then runs by gravity or a sump pump to a place away from the house where it can do no harm. Since a lot of stone is required, this can be somewhat expensive, so other less expensive systems have been developed. Special drainage mats or boards are used along the outside of the wall to direct any ground water down into a perforated drain tile.[5] These products must be combined with a waterproof coating applied to the wall; they are not a substitute for such a coating, they simply allow it to function better. These boards and mats are plastic products with a filter material to prevent the soil from clogging the system. Manufacturers include **BASF Corp.** (Enkadrain), **Eljen Corp., J-DRain Enterprises, Inc.** (J-Drain), and **Mirafi, Inc.** (Miradrain). Since all of these systems are made of synthetic materials that can bother some people, they should be chosen with care. It should be remembered that when the installation is complete, they will be underground with a much better chance of tolerability. Some type of system should be chosen with both basement and crawl-space construction to insure that these areas remain dry.

Interior waterproofing systems are available from a variety of manufacturers, but as a rule their effectiveness is not very great. The best place to install such a system is on the outside of the foundation wall. In new construction, this is relatively easy to do, but with an existing house it can mean costly excavation just to unearth the outside of the foundation. **Thoro System Products, Inc.** also produces a decorative "Thoroseal" Portland cement-based coating that can be used on interior walls in conjunction with an exterior system. It is sold in ten colors. Since it contains some minor acrylic additives, if used in the living space of a basement, it should be tested prior to use by a sensitive person. "Phenoseal Liquid Waterproofing," manufactured by **Gloucester Co., Inc.** is a vinyl-acrylic product that outgases relatively quickly. It is a water-based product designed primarily for interior use.

Radon

Controlling radon in new construction involves three basic principles: (1) eliminating the pathways for radon to enter the house; (2) reducing the vacuum effect that pulls radon from the soil into the house; and (3) incorporating additional features to remove radon if it is a problem after the house has been completed. Most of the control methods will be incorporated into the foundation system. In existing houses, there are several steps that can be taken, depending on the degree of the problem and the budget. More on all of these techniques can be found in publications available through the E.P.A.[6,7] Following is a summary of the things that can be done in existing houses.

Radon from the soil can enter a basement or crawl space through cracks or gaps in the structure. It can then pass from these areas into the rest of the house. Usually radon levels will be higher in below-ground areas than in above-ground areas. With a concrete slab on grade, radon can pass through any cracks directly into the living space.

Natural ventilation involves simply opening windows in a basement or adding vents to a crawl space. This has been shown to reduce radon levels, but will result in increased heating bills during cold months. It can also mean frozen pipes. *Forced ventilation* relies on the use of a fan rather than simply an open window or vent. This works even better to reduce radon levels but can mean even higher heating bills. By using a *heat recovery ventilation* system, the air can be changed more efficiently and the annual operating cost will be less. The initial equipment cost, however, can be high.

Appliances such as combustion-type furnaces, clothes dryers, and wood stoves need an air supply. In many situations, they create a vacuum effect in the house which causes radon to be pulled in. By creating *air supply* ducting, this can be minimized. An air supply duct, for example, could allow fresh air to enter near such an appliance, then pass through the appliance back to the outdoors.

Covering exposed earth in basements or crawl spaces will help block radon's entry. The best material to use would be a continuous layer of concrete, a somewhat expensive solution. Plastic barriers can help if they are sealed around the edges with caulking or tape. Sump pump pits should be fitted with a sealed cover. *Sealing cracks and openings* involves areas where plumbing or electrical lines enter the house, cracks in the wall or floor, or the open cores at the top of a concrete block wall.

If the house has a drain tile around the perimeter, then *drain tile suction* can be used. With this method, a fan is hooked up to the drainage system (which normally is not completely filled with water), and pulls air through the tile. This lowers the air pressure inside the tile and causes the radon to enter the tile rather than the house. It is then blown into the atmosphere, where it dissipates. Since concrete blocks are hollow, *block wall ventilation* can be used to intercept radon within the wall itself and blow it outside before it can pass the rest of the way through the wall and enter the house. *Sub-slab suction* can be used in a

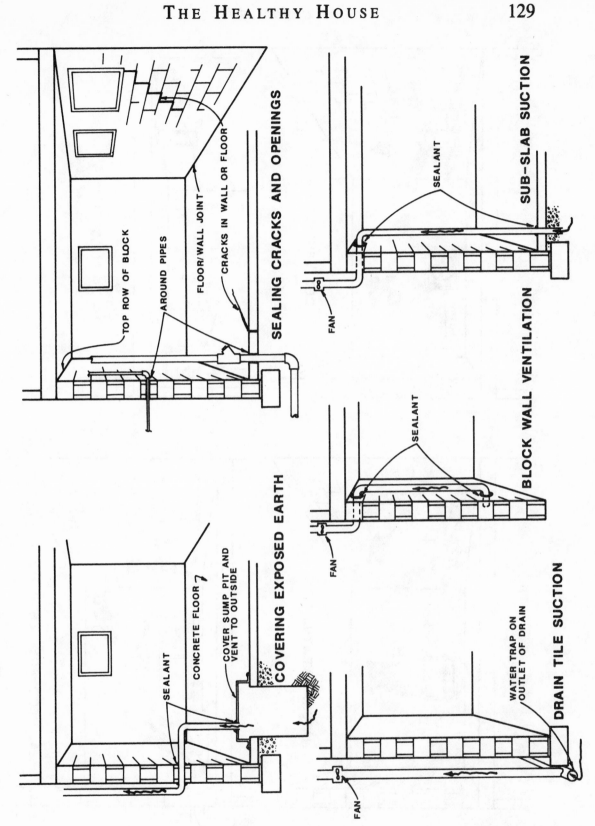

SEALING CRACKS AND OPENINGS

TOP ROW OF BLOCK

AROUND PIPES

FLOOR/WALL JOINT

CRACKS IN WALL OR FLOOR

SUB-SLAB SUCTION

SEALANT

FAN

BLOCK WALL VENTILATION

SEALANT

FAN

COVERING EXPOSED EARTH

SEALANT

CONCRETE FLOOR

COVER SUMP PIT AND VENT TO OUTSIDE

DRAIN TILE SUCTION

WATER TRAP ON OUTLET OF DRAIN

FAN

Radon Reduction Techniques

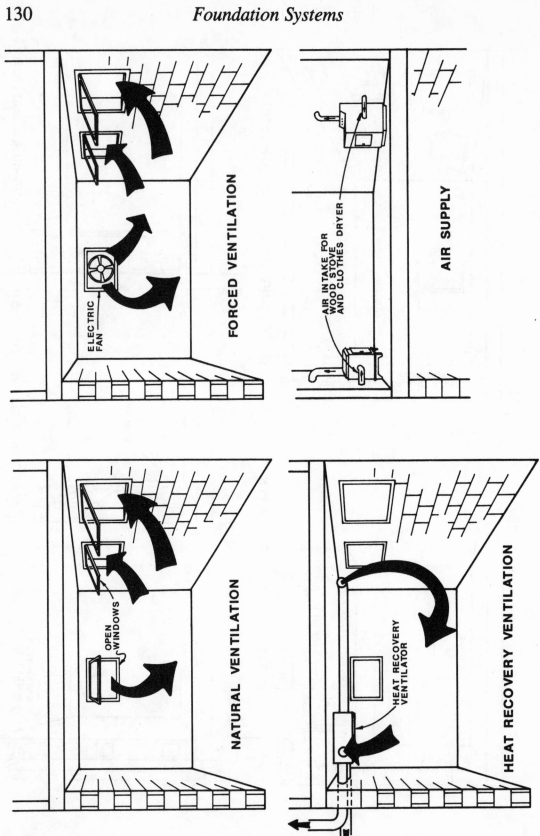

FORCED VENTILATION

ELECTRIC FAN

AIR SUPPLY

AIR INTAKE FOR WOOD STOVE AND CLOTHES DRYER

NATURAL VENTILATION

OPEN WINDOWS

HEAT RECOVERY VENTILATION

HEAT RECOVERY VENTILATOR

Radon Reduction Techniques

similar manner to pull radon from beneath a concrete floor slab and send it outdoors. In this method, holes are cut in the floor and ventilating pipes are run to the outdoors. While this can be very effective, it is also expensive.

These methods vary considerably in their installation and operating costs and they may not be applicable in all situations. In order to determine which method or methods are best for a particular situation, the E.P.A.'s Technical Guidance publication is a very good source.[8] It goes into considerable detail on the various techniques and is applicable to most situations.

Basement Construction

While all types of foundations can be constructed in a healthy manner, perhaps the most difficult and costly is the basement. In designing a basement, one should be concerned primarily with moisture and dampness, which result in mold growth, and with radon migration into the house.

The concrete basement floor should have at least a 6 mil polyethylene moisture barrier beneath it with any seams lapped at least 12″. This will keep ground moisture from coming through the slab by capillary action and will also act as a radon barrier if small cracks develop in the concrete. Care should be taken during construction so the moisture barrier is not punctured or damaged. Polyethylene is often problematic for sensitive persons, but in this location it will be separated from the living space by 4″ of concrete.

To minimize the chance of the concrete cracking, it should be mixed with the correct amount of water and be reinforced with steel mesh. Grade stakes used during the pouring of the slab should be removed because they will provide pathways for radon as the wood deteriorates. The joint between the slab and the basement wall should be caulked as an additional water and radon barrier, as should any pipes, wires, etc. that pass through the walls or floor.

A waterproofing and drainage system should be employed on the outside of the walls. It will help to block radon as well as ground water. In addition, an interior coating is also a good idea. One of the upper rows of concrete blocks above grade should be a solid block to prevent radon from rising up through the hollow cores into the basement. This also acts as a termite barrier, but an additional metal termite shield is also recommended. If a sump pump is used, it should

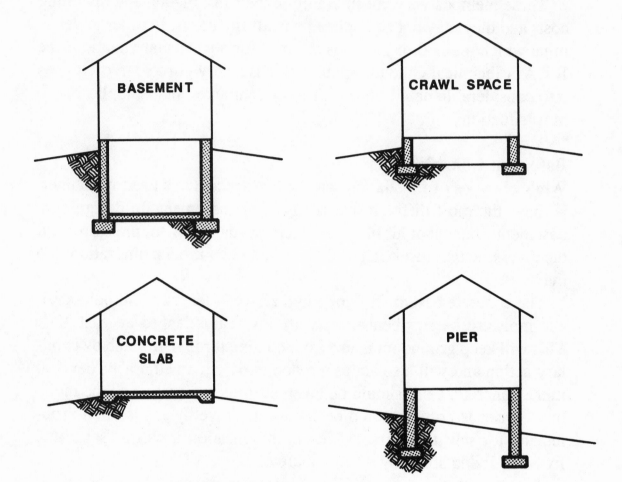

Basic Foundation Types

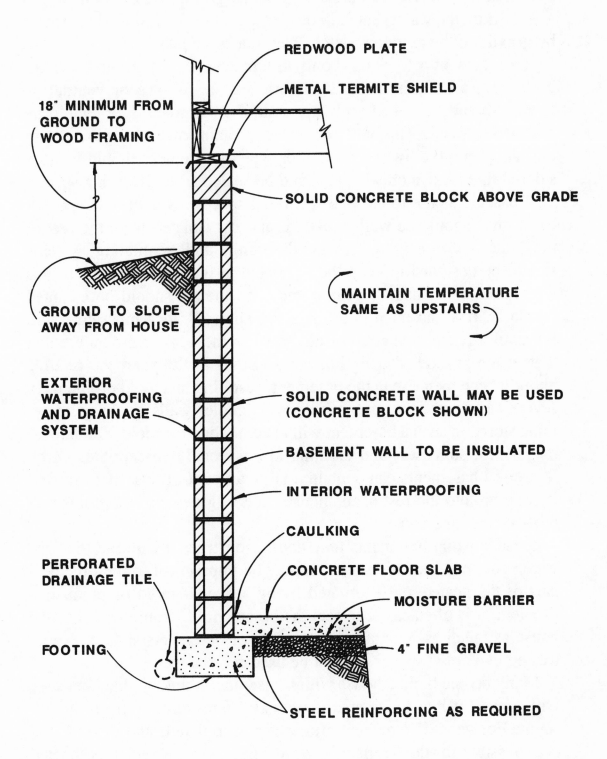

REDWOOD PLATE

METAL TERMITE SHIELD

18" MINIMUM FROM GROUND TO WOOD FRAMING

SOLID CONCRETE BLOCK ABOVE GRADE

GROUND TO SLOPE AWAY FROM HOUSE

MAINTAIN TEMPERATURE SAME AS UPSTAIRS

EXTERIOR WATERPROOFING AND DRAINAGE SYSTEM

SOLID CONCRETE WALL MAY BE USED (CONCRETE BLOCK SHOWN)

BASEMENT WALL TO BE INSULATED

INTERIOR WATERPROOFING

CAULKING

PERFORATED DRAINAGE TILE

CONCRETE FLOOR SLAB

MOISTURE BARRIER

FOOTING

4" FINE GRAVEL

STEEL REINFORCING AS REQUIRED

Basement Design Points

have a sealed cover. Radon exists in some ground water, so it can be given off by the water that is in the sump pit. Floor drains are best run by gravity to the outdoors rather than to a sump pit.

If a basement is to be used only as a mechanical room, and will not be heated, all seams in the ductwork for the furnace or ventilating system should be sealed with tape, and the basement door should be weather-stripped. This will prevent any radon or mold spores from migrating into the living space. This type of basement should be considered more like a crawl space, and be sealed from the living space.

If basements are to be used for living spaces, even on a temporary basis, they should be well insulated, and *not* isolated from the rest of the house. The heating, air conditioning, and ventilating systems should be designed to keep the basement at the same temperature as the rest of the house all year round, and the air should be changed regularly. If a basement is temporarily shut off, its temperature will fall until it reaches an equilibrium between the house temperature and that of the ground. During hot humid times of the year, the relative humidity can then rise in the basement, resulting in a mold problem. In severe cases, moisture can condense on cooler walls or floors. Anything stored in such a basement will become food for mold. Old books, magazines, suitcases, and clothing are especially susceptible. Dirty, little-used basements can contain a large amount of dust that can find its way up into the rest of the house, thus aggravating symptoms in a dust-sensitive person.

Since existing basements may not be constructed with the required waterproofing, insulation, etc., it may be impractical to treat them as part of the heated and ventilated living space. If mold or radon is a problem, it is often easier to seal the basement off from the rest of the house as much as possible. These types of basements should also be treated like crawl spaces and not be used for storage, etc.

Many people build a house with a basement, thinking that later they will convert it into living space, such as a family room or guest bedroom. For years it remains unfinished, uninsulated, and unused, except possibly for the washer and dryer that are inconveniently located there. It is basically shut off from the rest of the house, with a high potential for mold growth. Often when such a basement is finally converted to living space, the occupants will comment that it would have been nicer if the space was above ground, where it would be more airy, warmer, cleaner, more useful, better illuminated, and less musty (moldy) smelling. If the square footage isn't needed immediately for living, it may be better to eliminate a basement altogether and build an above-ground addition when needed.

There are some things which can be done during construction that will make it easier to control a radon situation should it become apparent after the house is occupied. It is not very expensive to do these things while the house is under construction and it can make a future radon reduction system more efficient and easier to install. A 4″ layer of gravel under the slab will facilitate the installation of a future sub-slab ventilation system, as will perforated drainage tiles inside or outside of the foundation perimeter.

Crawl-Space Construction

Crawl spaces are simply shallow basements that are not used as living spaces. They have most of the same requirements as basements as far as waterproofing and sealing radon entry points. Since they are not occupied, they should be well sealed from the living space and need not be insulated. The best place for insulation in crawl space construction is in the floor system. This helps further to separate the crawl space from the rest of the house. The access to the crawl space should be by way of an outdoor hatch or door, rather than a hatch in a closet floor which can allow mold spores to filter up into the closet.

Since there can be a certain amount of radon or moisture in a crawl space, the floor system should contain a well-sealed moisture barrier to keep both moisture and radon from entering the house. It will also prevent moisture in the house from passing into the crawl space. Any ductwork, plumbing lines, wiring, etc., passing through the barrier should be well sealed. It is usually possible to run many of these lines within the living space, and avoid most of the sealing requirements.

All ductwork located in this space should have the seams sealed with tape so contaminates do not enter them. This is especially important in the return-air lines because they have more of a negative pressure. The ductwork should be insulated for energy efficiency. If it is used for air conditioning as well as heating, it should have a moisture barrier on the outside of the insulation so that any moisture in the crawl space doesn't condense on the cooler surface of the ductwork.

The bare ground in a crawl space should always be covered with a moisture barrier. These barriers are usually covered with sand or a fine gravel to protect them from punctures when they are walked on or crawled on. Six mil polyethylene is commonly used, and it can help considerably, but it is rarely sealed around the edges sufficiently. This is necessary to minimize the chance of moisture or radon entering the crawl space. Since this type of sealing is usually not completely effective, plenty of vents should be provided so that any buildup of contaminants will be dissipated. The total area of required venting is determined by the area of the crawl space and the free area of the vents. "Free area" refers to the effective area of a ventilator after subtracting the effect of louvers or screening. This should be provided with the ventilator or it is available from the manufacturer. One source recommends that the ventilation area be $1/150$ that of the crawl-space area and the screening in the ventilators be no larger than $1/4''$.[9] As an example, a house having a 1500 sq. ft. crawl space should have 10 sq. ft. of ventilators spaced around the perimeter. (1500/150 = 10) This should be considered a minimum. While these vents are very important, the $1/4''$ screening can allow insects to enter. If a screen with smaller openings is used, considerably more ventilation area is required because of the increased resistance to air flow.

Vents should be located as high as possible on crawl-space walls and at opposite ends of the space to achieve proper cross-ventilation. If within three feet of corners, they will reduce "dead spots" where humid air could build up. In some cases it may be necessary to install vents in the rim joist, rather than in the foundation wall. This location is satisfactory from a ventilation standpoint, but it means that the floor cannot be insulated in that location. A cold spot on the floor above in winter will mean that the relative humidity will be higher in that area and mold growth could be a problem.

On hot, humid days when the outside air enters the cooler crawl space, there can be the danger of moisture from the air condensing on the cool below-grade walls. This is one of the drawbacks to installing vents in a crawl space. The problem can be alleviated somewhat by closing off the vents when the outdoor temperature and humidity get too high. This, however, can allow a buildup of radon to occur in the crawl space. In order to keep the radon and ground moisture out of the house, the above-mentioned floor moisture barrier should have all penetrations well sealed.

Crawl spaces should never be used for storage areas. The possibility of moisture on a humid summer day creating a mold problem is too great to take a chance on having your personal belongings become

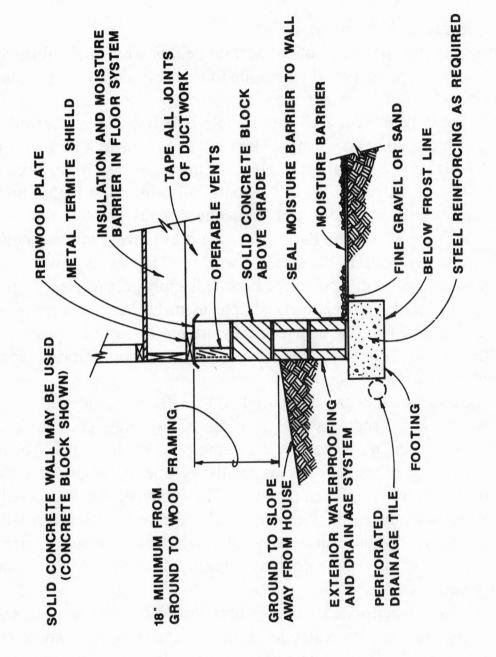

Crawl-Space Design Points

food for mold. Things stored even temporarily can be too easily forgotten, until it is too late.

Concrete Slab Foundation

A concrete slab can be poured as a single monolithic unit, forming an effective radon barrier. If expansion joints are required, they should be fitted with flexible water stops to prevent moisture and radon from passing through. The slab should be reinforced with a steel mesh to prevent cracking, and it should be insulated to make it more a part of the house than a part of the ground. An uninsulated slab can be considerably cooler than the air in the room, allowing for a higher relative humidity near the floor and consequent mold growth. Every slab should have a moisture barrier beneath it to prevent ground moisture from migrating up to the surface, with resulting mold growth. All of the requirements of a basement floor will apply here as well. Concrete slabs on grade are relatively simple to make healthy, compared to crawl spaces and basements, so they are preferred in healthy houses. They can easily have ceramic tile attached, but more effort is required with a wood finish floor.

A concrete slab can be poured so that it will be integral with the foundation that supports the house, or as a separate unit. Both types present difficulties when they are being properly insulated. The most effective use of insulation is around the perimeter, because it is closer to the extremes of air temperature. The center of the slab is only in contact with the earth. The earth under the center of a slab will be warmed by the house and will not be subject to extremes of temperature, so this area usually does not require insulation unless the climate is severely cold.

Perimeter-perforated drainage tiles should be used to keep excessive water away from a slab foundation and to provide a way of ventilating the slab, should radon become a problem for some reason after the house is complete. A 4″ layer of gravel under the slab will also facilitate the installation of a future ventilation system, and will also help to keep ground water from reaching the slab by capillary action.

Heating ducts imbedded in concrete slabs should be avoided because they can be difficult to clean, and if there is a water spill, they can become damp and harbor mold growth. Plumbing lines under slabs should be minimized because they are difficult to maintain. Be-

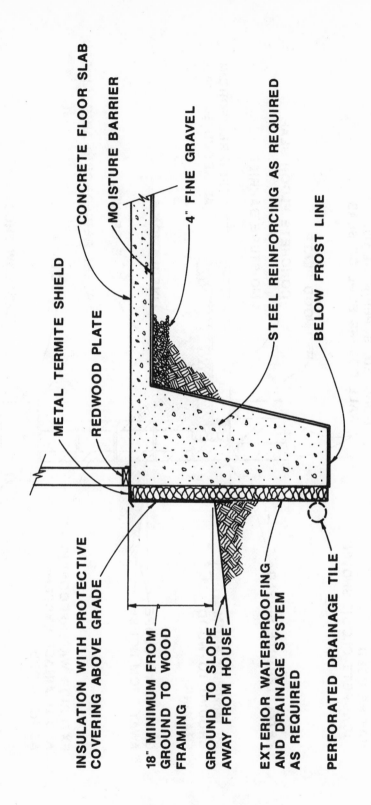

CONCRETE FLOOR SLAB

MOISTURE BARRIER

4" FINE GRAVEL

STEEL REINFORCING AS REQUIRED

BELOW FROST LINE

METAL TERMITE SHIELD

REDWOOD PLATE

INSULATION WITH PROTECTIVE COVERING ABOVE GRADE

18" MINIMUM FROM GROUND TO WOOD FRAMING

GROUND TO SLOPE AWAY FROM HOUSE

EXTERIOR WATERPROOFING AND DRAINAGE SYSTEM AS REQUIRED

PERFORATED DRAINAGE TILE

One-Piece Slab/Foundation Design Points

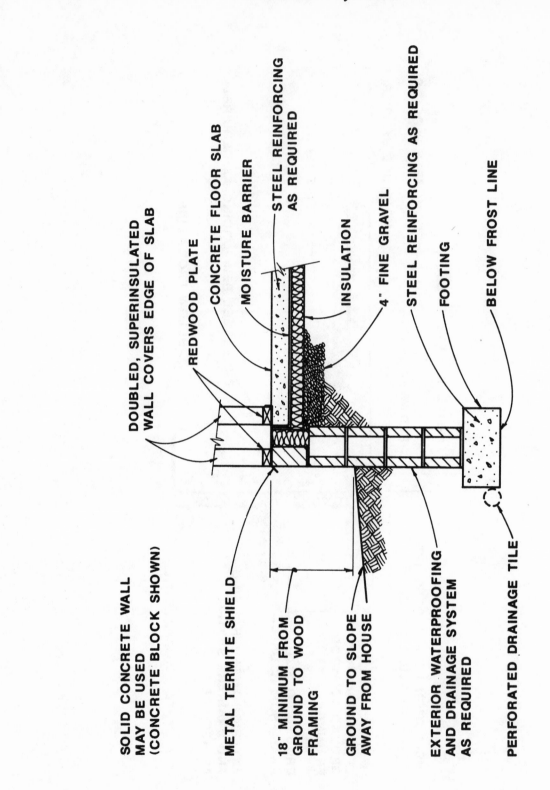

SOLID CONCRETE WALL MAY BE USED (CONCRETE BLOCK SHOWN)

DOUBLED, SUPERINSULATED WALL COVERS EDGE OF SLAB

REDWOOD PLATE

CONCRETE FLOOR SLAB

MOISTURE BARRIER

STEEL REINFORCING AS REQUIRED

INSULATION

4" FINE GRAVEL

STEEL REINFORCING AS REQUIRED

FOOTING

BELOW FROST LINE

METAL TERMITE SHIELD

18" MINIMUM FROM GROUND TO WOOD FRAMING

GROUND TO SLOPE AWAY FROM HOUSE

EXTERIOR WATERPROOFING AND DRAINAGE SYSTEM AS REQUIRED

PERFORATED DRAINAGE TILE

Separate Slab/Foundation Design Points

cause of this, extra cleanouts in plumbing drain lines should be installed.

If a slab has a good moisture barrier, it will not be as important to have a perfect waterproofing control system on the outside of the foundation, since small amounts of moisture under the slab should create no problems. It is, however, important to provide for proper drainage so that the structure remains reasonably dry in winter, and the ground moisture does not result in frost heaving. This is easily done with the perforated perimeter drain tile already mentioned.

Pier Foundations

By lifting the house up off the ground on piers, it will be well separated from both radon and ground moisture. From an energy standpoint, the floor in this type of construction should be well insulated. It will, in effect, function like an exterior wall and should be insulated and fitted with a vapor barrier accordingly. A pier foundation can support a variety of floor systems, such as metal or wood joists, with a wood or concrete subfloor. Since there is no direct connection with the ground, this will be the healthiest type of foundation from both a mold and radon standpoint.

It is important to provide proper drainage with this type of foundation also, in order to prevent frost heaving. The surface of the ground should slope away from the structure to prevent water from running under the house, forming puddles which will be havens for microorganisms.

The bare ground under a house built on piers can be somewhat unsightly and dusty. A covering of crushed stone or gravel will certainly improve the appearance and will help to control dust. Since this area is shielded from both the sun and rain by the house itself, weeds should not be a problem. However, if there is some concern, a plastic moisture barrier, if tolerable, can be used under the stone to minimize the growth of weeds. A latticework of wood or metal can also enhance the appearance, but if the space is totally sealed with a skirting material, much like a mobile home, it will begin to function like a crawl space and radon buildup can be a problem, so it should be kept as open as possible.

The tops of the piers should be capped with a metal termite shield so that the insects cannot sneak into the house through small cracks in concrete or through the hollow cores of masonry piers. Like basement walls, masonry piers should have solid blocks near the top to minimize the possibility of radon rising up through them into the floor system. Pier foundation systems are often used in hot, humid southern climates. They can be especially dramatic in other climates on hillside lots by lifting the house up in the air to enhance a view.

Termite Control

This should be accomplished by the use of metal shields in conjunction with solid masonry or concrete walls. Proper drainage is also important, because subterranean termites require damp soil to live in. If a house is framed out of wood, other precautions, as outlined in Chapter 11, may also be required. Under no circumstances should the backfill around a foundation contain any wood scraps. These will be the hors d'oeuvres that act as invitations for termites to eat the house as a main course.

Summary

Basements are probably the most difficult types of foundations to build in a healthful manner, but it certainly can be done. It is very important that basements in new houses be designed to be part of the living space. They should be heated and ventilated accordingly. Since crawl spaces are not used for living spaces, their requirements may not seem as severe, but in order to keep radon and mold from migrating up into the house, the should be constructed with care as well. Concrete slabs, however, are comparatively easy to construct in a healthy manner, the main requirements being a moisture barrier and insulation. Pier foundations, on the other hand, totally separate the house from the ground, so they should not be contributors to either radon or mold contamination of the house.

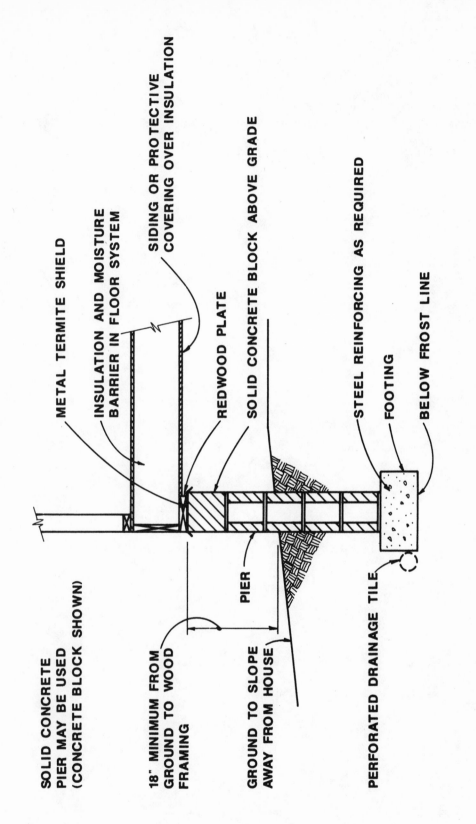

SOLID CONCRETE
PIER MAY BE USED
(CONCRETE BLOCK SHOWN)

METAL TERMITE SHIELD

INSULATION AND MOISTURE
BARRIER IN FLOOR SYSTEM

SIDING OR PROTECTIVE
COVERING OVER INSULATION

REDWOOD PLATE

SOLID CONCRETE BLOCK ABOVE GRADE

STEEL REINFORCING AS REQUIRED

FOOTING

BELOW FROST LINE

18" MINIMUM FROM
GROUND TO WOOD
FRAMING

PIER

GROUND TO SLOPE
AWAY FROM HOUSE

PERFORATED DRAINAGE TILE

Pier Foundation Design Points

Chapter 11

Wood and Wood Products

Wood is probably used in house construction more than any other material. It is certainly one of the most natural substances that is available. Yet wood can cause health problems in some individuals. For a few people, a house without any wood may be necessary. For others, careful selection will be sufficient to construct a tolerable house. In some cases the wood itself can be problematic, in others a glue or chemical treatment can cause symptoms.

Wood and Wood Products
Wood can be classified as being either a softwood or a hardwood. Softwood trees are evergreen or needle-bearing: pine, fir, spruce, redwood, cedar, cypress, hemlock, etc. The technical name for softwoods is "conifer," because many of them bear cones. Hardwood trees are known as "deciduous," or broad-leafed. Hardwoods are usually harder than softwoods, but not always. Balsa is classified as a hardwood because it does not have needles and isn't an evergreen. Some hardwoods that are often encountered are: oak, maple, birch, walnut, ash, poplar, etc. Hardwoods are usually slower-growing trees than softwoods. Since it takes longer to grow a hardwood tree, their cost is somewhat higher. Hardwoods are often known for their beauty and are used extensively in the furniture industry. Flooring and cabinetry are typical uses in the housing market. The framing lumber used in house

construction is almost exclusively softwood because it can be produced more cheaply.

It is very difficult to go to a lumberyard today and find anything but softwood lumber, most of which is grown in the South or the Pacific Northwest. Occasionally, a few hardwood boards will be stocked for hobbyists to use in the making of furniture. A hundred years ago, lumberyards stocked material that was cut locally from whatever trees happened to be growing in the vicinity. If there were a lot of oak or walnut trees in the area, oak or walnut boards were sold at the local lumberyard. There are barns built of oak, and walnut corn cribs are still dotting the countryside, built of native lumber. When they were built, oak and walnut just happened to be what was available. Today, walnut is relatively scarce because it takes so long to grow a walnut tree.

Plywood, particle board, flake board, and hardboard didn't even exist a hundred years ago. They have come into existence in order to lower the cost of wood construction. These products are somewhat cheaper than solid wood boards, and in some ways they have superior strength. However, they are often implicated in health problems, primarily because of the glues used in their manufacture.

All woods and wood products can be treated chemically for a variety of reasons. Since wood can burn, and is subject to fungus attack or to being eaten by insects, fire retardants, fungicides, and insecticides are popular treatments. For sensitive individuals, most of these chemicals can elicit symptoms.

Health Aspects

The health effects of different woods vary widely. In medical records of occupational diseases from the Pacific Northwest, there are numerous reports of "cedar poisoning," "pine, spruce, hemlock and fir poisoning," etc.[1] Allergic dermatitis is the most common problem in the forest products industry. Some woods are more problematic after they are dried because of the chemical changes that the wood goes through. Some are active allergens and some can cause systemic poisoning.[2] One article lists 220 different woods and documented sensitivities, primarily dermatitis, mucosal irritation, asthma, and general symptoms.[3]

A common problem in the wood products industry is wood dust, something not encountered in a completed wood frame house. This can settle on workers' skin or enter their sinuses. Long-term exposure to any kind of irritating dust can be harmful, and there have been reports of cancer affecting industrial workers after long exposure to wood dust. Hodgkin's disease is seen in woodworkers more than in the general population.[4] Illnesses have also been reported involving reactions to glues and to bacteria or fungi growing on wood.

There are a variety of constituents in wood that can affect human health: alkaloids, anthraquinones, benzo- and naptho-quinones, catechols, flavornoids, furocoumarins, glycosides, minerals, phenols, saponins, sesquiterpene lactones, stilbenes, and terpenes. Some are sensitizers and irritants, others cause cardiac and toxic effects.[5] The exotic tropical woods seem to be more of a problem than do the domestically used woods from the United States. Rosewood, teak, and other tropical woods are often found in the literature as causing various reactions. Violinists frequently place a handkerchief between their chin and the violin to avoid a skin reaction with the wood. For sensitive individuals, care should be taken in selecting woods because practically every wood in use has some recorded health effect.

For people concerned with using wood in the construction of a house, testing can be easily done. A sample can be obtained to see if it causes symptoms. Since interior woodwork will generally either be painted or varnished, any odor or irritating qualities can be sealed in, making the sample tolerable. Framing lumber will be inside of walls and may not be a problem unless very odorous. All woods have a characteristic odor, some much stronger than others. The softwoods commonly used in the United States are generally stronger-smelling than hardwoods.

Mold and Wood

When wood is freshly cut, it contains a large quantity of water. As a result, freshly cut wood can support mold growth. It must be dried until the water content is below 20 percent before mold growth is no longer a problem. Most of the commercially available lumber passes through several hands before it reaches your house. At different stages it can be sprayed with various water- or oil-based chemicals that, theoretically, can bother a sensitive person. Foresters can spray trees to control insects. Freshly cut logs can be subject to mold growth (decay) or insect damage and may be sprayed. The freshly cut surfaces of boards at the sawmill may need to be sprayed again to protect them. During storage, until the boards are dried to less than 20 percent moisture content, there is danger of a fungus attack and they might be sprayed once more.[6] When wood is dried in a kiln, the temperatures used are usually sufficient to stop any fungal growth, but not high enough to actually kill the fungus or the spores. Therefore, any subsequent moisture can trigger a renewed growth, requiring additional chemical treatment.[7] This spraying is a surface treatment, and when the boards are finally planed smooth the chemical residues probably remain only in the shavings, with the finished product containing little in the way of chemicals.

Once incorporated into a house, wood can again get wet and allow mold to grow. This can, on some occasions, result in severe decay and a weakened structure. For this reason, care should be taken to design the house so that it will remain as dry as possible.

Because of the various oils, resins, tannins, or other chemicals, some woods are naturally resistant to mold growth. These woods can be used where contact with dampness may be a problem. The heartwood from the center of the tree has the highest decay resistance, while the outer sapwood generally lacks decay resistance. Trees whose heartwood has exceptional durability even under conditions that favor decay are black locust, red mulberry, and osage-orange. Those of high durability include cedars, black cherry, chestnut, junipers, redwood, black walnut, and Pacific yew.[8] The various resins and oils in these woods that help them to discourage mold growth may also bother sensitive occupants. It may also be difficult to obtain some particular species. In order to minimize the risk of wood in a house being subject to mold growth and subsequent decay, it should be kept dry, below the critical 20 percent moisture content.

Weathering of unpainted wood outdoors is a result of the surface of the wood repeatedly expanding and shrinking as it gets wet and dries out. It does not always result in mold growth. If the wood has a natural decay resistance, has no pockets to collect moisture, and can completely dry out after a rain shower, it can last a long time without being painted. The weathering process does, however, result in surface deterioration. It can mean that up to a 1/4″ of the thickness of the wood will be lost per century.[9] In most situations, wood used outdoors should be protected with a coat of paint.

Under favorable conditions, some species of fungi can live in salt-treated lumber containing arsenic and release arsenical gases such as arsine.[10] To use this type of lumber indoors could result in an undesirable situation if one of these types of mold was allowed to proliferate.

Softwoods

If you go to your local lumberyard to buy a 2×4, you will likely receive one that was cut from a softwood tree, most often a pine tree. Lumber is usually marked with a stamp, specifying what species of tree it is from. The most common stamp is "S-P-F," meaning Spruce-Pine-Fir. Lumber with this marking can come from any of those three types of trees. "Hem-Fir" is another stamp that means the lumber is either from a hemlock or a fir tree. Sometimes a single species stamp will be seen, such as "Spruce." Redwood and cedar lumber are also often readily available because of their decay resistance. They are not often used for general construction because of increased cost.

For some sensitive people, softwoods can trigger symptoms. There are a variety of volatile compounds outgassed by the resins of softwoods, with hydrocarbon terpenes often being blamed.[11] Actually, there are a number of different chemicals given off as fumes that can be bothersome. The aroma from cedar or a Christmas tree can often elicit symptoms in sensitive people. Of the various softwoods that are usually available, fir, spruce, or hemlock are sometimes less bothersome than pine or cedar, but they may be more difficult to locate. For someone extremely sensitive, all softwoods can trigger symptoms and should be avoided.

It can be difficult to obtain lumber of a certain species, such as fir. If lumber is stamped "S-P-F," it can be any one of those species, and often only a wood scientist can tell the difference. Placing a special order could mean ordering a carload, not a very cost-effective idea when one is considering a room addition. Some lumberyards do, however, stock lumber of certain individual species. For example, they may handle spruce boards instead of those stamped "S-P-F" because they can obtain a more consistent quality.

The softwood framing lumber in a house can be separated from the living space by the use of a foil barrier, thus protecting a sensitive occupant from bothersome fumes. It is also possible to use less bothersome hardwood lumber for framing, or even eliminate wood completely and use steel framing. A combination of softwood, hardwood, and steel can often be an acceptable solution.

Redwood is often used for porches, decks, and in damp areas because of its natural decay and termite resistance, and it is readily available at most lumberyards. It has less in the way of volatile resins and oils found in other softwoods, so it may be a reasonably safe choice for someone sensitive to the odors of pine. When used outdoors, there may be enough fresh air to counteract any slight odor, but when in doubt, test first.

The woodwork, cabinetry, doors, etc., if made of softwood, should be sealed so that the smell of the wood does not escape into the house. Various paints or varnishes can be tested to see which performs this function the best. Generally, it will be better to select less offensive hardwoods for these interior applications.

Hardwoods

Hardwood lumber can be more difficult to locate for construction purposes. In some areas of the country, there are small sawmills that can supply lumber cut from locally grown trees. A difficulty in purchasing such wood it the fact that it is still "green." This refers to wood that is not dry enough to use. Its moisture content is well above 20 percent and it is subject to fungus attack and cannot be worked successfully. It is difficult to use for building purposes because it is also subject to shrinkage.

Wood will dry on its own over time if stored properly. This is known as air drying, and can be a slow process, taking a year or more. The process can be speeded up by kiln drying. If there happens to be a lumber kiln in the area of a local sawmill, this can be a good way to get workable wood, but of course, the kiln drying will add to the cost.

Another difficulty with sawmill lumber is its roughness. It will not have a smooth surface and its dimensions can vary as much as $1/4''$. A 2×4 directly from the lumberyard will measure $1^{1}/_{2}'' \times 3^{1}/_{2}''$ because it will have been planed to a smooth surface. Lumber purchased directly from a sawmill may seem to be priced reasonably, but by the time it has been properly dried and planed smooth, it can end up being quite expensive.

Because of the increased cost, hardwoods are generally only used for the finish wordwork in houses. A few lumberyards will be able to order hardwood trim or doors. In many areas there will be dealers of hardwood who supply furniture factories. Sometimes they will also sell to individuals, but without proper woodworking equipment, hardwood boards are simply boards. They can be transformed into trim, doors, and cabinetry by a local woodworker. For someone interested in using hardwood, this is the best route to follow. Look in the telephone book under "Woodworking" or ask the high school industrial arts teacher for a recommendation. There may be some local hobbyists willing to work with you. They will usually be able to supply you with small samples of various woods for testing purposes.

Hardwoods are not as odorous as softwoods, but they each do have a characteristic smell. Maple and birch are probably less odorous than some other varieties. Prices vary considerably for the different woods with walnut being relatively high and poplar being relatively low.

Man-Made Wood Products

Almost all of the plywood, particle board, and flake board being produced today is held together with a formaldehyde-based glue. There are a few other glues being used on a very limited basis such as caseines and isocyanates. Of the formaldehyde-based glues, there are two types: urea-formaldehyde and phenol-formaldehyde. Of the two, the outgassing characteristics of urea-formaldehyde are considerably greater, often by a factor of 10 or 20. Pesticides can sometimes be added to the glues. Products containing urea-formaldehyde glue should never be considered for use in an ecologically safe house, and those containing phenol-formaldehyde should be avoided if at all possible.

Plywood is a man-made product, usually sold in 4'×8' sheets. It is made of several layers, or plies, of wood glued into a sandwich, and can be used in a variety of places in house construction. Construction grade plywood is usually made from softwood trees while furniture grade plywood often is made from hardwood. Plywood has come into widespread use primarily because it is cheaper than solid wood and in some ways it is stronger. Almost all plywood made for construction purposes, both for interior and exterior applications, contains phenol-formaldehyde glue. Used as a roof deck, this material will be separated from the living space and may not bother a sensitive person. When used for a subfloor, it will be much closer to the occupants, and may prove troublesome to a someone sensitive to formaldehyde. A foil barrier can help to keep the formaldehyde vapors from entering the living space.

Plywood that is used for interior wall paneling can be made with the more volatile urea-formaldehyde glue. This material usually has a decorative hardwood surface layer and can be relatively expensive. It should be avoided at all costs because of the formaldehyde emissions. Warning labels are stamped on the back of these products, ironically just where they will *not* be seen after they are installed. The following is typical:

> Warning: This product is manufactured with a urea-formaldehyde resin and will release small quantities of formaldehyde. Formaldehyde levels in the indoor air can cause temporary eye and respiratory irritation and may aggravate respiratory conditions or allergies. Ventilation will reduce indoor formaldehyde levels.

Even though some plywood products contain a less volatile glue than others, they should all be avoided by someone with formaldehyde sensitivities, unless substantial measures are taken to seal them from the living space. In most situations, solid wood can be substituted, but care should be taken with solid wood as well, since it too may elicit symptoms. Plywood will outgas less and less over time. A piece of 25-year-old plywood will, therefore, pose less of a problem to a sensitive person than a new piece, so when found in an older house plywood may not be bothersome.

Particle board and medium-density fiberboard are made from wood chips and shavings, usually from softwoods that are held together with a glue. Most of the particle board produced today is made with a urea-formaldehyde glue. Particle board is often covered with a thin layer of attractive hardwood to improve its appearance. Some 4′×8′ sheets of wall paneling are made this way with an inexpensive particle board base, as are kitchen cabinets and much furniture. Particle board was developed because it is even cheaper than plywood. It is available in various thicknesses, with 1/2″ and 5/8″ being common. This material is used extensively in mobile homes and is one of the reasons for the often high formaldehyde concentrations in them. It can easily result in higher formaldehyde levels than in houses that are insulated with urea-formaldehyde foam insulation (UFFI). Pressed wood products containing urea-formaldehyde resins are among the strongest and most commonly used formaldehyde emitters in the indoor environment.[12] The particle board industry has reduced formaldehyde emissions considerably over the years on a voluntary basis, but the amount of formaldehyde released is still too high for this material to be considered in an environmentally safe house.

Flake board, oriented strand board, and some specialized types of particle board are made with the less offensive phenol-formaldehyde glue. They can be used in exterior applications because they are much more water-resistant. At least one company, **Boise Cascade Corporation**, sells a water-resistant particle board without any formaldehyde glue. They utilize an isocyanate glue and 100 percent ponderosa pine-wood chips. It has a very strong pine odor that can bother some people and isocycantes have been shown to cause irritation and immunologic sensitization of the respiratory tract.[13]

Hardboard is a harder, much denser product than particle board. It is usually medium to dark down in color and is generally sold in 4'×8' sheets, in thicknesses of ¼" or less. Pegboard is a hardboard product. "Masonite" is one particular brand produced by the **Masonite Corp.** Some hardboard products include interior wall paneling and exterior siding.

Hardboard is produced by pressing wood fibers into a dense sheet by means of heat and pressure, so that the natural lignin in the wood holds the hardboard together. While the lignin is the only glue required, formaldehyde and other chemicals are added to improve strength and moisture resistance. These can be bothersome to sensitive people. Hardboard is much less offensive than particle board, but should definitely be tested prior to using it. Sometimes the dense, tempered products are better tolerated than the standard grade. These are sometimes prefinished and used on bathroom or kitchen walls.

Treated Wood

Wood can be treated with a variety of chemical preservatives to make it resistant to fungal growth or termite attack. Log cabins are often routinely treated today. These chemicals are very toxic to humans as well as molds and insects. While research is being done into nontoxic alternatives[14], it is doubtful if they will find a ready market because of increased cost. Some less toxic do-it-yourself products are available but they will not be very effective in most situations. Both **Sinan Co.** and **Livos Plantchemistry** sell borax-based preservatives.

Wood preservatives can be easily applied by spraying, dipping, or soaking. Commercially, they are applied by a pressure process. Only by forcing the chemical into all of the pores of the wood under pressure can it be adequately protected. The other methods, that are usually done by homeowners, are much less effective at providing true protection for the wood. They should only be considered surface treatments. Surface treatments are ineffective for wood to be placed in contact with the ground. They can be very effective in protecting decay of end grain from fungus attack but less effective at protecting edge grain because there is less absorption by the pores of the wood.

Types of Preservatives

Although there are dozens of different preservatives made, only three basic types are commonly used in the commercial pressure treatment of wood that is encountered by builders and consumers: oily preservatives, solvent-soluble organic chemicals, and water-soluble salts. Creosote is an oily preservative. Pentachlorophenol is a solvent-soluble organic chemical. Common water-soluable salts include ammoniacal copper arsenate (ACA) and chromated copper arsenate (CCA). Because of recent restrictions by the E.P.A., it is more difficult to find anything but the salt-treated materials at local lumberyards.

Creosote is obtained from wood tar, often of the beechwood tree. It is dark in color, very oily, and is often used on utility poles. It is a complex mixture of phenols and their ethers and can be very odorous, especially on a hot day. Other oily preservatives can be obtained from coal tar. Breathing vapors on a hot day can bother some people. When chronically applied to the skin creosote has been shown to lead to lesions and skin cancer.[15]

Pentachlorophenol (penta for short), also dark in color, can cause several negative health effects. It is not only used as a wood preservative, but also in such varied products as paper, cleaning solutions, soaps, leather, and cotton. Penta is found in the urine of most human subjects in studies done in the United States. Because of its widespread use in Hawaii, Hawaiians have seven times that of the mainland population in their bodies. It can be absorbed by inhalation, ingestion, and through the skin. It has been shown to cause fetal death, and embryotoxicity as well as chloracne and significant liver damage in adults.[16] In one incident, three dairy farmers were poisoned by vapors from penta-treated wood and 600 cows died as a result of licking the wood.[17]

Water-soluable salts sound fairly innocuous. Wood treated with them is readily available today because it is less messy and cheaper than the alternatives. This wood has a greenish tint and it is widely used for decks and porches. There are several types available, but the most common, ACA and CCA, both contain arsenic compounds. Consumer information sheets are available at lumberyards that handle this material. They warn that it should not be used where it can contaminate food, as on countertops. Workers are cautioned to wash exposed areas thoroughly before eating and to wash their clothes separately from other clothing. Since this material is so resistant to fungus and termites, it is being used in basements. In such houses, traces of arsenic dust have been found in the basements.[18] The surface of the wood can often contain white arsenic powder.[19] The arsenic compounds can be leached out of the wood into the soil. Dangers to small children crawling around on a treated wood deck or chewing on a railing seem obvious, as do the dangers of constructing picnic tables of this material.

In summary, the treated woods that are commercially available are not recommended for use by sensitive people. Redwood will be a better alternative even though the cost will be higher. Of the three types of treatments, penta is probably the worst. Treated wood, especially water-borne salts, should never be used near gardens by anyone because of the danger of the chemicals being taken up by the plants. A new creosote-treated utility pole can be very bothersome to a sensitive person. Some utility companies use salt-treated poles which will not outgas like creosote and may be better tolerated, but it should be remembered that in choosing a treated wood, none are 100 percent safe.

Termites and Wood
Wood can be attacked by several different insects, but when told about a termite infestation, people often have visions of their house crumbling in a pile of sawdust. Not a very pretty thought when you realize that there are about 1500 pounds of termites for every person in the world. Termites can be dealt with in a variety of ways, some of which can not only be devastating to the insects but to the human occupants as well. Different types of termites will be dealt with in different ways, so it is important to know which kind of termite you have. There are a number of control strategies that are less toxic than the standard chemical treatment, but since no method will be 100 percent effective in controlling termites forever, regular inspections should be performed.

There are dozens of different species of termites in the world, with four major groups found in the United States. The subterranean group is by far the most widespread, with drywood, dampwood, and powderpost varieties confined to the southern and western parts of the country. A pest control professional can easily determine which variety is present. The homeowner can learn to identify them also.

Regular termite inspections are an important aspect of homeownership that are often ignored. It is almost automatic to notice when the roof needs replacing or a coat of paint is necessary, but termite inspections are usually only done when the house is being sold. By monitoring the house on a regular basis, an infestation can be discovered early. This means that a problem can be solved before it gets out of hand, usually with a less toxic method. Inspections can easily be done by the homeowner, thus avoiding the expense of a professional. An excellent source of information about do-it-yourself identifying, inspection, and monitoring is available from the **Bio Integral Resource Center (BIRC)**.[20] This is a very complete article and is well worth the nominal price. **BIRC** is a nonprofit organization dedicated to finding less toxic methods of pest control. Much of the information in this section is from their literature. They publish both the *Common Sense Pest Control Quarterly* (for consumers) and the monthly *IPM Practitioner* (for professionals).

Mechanical methods of termite control are always preferable to chemical means. Since subterranean termites must return to the soil to obtain moisture, they travel back and forth from the wood to the soil. They can travel through cracks in concrete as small as $1/32''$, or they can build mud tubes from the ground up to the wood. Whatever path they take, they must protect themselves from sunlight and air or they will die. To discourage them, wood should be at least $18''$ from the soil; however, this is rarely the case in existing construction where eight inches or less separation is common. Metal termite shields are used to block their paths. Termite-resistant wood is also used. None of these methods are foolproof, because termites can build their mud tubes around metal shields or treated wood to get at the "good stuff." This is a tremendous advantage to a homeowner, because the pathways will be very visible and with regular inspections will be noticed immediately, so large infestations can be avoided. Metal shields should be very tightly constructed with all joints properly sealed. The best method of sealing is done by soldering the joints, but a tar-like bituminous compound can also be used if it doesn't bother sensitive occupants. A metal shield will provide false security unless it forms a 100 percent continuous barrier, because the termites will simply travel through a small crack into the wood without a visible tunnel. It should be remembered that the main purpose of shields is to make the termites form visible tunnels; they are not true barriers.

In new construction, all lumber scraps, wood debris, stumps, etc. should be hauled away from the site. If this material is buried it will soon be devoured by termites. This will keep them busy for a while. Once the scraps are eaten, they will simply move on to the next food source—your house.

If a small colony of subterranean termites is discovered, it can be possible to dig them out. Ants have been used to eat termites since they are one of their natural enemies. The Argentine ant is especially good at feeding on them.

Drywood termites can enter a structure through breaks in the outer skin of the house. Any crack in exterior woodwork or siding can provide an entry point. Caulking, painting, and replacing defective or deteriorating materials will discourage them.

The "Extermax System" is an effective nontoxic method of killing drywood termites. Though not universally available, there are three distributors: **Michelin Canvas, National Bugmobiles,** and **Hydrex of San Diego**. This process involves the use of an "Electrogun," a hand-held device with a probe that is inserted into the wood to actually electrocute the termites.

A biological method of attacking subterranean termites involves the use of a particular species of nematodes to eat them. These microscopic worms are injected into the wood or soil in a water solution, where they enter termite colonies and destroy them. They will live for a maximum of two years depending on moisture conditions. Actual tests of nematodes have yielded mixed results with some applicators claiming to be 95 percent effective and other reporting 50 percent with follow-up visits necessary. Termite-eating nematodes are available from **N-Viro Products Ltd.**

Of the chemical treatments available for subterranean termites, **BIRC** has stated that "no single material can, in our opinion, be called significantly less toxic than any other."[21] If chemical means are required, spot treatment will significantly reduce exposure to potentially toxic chemicals. This involves simply treating the areas that are infested, rather than the whole house.

The dangers of the chemical chlordane were sufficient to have production stopped in August 1987. Unfortunately, there are thousands of houses already contaminated with this material. Once a home has been treated with chlordane, it will always be there, and it always outgasses.[22] Aldrin, dieldrin, heptachlor, and endrin are popular long-lived termiticides belonging to the same chlorinated hydrocarbon family as chlordane. Another popular chemical, said to be less toxic, is "Dursban." However, there are negative health effects associated with it as well. One report lists symptoms of drooling, sweating, nausea, diarrhea, abdominal pain, weakness, fatigue, and anxiety that occurred in office workers within a few hours of a building being treated.[23] This can usually be avoided if the Dursban is applied only to an empty building and reentry is delayed for a period of time after application. One material that has been tolerated by some sensitive individuals is "Ficam-W," manufactured by **BFC Chemical, Inc.** This is a relatively short-lived product, lasting approximately six months; so if this product is used, regular inspections are again recommended.

Drywood termites are often treated with a toxic fumigant such as methyl bromide. Alternatives exist in the form of desiccating dusts that can be used in both new and old construction. These materials cause the insects to lose the protective wax on their bodies, resulting in dehydration and death. "Dri-die" and "Drione" are available from **Fairfield American Corp.**

BIRC recommends the following program as being the least toxic method of control: 1. Monitor your building as least once per year. 2. Identify the species of termite. 3. Correct structural conditions that led to the infestation. 4. Apply physical or biological controls. 5. Spot treat with chemicals if necessary. 6. Check for effectiveness and repeat if required.

A method that has some potential for reducing the amount of chemicals required is the bait block technique. With this method, blocks of wood are strategically placed around a structure. These baits are treated with an attractant or feeding stimulant along with a termiticide. Thus, they draw termites away from a building and also kill them.[24]

One of the best methods of avoiding termites is to use building materials that termites cannot eat, such as concrete, masonry, metal, or termite-resistant woods. With these materials used in the structure of a building, it will not be subject to termite attack. However, the insects can still enter and attack nonstructural components such as cabinetry, woodwork, etc.

Summary

If wood is to be used in the construction of a house, one should first give careful consideration to a method of termite treatment, since in many areas of our country it will inevitably be required. Because of their potential to contaminate the indoor air with formaldehyde, most man-made wood products should be avoided. If softwoods are used, less odorous species such as fir or spruce should be selected. Hardwoods will be better choices, especially for exposed interior woodwork. When chemically treated wood is called for, redwood should be substituted.

Chapter 12

Steel Framing

Wood framing has a number of drawbacks when used in an ecologically safe house but can be eliminated by using steel framing. Unfortunately, it is little used in the single-family residential construction industry. Steel framing is often found in commercial construction, and is occasionally used in multifamily homes. It is a very inert material and is well suited to both prefabricated and conventionally built houses.

Steel was used in prefabricated houses in the 1930s. Pan construction and porcelain panels were used in some houses but eventually wood framing reigned supreme. Steel framing still has a place in the market, even though it is primarily a commercial material.

Advantages

Steel framing is often lighter in weight than wood framing, and considerably lighter than other relatively inert materials such as concrete or masonry. Quality control is consistently very good. Steel members aren't subject to twisting, shrinking, or warping. There is no need to search through a pile of studs to select the good ones. Steel studs have holes prepunched in them for electrical wires or plumbing lines. This saves time in that holes do not have to be individually drilled. Steel is noncombustible and some insurance companies will provide coverage at less cost. Steel framing is often galvanized, making it rustproof. It can accommodate virtually any type of interior or exterior finishing material: plaster, drywall, brick veneer, metal siding, stucco, etc.

For individuals with severe sensitivities, the primary advantages are that it has no outgassing characteristics, it is resistant to mold growth, and it will never need to be treated for termites.

Disadvantages

The big disadvantage to using steel is that most builders are unfamiliar with it. They can't cut it with a handsaw or nail into it, so they are at a loss as to what to do with it. Since it is routinely used in commercial buildings, it is often possible to find someone in that area to work with it. Drywall contractors may be familiar with it as well. Steel framing behaves differently than wood; thus, some special design details may be necessary for proper bracing or bridging. Most manufacturers have literature available that describes the various construction techniques.

Some special tools are required to work with steel. While cutting can be done with such things as a hacksaw, tin snips, or a portable circular saw with a metal-cutting blade, anyone contemplating building an entire house would be wise to invest in a power cut-off saw. Although the various members can sometimes be welded together, they are more often assembled with self-tapping screws. These can be installed with a power drill, but an electric screw gun will be more efficient. The addition of a few clamps will complete the list of special tools required.

For someone with sensitivities to petroleum products, it should be noted that steel framing materials often are coated with a thin oil film.[1] This is applied during the manufacturing process and can be easily washed off with a heavy-duty cleaner such as TSP (Trisodium Phosphate). One person can wash all of the framing for an average house by hand in a couple of days.

Types of Steel Framing

There are three basic kinds of steel framing. The average person may only be able to think of one: heavy-gauge steel. The most applicable to residential work is light-gauge steel, of which there are two types: load bearing and nonload bearing. All have the same basic advantages and disadvantages listed above.

Heavy-gauge steel includes such things as I-beams and angles, the heavy materials that skyscrapers are constructed of. Occasionally, a heavy steel beam or columns will be found in the basement of a house, supporting the floor. This is because of the superior strength of steel. A wood beam could easily be designed to perform the same function but since wood is not as strong, a much larger wooden beam would be required. Most heavy-gauge steel is painted with a primer to protect it from rust. This can sometimes bother paint-sensitive people.

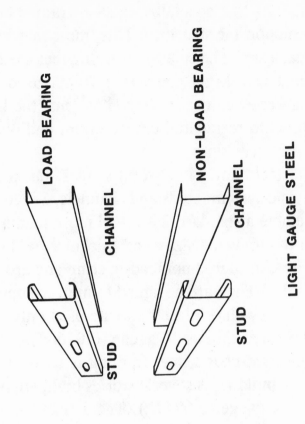

LOAD BEARING

CHANNEL

STUD

NON-LOAD BEARING

CHANNEL

STUD

LIGHT GAUGE STEEL

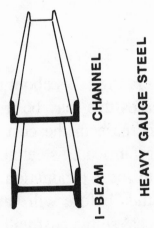

CHANNEL

I-BEAM

HEAVY GAUGE STEEL

Types of Steel Framing

A few companies that specialize in steel-framed houses use heavy-gauge steel to support the structure. This frame may have the members placed eight feet apart. The steel is so strong that closer spacing would be a waste of material. Light-gauge steel is then used to fill in between the heavier posts and beams. In most situations, the light-gauge framing is more suited to residential construction, and our discussion will be concerned primarily with it.

Light-gauge steel comes in several shapes, but there are only two that form the basic system: studs and channels. When these are assembled, they resemble a standard 2×4 wall more than a skyscraper. The studs come in a variety of sizes and thicknesses. The very thin and smaller sizes are considered nonload-bearing and are often referred to as "drywall studs." They are designed to merely support the finishing material such as drywall or plaster and are used only for interior partitions. They may be as thin as 26 gauge (0.0168").

Load-bearing light-gauge steel framing is used to actually hold up the structure. If a building is several stories high, slightly heavier studs are used, up to 14 gauge (0.0747"). The 3½" wide stud is common, with the larger sizes (up to 13½") being referred to as joists. These can be used in roof and floor systems. Several manufacturers will provide standard details for making roof trusses out of light-gauge steel.

Cost

The manufacturers' literature talks about steel framing being cheaper than wood. In some cases this may be true, but for most residential applications a slight increase in the cost of materials should be expected. A builder of prefabricated steel houses may be able to erect a lower-cost house due to mass production techniques. A builder who has never used steel studs before will have to pad his cost to cover unforeseen circumstances, so his cost will be higher..

Individual nonload-bearing light-gauge studs for interior walls are comparable in cost to wood studs, and can be priced slightly less, depending on their size. The load-bearing variety will be somewhat higher in cost; however, they can usually be placed on 24" centers instead of the common 16" centers used in wood construction, thus lowering the total cost.

Assembly

As mentioned above, heavy-gauge and light-gauge framing can be combined. Open-web steel joists may be combined to achieve wide spans. Wood and steel can also be combined. This may be a reasonable alternative for someone sensitive to softwood odors. A house can be framed out of wood in the conventional manner for all exterior load-bearing walls. These walls and the ceiling can then be drywalled and sealed per the airtight drywall approach, thus creating one large room whose interior space is protected from the softwood (and the insulation) by the foil-backed drywall. All interior walls can then be constructed out of inexpensive nonload-bearing studs.

One of the first questions that people ask about steel framing is, "How do you fasten everything to it?" Welding can be used with the heavier gauges but screws are more common. The thinner material is screwed together with pointed self-tapping screws by using a screw gun. Screw guns are made by many manufacturers of electric drills, but they are designed somewhat differently. They can have a magnetic chuck to hold a screwdriver bit, usually a Phillips bit. They will also have a clutch that disengages when the screw is seated. An electric drill, without a clutch, may prematurely wear out if used repeatedly for driving screws. Heavier gauges of steel framing are assembled with screws that appear to have small drill bits for points. These drill their own pilot holes and seat themselves very quickly. They are usually called "Teks" pointed screws. Teks is the trademark of one particular manufacturer (Shakeproof Co.). When selecting a screw gun, it should be noted that several models are available for various applications. Screw guns used with Teks type screws should run at a fairly low RPM.[2]

Drywall and plasterboard are attached with screws as well. In fact, much drywall is attached to wood framing with screws because it makes for a tighter installation and smaller dimples to finish with joint compound. Metal siding is also attached with screws. In this case it is important to use cadmium-plated screws, so they do not rust behind the siding and cause streaks of rust to run down the face. Interior woodwork is attached with what are called trim screws. These look like finish nails, with a small head, but they will accept a small Phillips screwdriver bit that is driven with a screw gun. Plywood roof decking or metal roofing can be screwed down as well.

Most manufacturers can supply a variety of screws as well as the

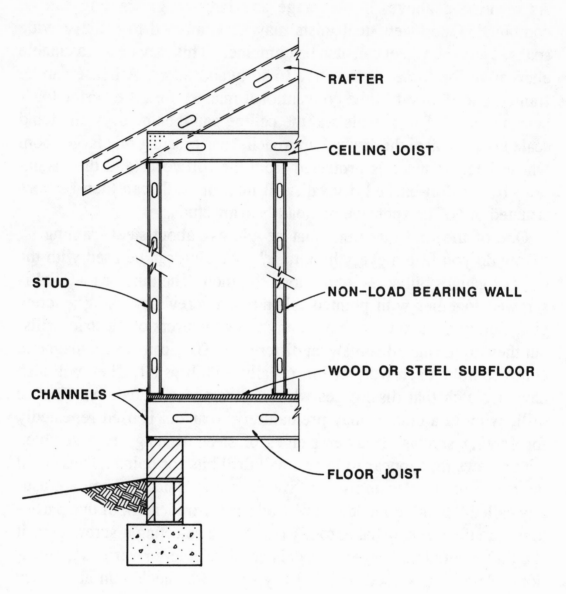

RAFTER

CEILING JOIST

STUD

NON-LOAD BEARING WALL

WOOD OR STEEL SUBFLOOR

CHANNELS

FLOOR JOIST

Steel Framing

metal framing itself. There are as many different kinds and sizes of screws as there are nails in a conventional house. It is simply a matter of learning to use a screw gun instead of a hammer.

Manufacturers

Steel framing is being promoted by the **Metal Lath/Steel Framing Association**[3,4] and the Zinc Institute, Inc. [5] They both have members who produce various types of galvanized (zinc-coated) steel framing. Listings can also be found in the telephone book's yellow pages under "Building Materials." Drywall suppliers often stock steel studs since some of the major drywall manufacturers produce steel framing and other building materials. They should probably be one of the first places to check when looking for a contractor familiar with using steel framing. Some commercial builders listed under "Buildings, Metal" in the telephone book may also be helpful.

A few companies exist that sell prefabricated steel-framed houses. For the most part, they use such potentially offensive materials as plywood, partial wood framing, or foam insulations. However, they may be able to supply a shell that could be completed with nontoxic materials. **Tri-Steel Structures** is one such producer, with distributors nationwide. They have a number of basic plans and can provide custom designs, utilizing both heavy-gauge and light-gauge steel framing. A book is available that discusses these houses as well as steel framing in general.[6]

There are many manufacturers who produce light-gauge steel framing. Some are local firms and some distribute their product nationally. They have literature available describing their product, most of which is geared to the needs of architects and engineers. Strength tables are most helpful to the designer, but may not be of interest to the consumer. Most will help designers with specific questions, but generally they are not geared to work directly with consumers. They can, however, often recommend contractors in the area familiar with using their products. **U.S. Gypsum Corporation**, one of the larger manufacturers, has a good publication that deals with load-bearing applications and contains not only technical information but also descriptive photographs that can be helpful to the do-it-yourselfer.[7] Similarly, **Gold Bond Building Products** has a good publication describing nonload-bearing applications.[8]

Following is a partial list of manufacturers of light-gauge steel framing materials:

Amico/MAS, Inc.
Angeles Metal Systems
Chicago Metallic Corporation
Dale Industries, Inc.
Gold Bond Building Products
Harrison Manufacturing Co.
InCor, Inc.
Marino Industries, Inc.
U.S. Gypsum Corporation
Western Metal Lath Co.

Summary

Steel framing is an excellent material to used in an ecologically safe house. Its primary drawback is the fact that it is unfamiliar to most residential builders, but it requires no great skills to master and any special techniques can easily be learned with practice.[9] The advantages for a sensitive person will outweigh the slight increase in cost. It is widely available from a variety of suppliers, coast to coast.

Chapter 13

Roofing Systems

Even though roofing is on the outside of a house, it should still be considered as far as nontoxic construction is concerned. Some materials can emit fumes that will seep into the attic and the house, or bother sensitive people walking around the outside of the house. A mild outdoor breeze may not be enough to carry away any offensive fumes, especially on a hot day when the sun's energy causes outgassing of the roof. There are several materials available for roofing, although some, such as asphalt shingles, seem to dominate the residential market. Wood singles, clay tiles, and metal panels are also used. All types have certain advantages and disadvantages that will be discussed.

Roof Decking
The actual roofing material is attached to the roof deck, which is also called sheathing. Most of the decking material used today is plywood or flakeboard, both of which can emit formaldehyde fumes from the phenol-formaldehyde glue. Even though the decking is separated from the living space of the house, some sensitive people should be concerned with having any formaldehyde sources in the construction. 1×8 solid boards can easily be substituted.

On roofs with shingles or shakes, solid boards are a better choice than sheet materials such as plywood. The boards should be spaced a few inches apart to allow for better air circulation and drying of the wood shingles. This is called skip-sheathing.

Individual shingles must often have an underlayment between them and the decking. This material is usually an asphalt-saturated felt paper (sometimes called tar paper), which can bother some sensitive people as the asphalt outgases, especially on a hot day. It has been suggested that polyethylene or polyester be substituted for the asphalt-saturated underlayment. This is a method of reducing asphalt outgassing; however, these alternate materials can be subject to deterioration when exposed to the heat of a roof.

It should be remembered that the tighter the house, the less likely fumes from the roof system will filter through cracks, electrical outlets, etc. In all types of construction, roof systems should be ventilated to remove excess heat and moisture from the attic space. This will also vent any minor fumes from the decking material and underlayment to the outside. Fumes can enter through the fresh air intake of a general ventilation system if it is located near an outgassing roofing material.

Sheet metal roofs are typically attached to wood or metal purlins that are spaced 24″ to 60″ apart. This forms a ladder that installers find convenient to use on steep roofs during construction. Wood purlins are usually 2×4s. Metal purlins are made in a variety of sizes and should be designed for each particular application. A few sheet metal roofs need to be installed over solid decking to provide more support, but most can be attached to purlins.

Composition Shingles

Asphalt shingles are more correctly known as composition shingles. They are made of asphalt-saturated felt with a mineral granule surface. Fiberglass shingles are composition shingles composed of asphalt-saturated fiberglass with mineral granules on the surface. The fiberglass is stronger than the felt, and fiberglass shingles do not contain as much asphalt. Most of the composition shingles used today are the fiberglass variety. These shingles are by far the most commonly used roofing material found on houses. They are typically nailed to a solid roof deck of plywood or solid boards. An underlayment material is usually installed between the deck and the shingles.

Many sensitive people react to asphalt materials when they are warm. Since a roof can get very hot on sunny summer days, it can definitely bother some people. A roof outside a bedroom window can be especially bothersome. Sitting outdoors on a patio when the wind blows asphalt fumes down from the roof can also be a problem. As these roofs age, they will outgas less, but may still bother those with asphalt sensitivities. It has been recommended that fiberglass shingles be substituted for asphalt shingles. This is a step in the right direction,

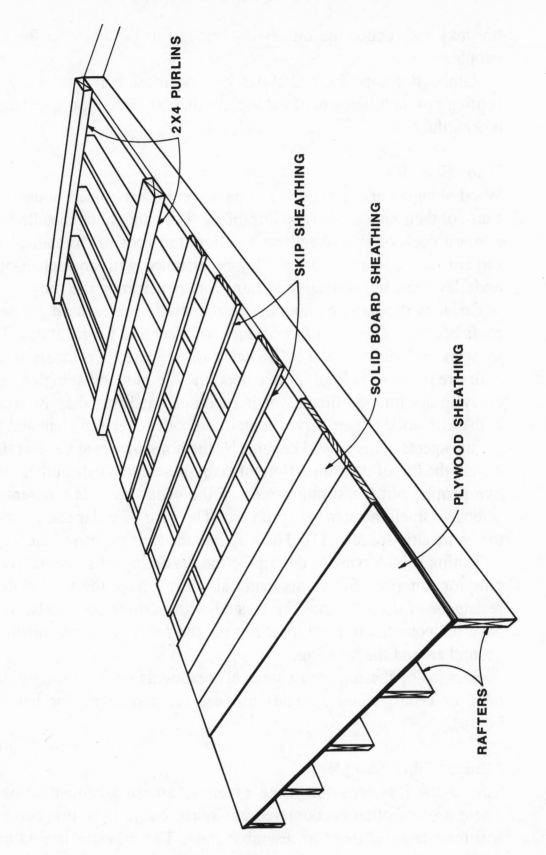

Roof Construction

but may not reduce the outgassing enough to be tolerable for some people.

Although composition shingles are the most common residential roofing product, because of the asphalt they are also a poor choice for a healthful house.

Wood Shingles

Wood shingles and shakes are popular on higher-priced housing because of their appearance and durability. They should be installed over a board deck of skip sheathing to allow the roof to "breathe." It is sometimes recommended that they be installed with an asphalt-based underlayment, to keep blowing rain from penetrating the roof.

Cedar is the most commonly encountered species used for wood roofs because of its natural resistance to insect and fungal attack. Both shingles and shakes are sold in the natural state or pressure-treated with fire retardants. In order to extend the life of wood shingles, especially in hot humid climates, it is recommended that they be treated with clear wood preservatives containing both water-repellent and fungicidal agents. This should be done by the homeowner at various times during the life of the roof.[1] Not only can these chemicals bother sensitive people, but the strong aroma of the cedar itself is a potentially offensive smell that can be a problem. The odor of cedar can permeate the entire attic space and find its way into the living space of the house.

Testing is underway to determine the feasibility of southern yellow pine for shingles.[2] Since this material doesn't have the natural decay resistance of cedar, it must be treated with various chemicals. These have the potential to leach out, run off the roof, and contaminate the ground around the building.

Because of the required chemical treatments or the strong natural odor of cedar, wood shingles are not recommended for healthful houses.

Mineral Fiber Shingles

This is the less ominous name given to asbestos cement shingles. These are not often encountered anymore, but at least one company still manufactures them to resemble slate. The asbestos is said to be "locked-in" a cement base, and is not considered a health hazard. However, these products can release asbestos fibers when cut during installation or broken during demolition. A future homeowner could have them removed during remodeling or repair and not realize that they contain asbestos. They can contain up to 20 percent asbestos fibers; therefore, they are not good choices for a roofing material.

If encountered on an existing house, it should be remembered that the greatest danger is when they are broken. If removal is necessary, the precautions required with any asbestos-containing product are strongly recommended.

Slate

Slate is a durable roofing material, often found on churches and occasionally seen on older houses, especially in the Northeast. It is an inert product and should be well tolerated by most people; however, because of its expense, it is rarely seen in new construction. Despite its high initial cost, it can be cost-effective during the life of the building, since it will last over 100 years. It is not difficult to apply, although most builders will need to do some reading before tackling a slate roof.[3] Slate is very heavy, and it will require a stronger roof system than some other materials.

Occasionally, used slate can be found at local salvage yards at a reasonable cost. New slate can be purchased from **Buckingham Virginia Slate Corporation**, **Rising and Nelson Slate Co.**, **Structural Slate Co.**, and **Vermont Structural Slate Co.** As mentioned above, at least one company (Supradur Manufacturing Co.) manufactures an asbestos cement product that resembles slate. It should be avoided.

Clay Roof Tiles

Clay roof tiles are often seen in hot climates, especially in Spanish architecture. This is a very heavy material and the house must be designed to withstand the extra weight; therefore it is not a good choice for retrofits. Clay tiles can be fairly expensive, depending on the style, but will generally last for the life of the building. It is often recommended that they be applied over an asphalt felt underlayment, which is their only drawback for sensitive people.

This material is available in several styles from the traditional reddish-colored roll type to contemporary glazed flat tiles in a variety of colors. Manufacturers include **Gladding, McBean & Co.** and **Ludowici Celadon Co.**

Concrete Roof Tiles

This material is seen in some hot climates in residential construction. The concrete is porous and subject to mildew growth. It must be periodically painted with a waterproofing paint to retain its integrity. The painting requirement will make it less than desirable for a paint-sensitive person.

Built-Up Roofs

Built-up roofs are made of layers of hot asphalt and roofing material. They are used extensively on flat roofs. Because of the asphalt they can bother some people. Sometimes they are covered with a gravel ballast, which can help to contain some of the asphalt odor. Today, synthetic membranes are rapidly replacing asphalt built-up roofs because they are much more durable. These roof systems can easily bother sensitive people because of outgassing, so the materials should definitely be tested prior to use. Since flat roofs can be prone to leaks, it may be desirable to consider building a sloping roof system over a flat roof to better shed water and then use a less offensive roofing material.

Metal Roofing

Metal roofing is made from a variety of different materials including copper, aluminum, steel, and stainless steel.[4] Stainless steel and copper are fairly expensive and are not often encountered in residential construction. Aluminum and steel roofs usually have a protective coating such as paint, zinc (galvanizing), or terne metal (an alloy of lead and tin). Some rely on a controlled oxidation process to provide a protective coating. This process is chemically similar to rusting but it actually helps to protect the roof. Steel is probably the most encountered metal with a galvanized steel roof having a colored baked-on paint coating being quite durable and attractive. Long sheet-metal panels that run from the ridge to the eave are commonly available but individual metal tiles can be purchased that resemble wood shakes and clay tiles. In general, metal roofs with baked-on paint films will be well tolerated by sensitive individuals, and are good choices for ecologically safe houses. There is a wide variety of different paints being used; for very sensitive people, it would be wise to obtain a sample prior to installation. Since most paints are baked on, any outgassing should be minimal.

The gentle sound of rain on a metal roof is viewed as a positive point by some people. Others consider the noise to be a drawback. In a well insulated house the sound will, in fact, be minimal, but in an uninsulated garage with no ceiling, it can be quite loud.

Sheet metal roofing is often used on agricultural buildings. It can easily be used on a house, and with a little planning does not have to look like a barn roof. Usually all that is necessary to achieve a striking residential look is to pay attention to designing an attractive eave detail and selecting an appropriate color. Metal roofing is often preferred by architects and developers because of its long life, esthetic qualities, and ease of installation.[5] Most sheet roofing is available in several ribbed or corrugated shapes, but three manufacturers (**Met-Tile, Inc.**, **Metal Sales Manufacturing Co**, and **Berridge Manufacturing Co.**) have a sheet product that is formed to resemble curved clay tiles. By forming ribs or other shapes into the sheets, the relatively thin metal gains a great deal of strength and rigidity.

Higher-priced sheet roofing is used extensively in commercial buildings, and lower-priced materials are seen on old deteriorating barns. The quality and the price are closely related. It is possible to pay very little and have a rusty roof in just a few years. Depending on the particular product, sheet metal roofing may be applied over 2×4s or metal members (purlins) that are spaced 24″ to 60″ apart. A plywood roof deck is usually not needed, so the total material cost of a sheet metal roof with purlins can be comparable to a roof of asphalt shingles over a solid wood deck. Due to the large size of the sheets, installation costs will be less as well.

Sheet metal roofing can be installed in several different ways. The best method is called a standing seam roof. It is usually only seen on commercial buildings because of its increased cost. A standing seam roof utilizes hidden fasteners so that there are no holes placed in the roof itself. Less expensive installations utilize nails with rubber washers under their heads to simply nail the roofing down to the wooden purlins. A drawback to using nails is the fact that they can work their way out slightly allowing for a possible leak. Intermediately-priced installations rely on screws with rubber washers to attach the roof. Properly installed, they should not result in leaks. Special flashings are required in some locations where roofs abut walls or for plumbing vent stacks. These will generally be available from the roofing supplier.

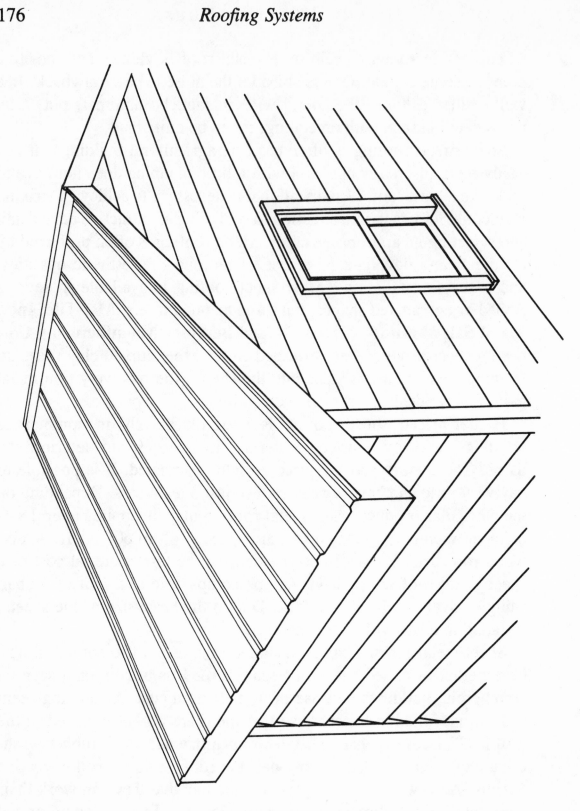

Ribbed Sheet Metal Roofing

To find a supplier or installer familiar with metal roofing, you should check in the telephone book under "Buildings, Agricultural," "Buildings, Metal," or "Buildings, Pole & Post Frame." A good quality residential roofing will be a little better than the standard for agricultural buildings but will not need to be of the standard used on commercial buildings. As with many things, "you get what you pay for." An expensive commercial roof will be of a heavier material with a better coating system and can usually be expected to last longer. When comparing prices, ask the supplier for an expected life of the roof. It can then be compared to the commonly used fiberglass shingles which will last only 15–20 years.

There are many small suppliers of metal roofing, but if none are to be found locally, some national manufacturers of ribbed metal roofing include:

ASC Pacific Inc.
Berridge Manufacturing Co.
Georgia Pacific Corporation
McElroy Metal, Inc.
Metal Building Components, Inc.
Metal Sales Manufacturing Corporation
Rib-Roof Industries, Inc.

Berridge Manufacturing Co. also sells a variety of individual metal shingles that resemble wood shakes, Victorian metal shingles, and fish-scale shingles. These all utilize hidden fasteners and must be mounted over a roof deck of solid boards or plywood with an asphalt felt underlayment.

Aluminum shingle-shakes are manufactured by **Reynolds Metals Company** and **Alcoa Building Products** in several colors. These are seen on some fast food restaurants. An attractive individual steel roofing tile is made by **Steeltile Company** that relies on a natural oxidation process to obtain a dark earthy color. Both products are attached with hidden fasteners over solid decks with a layer of asphalt felt paper.

Mold on Roofs

Moss, algae, mold, and mildew can grow on many types of roofs, especially in damp shaded locations. This can not only be unattractive, but also unhealthy as spores blow down on sensitive persons. The best remedy is to remove any overhanging branches so the sun and wind can work to keep the roof dry. North slopes are especially susceptible because they do not receive very much sunlight, of which the ultraviolet portion will help to kill the mold and mildew. One method for controlling moss on a wood roof involves stretching bare copper wires across the roof every ten feet horizontally along the butt ends of shingles. The normal corrosion of the copper will help to poison the moss. A copper or galvanized ridge will also be effective for about ten feet down the roof.[6]

Gutters and Downspouts

The function of gutters and downspouts is to divert water away from a building. Without them, excess water would run off the roof and saturate the ground, resulting in a wet foundation, crawl space, or basement. Plastic gutters should be avoided by sensitive people because of the outgassing potential, especially on hot days. Gutters can be havens for mold to grow, because of accumulating leaves and debris. Therefore, they should be cleaned regularly. It may also be a good idea to rinse them out with a garden hose. If the ground surface has a steep slope away from a house with a wide overhand, there may be little danger of water saturating the ground near the foundation. In this situation, it may be possible to eliminate gutters. However, this can result in erosion of the ground under the eaves.

Roof Ventilation and Moisture Control

The structure of a roof system must be designed to breathe. One way to accomplish this is to have vents at the eaves and ridge. This allows air to enter at the eave and rise up through the ridge, removing any excess heat and moisture from the attic space. In order to prevent condensation, the basic rule of ventilation states that the attic temperature should be as close to the outside temperature as possible at all times.[7]

There is a wide variety of methods used to vent roof systems: louvers, ventilators, fans, grills, etc. Venting must be done with cathedral ceilings as well as attics. Even though a moisture barrier is used in a ceiling system, a certain amount of water vapor can get through and condense on the underside of the roof deck. Moisture and heat are two things that can shorten the life of a roof and they can easily be controlled by proper venting.

Many venting products are sold through local lumber or building materials suppliers. Roofing installers should be familiar with local sources and types.

Summary

There is a wide variety of materials used for roofing. Because of the outgassing characteristics, the asphalt and wood products will generally be poor choices for a healthful house. Other materials such as slate and clay tile are fairly inert, but they are also higher in cost and add a considerable amount of weight to the roof. One of the safer materials that is cost-effective as well is a sheet metal roof. They are being seen more and more as designers realize that they can yield a very attractive and lasting roof. For someone seeking an ecologically safe roof, they can be an excellent choice.

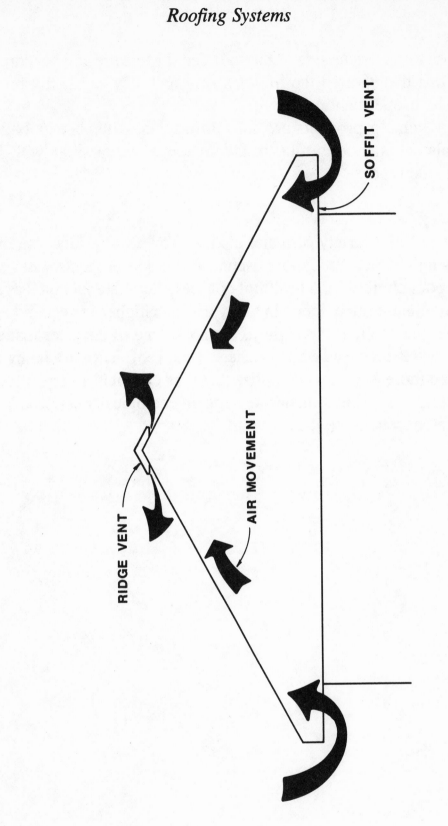

Roof Ventilation

Chapter 14

Exterior Siding

Exterior siding materials can be part of the structure itself, such as concrete or masonry, or they can be affixed to the structure, as is the case with various wood or metal sidings and stucco finishes.

For sensitive persons, the material on the exterior of the wall will be of less concern than the interior wall finish because there is less direct exposure. Any outgassing will be diluted by the outdoor air. The outgassing products can, however, be brought indoors through an open window. It could also be problematic for someone sitting outdoors near the siding on a deck or patio. Outgassing will be more pronounced when the siding is warmed up by the sun, so materials used in hot climates should be chosen with more care.

Besides the siding, the sheathing used under the siding can elicit symptoms if it is not considered. Some plastic wind barriers are also subject to outgassing. There are alternatives to these materials, but since the outside of the house is subject to severe weather conditions, you should consider their function before simply switching materials.

Sheathing and Wind Barriers
When 2×4 construction came into existence in the early 1800s, sheathing was not used. As a result, some of these old buildings began to lean because there wasn't enough bracing to keep them square. They were not very resistant to the wind, and in a storm the air simply blew right through the cracks into the house. Solid board sheathing helped somewhat, but there were still a lot of cracks. Diagonal wood bracing was developed to help keep the structure square.

Eventually, when plywood and other larger sheet materials came into use, they were used for sheathing. Because of their strength, when plywood or waferboard was used on the corners of the walls, the diagonal wood bracing could be eliminated. Less expensive sheathings, like asphalt-impregnated fiberboard, could be used on the rest of the wall, providing a reasonably good wind barrier.

As the country found itself in the middle of an energy crisis, better insulating boards were developed and used for sheathing. Since plywood wasn't a particularly good insulator, it was eliminated as a sheathing material, and the new insulating boards were used all around the house. In order to keep the building from leaning because of the force of the wind, some builders went back to using the diagonal wood bracing. Others began using a metal scrap for this necessary component. Both perform the function well.

From a health standpoint, most sheathings are problematic. The asphalt-impregnated fiber products can outgas asphalt fumes, and the various insulating boards, being plastic products, outgas as well. They also emit noxious fumes when burned. Gypsum sheathing utilizes a specially treated water-repellant paper facing that many sensitive people find bothersome. There are some heavy laminated cardboard sheathings with aluminum foil on both sides that are generally quite tolerable. These products are surprisingly strong and some grades can actually be used instead of diagonal bracing. However, they are not readily available in all parts of the country. Since the aluminum foil is a good vapor barrier, the use of this type of sheathing on the outside of the wall in cold climates can lead to moisture problems inside the wall cavity. (See Chapter 7.) They should cause no such problems in warm climates.

These foil-faced sheathings are made by several manufacturers. "Thermo-ply" sheathing is distributed by **Simplex Products Division**. "Dennyboard" is available from **Denny Sales Corporation** and is manufactured with three different facing combinations: (1) foil on both sides, (2) foil on one side and aluminized poly on one side, and (3) aluminized poly on both sides. Sensitive individuals should choose the product with foil on both sides. **Shepherd Products Co.** has a sheathing called "Thermo-bar." There are other sheathings of this type available, but since they utilize an aluminized poly facing, they are not recommended.

Since these foil-faced products should not be used in cold climates, something else can be done. If we examine the function of sheathings, it will be apparent that they are not necessary in many situations. The reasons for using a sheathing are: (1) to act as a wind barrier, (2) to strengthen the structure, and (3) to provide additional insulation. We have seen that either wood or metal diagonal bracing can easily provide the necessary strength, and if the wall system is designed with sufficient insulation in the cavity, the additional insulating ability of the sheathing is not required. Wind barriers are available made out of foil, as discussed in Chapter 16. If these three functions, often performed by sheathing, are handled in other ways, the sheathing may not be necessary.

Sheathing can also function to keep wind-driven rain from penetrating through a loose-fitting siding and getting the insulation wet. For this reason, a wind barrier of some type is necessary. Tighter fitting sidings can also be a good idea. However, siding that is too tight can function as a moisture barrier, preventing moisture from escaping from the inside of the wall. For problems with an incorrectly located moisture barrier, see Chapter 7.

Masonry Siding

Concrete blocks, brick, and stone make acceptable siding materials. The main precaution is in using a mortar without chemical additives, as noted in Chapter 9. Since sensitive people often react to paint, it would be wise to select materials that do not require painting, such as harder, nonabsorbent bricks or stone. Concrete blocks and some softer bricks tend to retain water for a certain period after becoming wet during a rain. This can result in mold growth on the surface. Sometimes a Portland cement-based sealer will help, such as the "Thoroseal" products discussed in Chapter 10.

Wood Siding

Solid wood siding can be applied either horizontally or vertically, but horizontal siding that is lapped is probably superior in shedding rain. Wood shingles can also be used for siding. Often a wood such as cedar or redwood is used because of its natural ability to resist insect or fungus attack. For sensitive people, cedar should be avoided because of its strong fragrance, and redwood should be chosen only after testing. Other woods can be used for siding, but they may not be widely available. Local mills may, however, be able to produce siding out of any species of wood, but the cost could be higher.

Plywood siding is seen more and more, primarily because of its lower cost or rustic appearance. As with most plywood products, the glues used will emit formaldehyde, so these materials should be avoided. Hardboard siding uses less glue than plywood and is a much denser product, hence it is subject to less outgassing, yet some people can still find it troublesome.

The big problem with wood siding is the need to paint it. Exterior paints will generally have more additives, like fungicides, than interior paints because they have a tougher job to do outdoors, being exposed to weather. In some instances, paint can be eliminated. Many people prefer the look of weathered wood; however, as the wood is weathering, the surface is slowly deteriorating. Unpainted wood must be able to dry out fairly quickly after a rain shower or mold growth can result. A house that is shaded from the sun by large trees, and protected from a drying breeze, can remain damp long enough to result in dark mold or mildew growth. This can be a problem in a wooded area where the building site isn't cleared out sufficiently.

Metal Siding

Aluminum and steel siding are widely used in the residential market. Both horizontal and vertical styles are available in several patterns and colors. The various manufacturers use different types of paints on their products, most of which are baked on. Polyvinyl chloride (PVC) finishes seem to be more and more popular because of their durability, but polyesters, fluorocarbons, acrylics, and enamels are also used. Sometimes a different finish is used on the back of the siding as a cost-cutting measure. Some manufacturers offer two different options, such as a PVC finish and an enamel finish. Baked-on finishes are often well tolerated by sensitive people because the outgassing period has been accelerated; however, since these are usually synthetic finishes, they should definitely be tested prior to use. In hot, sunny climates, continual outgassing can be more of a problem than in milder climates, where the siding doesn't get as warm. Of the different finishes, the vinyl coatings will generally be the most problematic, but there are enough variations in the different formulations to warrant testing several different products.

Following is a list of the larger siding manufacturers. There will be other smaller producers in different parts of the country.

Alcan Aluminum Corporation (aluminum, steel)
Alcoa Building Products (aluminum)
Alside (aluminum, steel)
Alumark Corporation (aluminum, steel)
Berridge Manufacturing Co. (steel)
Reynolds Metals Co. (aluminum)

Besides the standard horizontal and vertical patterns, **Reynolds Metals Co.** and **Alcoa Building Products** have aluminum shingle shakes that can be used for either roofing or siding. The metal sheet roofing panels discussed in Chapter 13 can also be used as a vertical siding material, as is often seen on commercial and agricultural buildings. Some of these use protective coatings other than paint, such as a zinc coating or controlled oxidation.

Metal siding is easily attached to wood or steel studs with nails or screws. When attaching aluminum siding to steel studs there can be the possibility of corrosion between the two different metals. If the metals are kept completely dry, there will not be the possibility of corrosion taking place. According to the Aluminum Association, where moisture is present or where condensation could occur, there can be corrosion between steel and aluminum, and it is recommended that the steel be painted. However, if the steel is galvanized (as most steel studs are) then corrosion is insignificant, because the zinc coating tends to protect the aluminum.[1] Cadmium-plated screws are recommended so that any minor amount of moisture that comes in contact with them does not cause rusting. Siding contractors routinely use aluminum or galvanized nails for this reason.

Radiation Shielding

There has been some concern expressed about metal siding shielding the beneficial effects of natural background radiation from the occupants of a house.[2] While it may, at first, seem wise to avoid all forms of radiation, research has shown that some forms of radiation are beneficial. One scientist, after shielding test subjects from all outside influences, including electrical background radiation, found that their biological rhythms became completely desynchronized. It was determined, after further experiments, that the part of the weak background radiation that pulsed at 10 cycles per second was a natural biological timer.[3] Of course, there are some forms of radiation that should definitely be avoided, such as X-rays or gamma rays. There has been less research done about the health effects of radio waves and visible light, but these are forms of radiation also. (See Chapter 15 and 21 for effects of light.)

In order to block out radiation, both natural and man-made, an enclosure known as a Faraday cage is needed. This can be made of either metal screen or metal sheets that are grounded. The grounding can be accomplished by firmly attaching a wire between all of the metal sides of the enclosures and a good electrical ground. In order to block out radiation, the ground connection must be very secure. While this is certainly possible when using metal siding, it is unlikely that adequate grounding is achieved in most installations. Since most metal siding is painted, the paint will tend to insulate the individual pieces of siding from each other. Furthermore, metal siding should not be installed tightly to the framing to allow for expansion and contraction as the temperature changes throughout the year. Unpainted aluminum foil will quickly form an oxide on the surface that will provide some insulation properties, thus making a grounded connection difficult when it is used as a wind or moisture barrier.

Different types of metals will block different wavelengths. For example, radio waves can be blocked by aluminum or copper, while X-rays require denser lead shielding. Steel is effective at lower frequencies because of its magnetic character.

Therefore, in the average installation, even though a few pieces of siding or sheathing might become grounded, many others would not. Background radiation would, therefore, pass through all of the pieces of metal siding, sheathing, or roofing that were not securely grounded. Some radiation would also pass through windows unless they were covered with securely grounded metal screening. It is doubtful that by using conventional construction techniques, a house with metal siding would act as a Faraday cage, and in any case, the occupants would occasionally be outdoors where they would be exposed to any radiation in the vicinity.

Vinyl Siding

Since solid vinyl siding is a plastic that is subject to outgassing, especially when warmed by the sun, its use is not recommended in healthful housing.

Stucco

Traditional stucco finishes can result in a very inert and well tolerated exterior wall finish; however, there are many synthetic resins being used in stucco mixes today. Some of these do not contain any Portland cement at all. For sensitive persons, only the basic Portland cement and lime mixtures are recommended.

Stucco, like plaster, has been traditionally applied in a three-coat system, but two-coat systems are also used. These will be 7/8" and 5/8" thick respectively. Thinner veneer systems are available, but they rely on various synthetic resins that can outgas undesirable chemicals. The traditional mix contains Portland cement, lime, sand, and water. Other aggregates besides sand are sometimes seen, such as expanded shale, clay, slate, or slag. Plastic cement, a Portland cement product containing several admixtures, is used in some parts of the country. Admixtures in stucco mixes have included asbestos, glass fibers, accelerators, retarders, etc. If anything other than the basic mixture is contemplated, testing should certainly be done.

Stucco is applied in a manner similar to plaster, with the three-coat system consisting of a scratch, brown, and finish coat. The two-coat system is comprised of a base coat and a finish coat. The texture of the finish coat can be varied to achieve a number of different effects. The material can be applied by hand or sprayed on with a machine.

Stucco can be applied directly to concrete and masonry surfaces only if a sufficient bond can be achieved. Otherwise a layer of metal reinforcing should be used. Expanded metal lath, similar to that used in plaster work, or wire lath can be used. These reinforcing materials are required in all installations over wood or metal studs, and over various sheathing materials. Since stucco is exposed to the weather, any cracks that develop could allow moisture to penetrate the wall. For this reason, an asphalt-impregnated felt paper is used behind the reinforcing steel to act as a secondary weather barrier. The paper also helps to separate the stucco layer from any sheathing or other base, so that they can expand at different rates, minimizing any cracking. Since the stucco forms a good barrier between the asphalt-impregnated paper and anyone walking around the outside of the house, it is doubtful that asphalt fumes will penetrate the stucco enough to be a problem. Aluminum builders foil could probably be used as a substitute, but it could be damaged much more easily during construction. If you are concerned about the use of the asphalt-containing felt paper, a visit to a house that has a new stucco finish will reveal any tolerability problems.

Metal casing beads and drip screeds are used at edges of stucco. In order to control cracking, metal or plastic control joints can be used to relieve stresses. Caulking may also be required in some situations. In order to harden correctly, stucco must be allowed to cure properly. Generally this involves occasionally misting water on the wall. Methods employing some admixtures or synthetic resins do not require such damp curing, but they should be avoided by sensitive people.

Columns and Shutters

As with many common building materials, exterior columns and shutters are being made of plastic, a material that can outgas undesirable odors. Fortunately, there are companies that make these items out of metal. **Moultrie Manufacturing Co., Reynolds Metals Co.,** and **Alcoa Building Products** sell colonial aluminum porch columns, caps, and bases in a variety of sizes with either a primed or baked-on finish. Aluminum shutters and cupolas are available from **Lomanco, Inc.** Of course, wood columns and shutters could be used to avoid outgassing from plastic.

Older Siding Materials

There are many older homes that have been re-sided with an asphalt-based product that resembles bricks. This material is very similar in composition to asphalt roofing singles, although it has not been manufactured for a number of years. Since outgassing decreases with time as the siding ages and becomes more brittle, most of this siding may be old enough to be tolerable for sensitive people; however, it may still outgas a little on a hot day.

Asbestos cement siding is another product that was once popular as a re-siding material. When it is undisturbed on the side of a house, it should be quite inert; however, sanding and scraping prior to repainting can abrade the surface sufficiently to liberate some asbestos fibers. Similarly, when removing the siding during remodeling, restoration, or demolition, it can become broken, resulting in fibers being released.

Care should be taken when scraping any old painted surface, because of the danger of the old paint containing lead. Lead-based paints were once quite common, so many old houses still have one or more layers of lead paint on them. A good quality dust mask is highly recommended.

Summary

Stucco is usually a well tolerated wall finish, although it can be fairly expensive. Masonry walls are also fairly inert. Wood siding, while popular from an esthetic standpoint, usually has the major drawback of requiring periodic painting. If the baked-on finish of the various metal sidings causes no problems, they make an attractive and tolerated exterior wall siding.

Chapter 15

Windows and Doors

Modern technology has had a major effect on how doors and windows are being manufactured. Wood is increasingly being replaced with metal or plastic. The energy crisis dictated new and tighter designs to keep cold winter air outside. While energy efficiency is certainly a desirable feature, health should not be sacrificed to save money on a heating or cooling bill. Some window and door installations can result in ill health unless care is taken in material selection and proper ventilation requirements are followed.

Besides providing security, doors often are the focal point of the exterior of the house. A well chosen entry door will enhance the appearance of any home. Sometimes a double door system or vestibule will be used to provide extra protection from the weather. Exterior doors allow for privacy from neighbors and interior doors privacy between rooms. Sliding doors or pocket doors can be used where space limitations are a concern. From a health standpoint, doors can isolate undesirable odors either outdoors or confine them to certain rooms. If closets are used to store odorous belongings, tight-fitting hinged doors should be used rather than sliders or bifolds. In some instances it will be advantageous to use weather-stripping on an interior door to isolate smells. This may be important for basement doors or a door leading to a utility room. Doors to an attached garage should always have well sealed weather-stripping to minimize the amount of exhaust fumes that enter the house.

Windows provide both security and light from the sun. At the same time they create a view that helps the occupants to feel less closed in. The psychological benefits of looking out of a window and watching birds, trees, and sunsets can be enormous. Properly designed windows allow heat from the sun to keep a house warm in the winter. An important aspect of windows in bedrooms is to provide a means of escape in the event of a fire. Open windows are also a prime source of fresh air.

There are too many different window and door manufacturers in the country to single out a few as being less toxic than others. Instead we will discuss the various types, listing pros and cons. In this way, you can easily evaluate the windows and doors available at a local lumberyard, glass supplier, or building materials center.

Window Construction

Windows are manufactured in a variety of styles: single hung, double hung, slider, casement, projected, fixed, etc. New windows come in standard sizes but replacement windows can be made in any size to fit existing openings. Their cost will be higher because of special handling. There are no particular health advantages to any one type, except that casement windows will generally seal the tightest and the traditional double-hung windows will form the loosest seal. Of course, the products of different manufacturers will vary considerably.

Window frames have been traditionally constructed of wood with a single pane of glass held in place with putty. Today, frames can be either wood, metal, plastic, or a combination of materials. The putty may be replaced with an extruded synthetic rubber material. The single pane of glass is increasingly being replaced with two or three panes to achieve greater year-round energy efficiency. Sometimes, plastic is used in place of glass. The storm windows that were taken down in the spring and put up again in the fall are now built into the window unit.

Many of the materials used in window construction can bother sensitive people. Wood windows may be chemically treated. Plastic windows can outgas offensive odors as can rubber seals. Improperly designed windows can allow moisture to condense on them, resulting in mold growth. Solar energy entering a window can cause outgassing of draperies or carpeting as it warms them. Loose-fitting windows can allow unwanted outdoor air pollution to enter the house.

When windows are installed, it is common practice to use caulking on the outside as a barrier against the weather. The gap indoors between the rough framing and the window unit can be stuffed with fiberglass insulation or filled with a foam insulation dispensed from an aerosol can. They both can result in tolerability problems. Sealing them from the living space can be accomplished by covering the insulation with aluminum foil tape.

Glass

Glass itself is a relatively inert material, and is well tolerated by most people. A disadvantage of glass is the fact that it blocks a certain portion of the ultraviolet light that is a natural part of sunlight. Someone who rarely goes outdoors will be lacking in this exposure.

It has been demonstrated that when people look at light sources lacking the ultraviolet portion of the spectrum that is near visible light, their muscle strength is weakened.[1] There are a wide range of wavelengths that are classified as ultraviolet light, not all of which are desirable. For example, some wavelengths are more closely related to X-rays than visible light and are harmful. Fortunately, there are few of these dangerous wavelengths present in the sunlight reaching the earth, most having been filtered out by the atmosphere.

Some types of plastic windowpanes will allow the beneficial ultraviolet light to pass through, but they may be subject to outgassing when warmed by the sun. Manufacturers of this type of plastic include **American Cyanimid** and **Rohm and Haas**. There is a very specialized type of glass called quartz glass which will also allow the beneficial ultraviolet light to pass through, but it is considerably more expensive than ordinary window glass and very difficult to obtain.

Insulated glass consists of two or more panes that are separated, usually by a sealed metal frame. The resulting airspace will be between 1/4″ and 3/4″ thick depending on the manufacturer. The metal frame often contains a drying agent sealed inside to prevent fogging between the panes. Sometimes a plastic film will be suspended between two panes of glass to provide extra airspace. Multiple airspaces are highly desirable from an energy-saving standpoint. The number of airspaces is more important than the thickness of the airspace. For example, two 1/2″ airspaces will be more energy-efficient than a single 1″ airspace. Sometimes an insulating glass unit will be combined with an additional permanently-mounted storm window. Two panes of glass are becoming the industry standard with three panes being encountered in colder climates. Occasionally in very cold areas four panes may be seen. If the window units are not properly sealed or are poorly constructed, moisture can leak between the panes of glass and condense. A reputable window manufacturer should stand behind his product and replace a defective unit within a reasonable time period.

Coated glass and plastic films are available from a number of manufacturers to make glass more energy-efficient. These materials are designed to allow sunlight to pass through the window into the house, but they block radiant heat from leaving the house. The plastic films suspended between two panes of glass should pose no problem for sensitive people because they are usually well sealed, but some of the glass coatings have the potential to outgas depending on their composition. These should be tested by sensitive people prior to use.[2] Energy-efficient glass containing a low E infrared film will block virtually all of the ultraviolet light. This can be advantageous, since the ultraviolet light is responsible for material degradation and fabric fading.

In some window and door applications, unbreakable glazing is required to prevent occupants from being injured by broken glass if they should fall against it. The glazing material can be acrylic or polycarbonate plastic sheets or tempered safety glass. The plastic materials should be avoided because of outgassing potential.

Seals and Glazing Compounds

The traditional material used to hold glass in a frame is glazing compound or putty. This will be either a vegetable oil-based material or a plastic or rubber-based material, that usually requires painting. For a sensitive person, the glazing compound or the paint can be problematic. Occasionally, glazing compound is applied to the inside portion of a window, but generally it is on the exterior, where it will be unlikely that any outgassing will contaminate the indoor air, unless the window is opened. Increasingly, an extruded synthetic rubber seal is used instead of a glazing compound, especially on metal windows. This, too, is subject to outgassing and can bother some people, especially when heated by the sun. As with many materials used in house construction, there is no single material that is 100 percent safe. For this reason, a sensitive person should select the window unit with the least total potential for outgassing. Bothersome seals or weather-stripping can sometimes be coated with a sealant to make them tolerable. One of the clear finishes discussed in Chapter 19 will usually work fairly well, but for very sensitive people, testing is always recommended. The sealant can be applied with a small artist's brush.

Window Frames

Wood, metal, and plastic are the primary materials used in window frame construction. Sometimes, wood is clad with plastic or metal to increase its durability. Other combinations may also be seen, such as an aluminum window being used with a plastic track for a storm unit or a wood window with a metal exterior.

Plastic window frame components should generally be avoided by sensitive people because of their outgassing potential. A hot sunny day will be more likely to result in the plastic giving off bothersome fumes. This is also the time when a window will likely be open in a house that is not air-conditioned, resulting in the odors entering the living space.

Wood window frames have been the traditional choice for residential windows. In fact, for years they were the only choice. Today, the majority of the wood windows manufactured in the United States comply with the NWWDA Wood Window Standard I.S.2 of the **National Wood Window & Door Association**. This requires that all wood parts (except interior trim) be water-repellant preservative treated to reduce water absorption and attack by molds or mildew. Most often, the water-repellant is a paraffin wax and resin in mineral spirits. Popular fungicides include: Pentachlorophenol (Penta), Tri-N-butyltin oxide (TBTO), and 3-ido-2-propynyl butyl carbamate (IPBC).[3] Penta has many well documented health effects, as was discussed in Chapter 11, and should be avoided. Because of new EPA regulations, its use is being phased out. Both TBTO and IPBC are listed as being toxic to fish, wildlife, and domestic animals and overexposure in the workplace can result in eye or skin irritation, nausea, dizziness, or headache.[4,5] Windows that are chemically treated should be avoided by sensitive people, although in some cases they have been coated with a paint or sealant and made tolerable.

Wood windows that are not chemically treated can sometimes be specially ordered from a window manufacturer. Small, local companies will be easier to deal with than large firms. Softwoods are the most commonly used woods in window construction, but a manufacturer willing to use untreated wood may also be willing to use a specified hardwood. Of course, any window requiring special handling will result in increased cost, and delays in shipping. If a wood window is properly painted, there should be no real need for it to be chemically treated. However, the paint could be problematic for sensitive people.

At least one company (**Benchmark Windows**) manufactures solid redwood window frames for those who desire a wood window but are concerned about moisture absorption or fungus attack.

Metal window frames are usually made of steel or aluminum. **Ampax Aluminum Co.** will custom make windows out of stainless steel, copper, or brass but the cost can be quite high for most residential applications. Metal frames can result in moisture condensing on them unless they have a thermal break. When the temperature difference is high enough, a metal frame can become cold, allowing humid air to condense on it. A thermal break effectively insulates the indoor portion of the frame from the outside of the frame, eliminating condensation or "sweating." The material used for the thermal break is usually a synthetic rubber or plastic material that theoretically can outgas and bother sensitive people; however, its exposure to the living space is usually minimal. Because of the potential condensation problems, thermal breaks are very desirable features.

Steel window frames are often confined to commercial applications, but residential steel windows are also available in a variety of attractive styles. Steel frames are usually fitted with single-pane glass for use in moderate climates, but insulated glass is also available. A variety of finishes can be provided, including a factory-applied primer, zinc galvanizing, or special coatings. The zinc galvanizing would be a well-tolerated finish for most people, as would a baked-on finish. Although steel windows can be made with thermal breaks, they are usually supplied without them, because of their use primarily in mild climates. Steel windows are not as readily available as aluminum windows for the residential market and their cost may be higher. The strength of steel allows for thinner frames to be used than in aluminum windows. A manufacturer of steel windows is **Torrence Steel Window Co. Inc.** and **Coast to Coast Manufacturing Co.** A list of other suppliers can be obtained from the **Steel Window Institute**.

Aluminum windows are made by many different companies. The **American Architectural Manufacturers Association** lists dozens of different manufacturers of both commercial and residential aluminum windows.[6] Many do not distribute their products to all parts of the country, so someone desiring an aluminum window should check at local suppliers to see what is available in their area.

Most residential aluminum windows are available with either a white or brown baked-on finish, which is usually well tolerated. Some

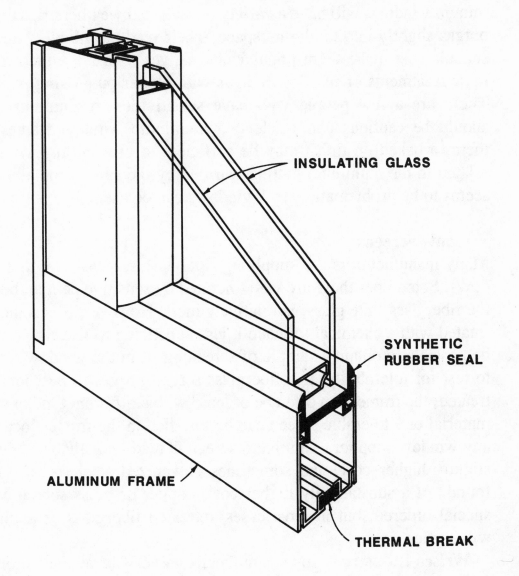

INSULATING GLASS

SYNTHETIC
RUBBER SEAL

ALUMINUM FRAME

THERMAL BREAK

Energy-Efficient Window

are anodized in various colors by an electrolytic process that is also well tolerated. The glass is set in an extruded seal of a synthetic rubber or plastic. This can bother some sensitive people. Quality airtight aluminum windows will have a variety of seals and weatherstrips that can outgas slightly into the living space. Their ready availability and reasonable cost make them popular alternatives to wood windows with toxic treatments or plastic windows with higher outgassing potential. There are a few people who have sensitivities to aluminum; they should be cautious about selecting aluminum window frames. For them, a baked-on finish may be sufficient to prevent any symptoms related to the aluminum getting warmed by the sun. If the aluminum seems to be problematic, steel windows can be used.

Window Screens

Many manufacturers are supplying fiberglass screens with their windows. Sometimes these are well tolerated by sensitive people, because the fiberglass, like glass, is relatively inert. However, it is sometimes treated with a chemical to make it less appetizing to insects. It should be possible to obtain a sample of screening from the window supplier to test for tolerability. If a fiberglass screen proves to be chemically treated, the frames can often be ordered with a different type of screen material or a tolerable screen can be installed in the frames locally by any window supplier. Aluminum screen is readily available, only at a slightly higher cost, and sometimes galvanized steel screen can be found. At a substantially higher cost, copper or brass screen can be special ordered, but in most cases untreated fiberglass or aluminum will suffice.

Wrisco Industries, Inc. manufactures a very attractive aluminum-framed screen room kit in white or brown. It can be purchased in a variety of sizes, with or without an aluminum roof. Fiberglass screening that is chemically treated is usually furnished, but the kit can be purchased without screening and then metal screening can be inserted in the framework.

Other Windows

Skylights are simply roof windows. While they will admit more light into a room than a wall window, they also will be rather inefficient from an energy-saving standpoint and extra sunlight may not be welcomed on a hot summer day. Many skylights do not provide for a very interesting view, and one's neck will get stiff after a period of looking up. On a steeply sloping roof, however, they can provide both light and a view if placed at a comfortable height. Skylights are made of the same materials as regular windows, and can be obtained with multiple panes of glass. It has been said that skylights always leak, but many new models have been developed that minimize any leakage problems. It should be remembered, however, that anything that penetrates a roof is a potential leak that can result in mold growth. Skylights have been somewhat overrated and used in inappropriate areas where they are hardly even noticed until they are pointed out by the homeowner.

Interior windows can help to open up rooms while keeping odors isolated from the rest of the house. For example, a fixed window between the kitchen and family room or dining room will help to open up the kitchen. At the same time it will prevent cooking odors from permeating the whole house, something that can bother an occupant with various food allergies.

Traditional stained glass windows are made with lead dividers between the pieces of glass. Lead poisoning can be a problem with some craftsmen. Lead oxide on the fingers can be ingested when eating, lead fumes can be inhaled when soldering, or it can be absorbed through cuts in the skin,[7] but these exposures will not be encountered by a homeowner with a stained glass window. Hands should be washed, however, after cleaning a stained glass window. A linseed oil-based putty is often used in stained glass work to keep the individual pieces from rattling in the dividers. This can be bothersome to some sensitive people. If you are working directly with a stained glass craftsman, you can request that putty not be used.

Window Locations

In cold climates it is advisable to have a large percentage of windows on the south side of the house to take advantage of the free solar heat. If the roof overhang is properly designed, the south-facing windows can be shaded in the summer and exposed to the sun in the winter. In warm climates it will be desirous to have the windows shaded all year long.

Bedrooms should have at least one window that can be used as a means of fire escape. Two bedroom windows on different walls can allow for fresh air to easily pass through the room on nice days. This should not be a substitute for mechanical ventilation because an airtight house will not always have the windows wide open.

Building codes usually do not require a bathroom window if an exhaust fan is used. However, it is a good idea to have a window in every room of the house so that if unusual odors are generated, say from painting, a window fan can be used to pull air through the room until the outgassing is complete.

Where possible, windows should be located away from kitchen, dryer, or ventilation system exhausts. They should not be placed near plumbing vent stacks nor near garages or parking areas because of the danger of fumes entering the house when windows are opened. An asphalt roof near a window can also allow undesirable odors to enter the house as the roof heats up during the day and outgasses. With a knowledge of the local wind directions, it should be possible to locate windows so that a gentle breeze will flow through the house.

Window Coverings

Synthetic curtains and draperies can be the cause of outgassing when heated by the sun. Natural fabrics such as cotton or linen can easily be substituted. Fabric curtains can generate dust that will bother some sensitive people. If one is allergic to dust, metal Venetian blinds are available that will provide privacy while being relatively inert. They have the advantage of not creating dust, but they can collect dust that already exists in a room. They can be vacuumed as necessary. A properly designed window will not require curtains to dress it up, so they may not be necessary at all in some rooms, unless privacy is required.

Curtains or draperies that are closed in the winter to keep the heat from escaping can result in a moisture problem. The airspace between the window and a curtain will be colder than the rest of the room. This causes moisture-laden interior air to travel behind the curtain and condense on the colder glass, resulting in a potential mold problem. If this happens, curtains should be kept open in winter. It is for this reason that energy-saving window quilts should have a vapor barrier inside them and be securely sealed at the edges.[8] This prevents the moisture from getting between the quilt and the glass.

Interior Doors—Wood

Hollow core-wood interior doors are common in residential construction because of their low cost. They are available in flush styles that have a thin skin of plywood and a core of a paper honeycomb material, or they can be molded of hardboard to resemble a paneled door. The paneled types will emit less formaldehyde than the flush styles because of less glue, but both should be avoided by sensitive people. Some fire-rated interior doors have a particle-board core which can outgas considerably. Doors that appear to be wood can, in fact, be plastic with a wood-grained finish. Plastic doors should be avoided because of their outgassing potential.

Solid wood interior doors are usually of the frame and panel type and are available in several different patterns. Most of these that are stocked by building materials suppliers are made of softwood, often pine. Less odorous fir or hemlock doors can be especially ordered. It is also possible to order solid hardwood doors out of oak. Some doors that look like solid hardwood, on close examination can be veneered, so you should make sure that they are what they appear to be. The glues used to assemble wood doors are often formaldehyde-based, but very little glue is required in a panel door, as compared to a flush door, so outgassing from the glue will be negligible.

Most woodworking shops can easily make doors to your specifications, out of any type of wood or glue that you prefer. Sometimes the cost will be less than the cost of a factory-made door that must be especially ordered. Attractive, yet inexpensive woods such as poplar can be used instead of more costly woods such as walnut or oak. A simple style can be selected to reduce labor costs, making custom made doors even more affordable.

Another source to consider for interior wood doors is the local salvage yard. Used doors and antique doors are available in many different styles and woods. Older softwood doors should not be as offensive as new doors for sensitive people. Some people enjoy having each door in the house of a different type. In this way each room can have its own character. A beveled glass door can be used for the dining room, French doors for the family room, and various paneled doors for bedrooms. If the salvage yard has all of the doors from a school or a hotel, matching doors can be used throughout the house. It should be remembered that it will usually not be possible to choose from a variety of sizes, and in the case of building a new house, the doors should be selected before rough framing of the openings so that they will fit. If stripping of an old finish is necessary, care should be taken to use less-toxic strippers. Shellac finishes can be removed with alcohol. Other finishes can be removed with alkali paint strippers such as the

"Brookstone Paint Stripper" sold by **Brookstone Co.** either by mail or through one of their retail stores. This is a powdered product that is mixed with water. Other sources and do-it-yourself recipes are available.[9]

Interior Doors—Metal

Hollow metal interior doors are commonly used in commercial applications. They can be hung in either metal or wood frames. Some have a corrugated fiber core that adds rigidity to the door and can contain formaldehyde-based glues. Others utilize an asphalt-based sound-proofing sprayed inside the door. By reading manufacturers' literature at a local supplier, you can determine whether or not a door is all metal. **Fenestra Corporation** makes a "Presidential" series all-metal interior door that can be especially ordered without soundproofing. Metal doors are usually shipped with a primer finish, but can sometimes be ordered with a factory-applied finish coat. Baked-on finishes will be the best tolerated.

"Benchmark" metal bifold doors are available from **General Products Co., Inc.** in louvered or raised panel designs or with full-length mirrors mounted to metal frames. These are well suited for closets. They are also available by mail order through **Sears, Roebuck and Co.** catalogs. They are made in several different widths and heights and have a factory-applied white finish. The finish will require some outgassing time before it will be tolerable for very sensitive people.

Exterior Doors—Wood

Flush exterior wood doors are similar in construction to interior doors. They have a core of either wood or corrugated fiber with a thin plywood skin, held together with a formaldehyde-based glue. Most panel doors are softwood, usually pine. Exterior pine panel doors that meet the **National Wood Window and Door Association** Standard NWWDA I.S.6 will be treated with the same chemicals as are wood windows. Fir and hemlock exterior panel doors are not routinely treated, although a manufacturer may elect to treat all exterior doors.

Because of the temperature and weather extremes that exterior doors are exposed to, they receive a lot of abuse and are subject to warping. The required routine painting can be a problem for someone sensitive to paint odors. Because they will slightly change dimensionally as the seasons change, they often do not seal as well as metal doors.

Exterior Doors—Metal

Most exterior metal doors are insulated for energy efficiency. The insulation will usually be polyurethane or polystyrene. A metal door will likely seal in any outgassing fairly well, especially if there is metal on not only the faces but also the four edges. Most metal doors use wood or plastic at the edges to act as a thermal break, reducing the likelihood of "sweating," although condensation is much less a problem with insulated doors than it is with windows. Even though the insulation material would be problematic for a sensitive person when exposed directly, the insulation sealed inside a metal door will often be tolerated.

Doors can be embossed to resemble panel doors or they can have moldings attached for decoration. Often the moldings are plastic which have the potential to outgas. Moldings around glass in doors can be either wood or plastic. Flush or embossed doors without moldings will be less offensive for sensitive people.

Residential exterior doors usually are mounted in softwood frames while commercial door frames are generally metal. At least one manufacturer (**General Products Co. Inc.**) makes a residential door for new construction with an all-metal frame. Their "Adjusta-Fit" steel frame is a two-piece system. Several residential replacement doors are made with metal frames that slip into an existing wood frame. (**General Products Co. Inc., Stanley Door Systems,** and **Steelcraft**.)

Steel doors are usually galvanized with a primer finish supplied from the factory. Most manufacturers do not apply a finish coat, so they must be painted prior to installation. For paint-sensitive persons, doors should be purchased and painted early in the construction process so they can have sufficient time to outgas. Aluminum sliding glass patio doors are usually finish-painted or anodized. They are often made by window manufacturers.

Other Exterior Doors

Garage doors can be made of the same materials as other doors: plastic, softwood, hardboard, etc. All-steel uninsulated garage doors are available from **Clopay Corporation** and **Stanley Door Systems. Taylor Building Products** and **Clopay Corporation** have insulated steel garage doors with a polystyrene core. The Clopay doors come with a finish coat of brown or white and the others are primed only. All are available in a variety of styles and sizes.

Bilco Company manufacturers an outdoor steel hatch-type basement door in a variety of sizes. These are weatherproof and secure, and have a baked-on primer finish. They are uninsulated.

Weather-Stripping

Most weather-stripping today is made of some type of synthetic plastic such as vinyl, a type of foam, or a fabric pile. The purpose of weather-stripping is to control air infiltration and rain penetration. This limits the amount of undesirable odors, pollens, and mold spores entering the house. Steel doors often utilize a magnetic, vinyl weather strip somewhat like a refrigerator door. This provides for a very tight seal. Some sensitive people have had luck coating weather strips with a clear sealant to make them tolerable. Others need to remove the synthetic material and replace it with a metal product. Brass or stainless steel weather-stripping is manufactured by **Pemko, Inc.** and is available in many hardware stores.

"Tygon" tubing is manufactured by **Norton Performance Plastics** and although it is a plastic product, it is often well tolerated by sensitive people. Available in many sizes and grades, it can be slit and tacked in placed for use as weather-stripping. It is available from laboratory supply houses and small quantities can often be purchased through individual laboratories.

Thresholds can be made of wood (usually oak), metal (usually aluminum), or plastic. Most exterior steel doors are supplied with aluminum thresholds. These should have thermal breaks in cold climates to prevent moisture from condensing on them. In order to provide a seal, thresholds are usually fitted with a vinyl weather strip. **Pemko, Inc.** makes aluminum thresholds that utilize metal hooks or spring seals but these may be difficult to locate through retail suppliers.

Summary

Windows and doors can cause a variety of health effects because of outgassing from the materials of which they are constructed or because of their location. No window or door is 100 percent inert; all will have some minor drawbacks. For most people, aluminum windows with insulating glass will be the best choice from a health standpoint, although there may be some minor outgassing from the seals. Metal or hardwood interior doors will be healthier choices than softwood doors or hollow core doors. Exterior insulated steel doors should be fairly well tolerated because they tend to seal in any outgassing of insulation, but in mild climates hardwood doors may be a reasonable choice.

Chapter 16

Insulation Products

Insulation is used in a variety of locations in houses: inside walls and roof systems, under floors, and around foundations. Water heaters and heating ductwork are also commonly insulated. Insulation is required in warm climates to keep the heat outside and in cold climates to keep the heat inside. There are available a variety of different types and forms that are suited for use in specific areas. Nearly every type of insulation has been implicated in some health problem, yet with care in installation and material selection, a healthy house can be properly insulated.

Insulation should always be installed in conjunction with a moisture barrier of some type because when a house is insulated, two different climates are the result—one indoors and one outdoors. These two different climates will have different humidity levels as well as temperature levels. Without a proper moisture barrier, moisture will attempt to travel through the insulation from the climate with high humidity to the climate with low humidity. This can result in a moisture buildup inside the wall and a possible mold problem. When some insulations take on a small amount of moisture, they lose a great deal of their insulating ability, so a moisture barrier is an energy-efficient investment as well.

Background
All materials will resist the flow of heat to some degree. Insulating materials tend to resist the flow of heat very well. Solid materials such as steel and concrete will resist the flow of heat, but they do a poor job of it. Most of the substances that are used specifically for insulation,

resist the flow of heat by trapping different layers of air within their structure. They can sometimes be compared to a sponge with many spaces to trap air. Insulations are compared by their R-value (Resistance-value). The higher the R-value, the better the insulating ability. A common brick has an R-value of 0.20 per inch while fiberglass batt insulation has an R-value of 3.17 per inch. Both materials can be used to insulate a house, but fiberglass does a much better job, in fact it is over 15 times better.

Historically, natural materials were used as insulations. Such things as cotton, straw, sawdust, feathers, moss, and cork were common. Today, most insulations that are commercially available are man-made. Rock wool and fiberglass were two of the first to be developed. These were followed by perlite, cellulose, and various plastic foams. Asbestos was used in the past in some insulations.[1] It was not as common in residences as in other buildings; nevertheless, asbestos can be found in some houses, especially around older heating systems.

Health Problems

There is a variety of health problems associated with insulating materials. Some illnesses have been reported in the factories that manufacture various products. Sensitive individuals report symptoms related to outgassing. Urea-formaldehyde foam was banned for a time because of adverse health effects. These problems can be minimized in a house by careful material selection. It is also important to install insulation correctly to avoid outgassing into the living space.

Many of the synthetic insulating materials release extremely toxic gases when they are heated and burned. Fire departments are well aware of this and most routinely wear oxygen masks when entering a burning building. For the occupants of a burning house, oxygen masks are rarely available. To them, smoke inhalation means toxic vapors that cannot easily be avoided. In most fires, deaths are due to carbon monoxide and other noxious gases and vapors, not flame contact.[2] Since totally incombustible materials are not available, you should select those providing the least hazard. Many building codes require that flammable foam-insulating materials be separated from living spaces by fire-resistant materials such as drywall or plaster.

Improper installation of insulation can cause some electrical fixtures to overheat and, as a result, can contribute to a fire starting. This can be especially dangerous when recessed ceiling lighting fixtures are covered with attic insulation. Instructions supplied with insulation will specify proper clearances to be maintained between the insulation and lighting fixtures, furnace flues, water heaters, etc. If a device isn't specifically designed to be in contact with insulation, three inches of clearance should be provided to minimize the chance of fire.[3]

The energy conservation movement has been implicated in causing increases in indoor air pollution and consequently ill health. This is primarily due to excessive tightening of houses rather than the insulating material itself, although there are certainly some unhealthy materials being used for insulation. If fresh air is introduced mechanically, excessive tightening does not have to result in poor indoor air quality. The house must be viewed as a whole, with all of the separate parts working together. In this way an energy-efficient *and* healthful house can be built.

Since the health effects will vary depending on the type of insulation used, a more complete discussion is necessary with the material descriptions.

Batt Insulation

Batt or blanket insulation is probably the most commonly used today. It is a fluffy product that can be purchased in different colors, depending on the manufacturer, and in different thicknesses and widths. There are two basic types: rock wool and fiberglass, although there are other specialized kinds used in industrial applications. While rock wool was very popular before World War II, today fiberglass is more often encountered in residential construction. Both types are considered man-made mineral fibers and can be referred to as "mineral wool."

Residential batt insulation is available with a kraft paper, aluminum foil, or plastic facing which is designed to be a moisture barrier. These facings may be coated with asphalt, which can outgas for a long period and be bothersome to some sensitive people. There will be seams between batts that will need to be taped in order to form a continuous moisture barrier. A better, more tolerable moisture barrier can be obtained by other means, so it is often advisable to order batt insulation without any type of facing material.

Installers of both rock wool and fiberglass often complain of itching due to small cuts from the fibers. Itching can also be due to a reaction with the binder used to hold the insulation together.

Recent medical reports have indicated that man-made mineral fibers such as rock wool and fiberglass can cause cancer in production workers.[4,5] Illnesses reported included cancer of the upper respiratory and alimentary tracts and digestive system as well as nonmalignant respiratory disease. Production workers are usually exposed to higher concentrations than homeowners, but installers and builders can be exposed to even higher levels.

The increased cancer risk may be attributable to the small diameter of the inhaled fibers that are similar in size to asbestos fibers.[6] One report suggests that these man-made mineral fibers "appear to be more potent than asbestos with regard to chronic pulmonary disease."[7] Further information about the dangers of mineral fiber insulations can be obtained from the **Victims of Fiberglass**.

Rock Wool

Rock wool is produced by heating natural rocks or industrial slag in a furnace. As the material melts, it is drawn out into fibers and formed into felts, blankets, or batts. Today rock wool has been generally replaced in residential construction with the less expensive fiberglass insulation.

Rock wool is often contaminated with lignite, a type of coal, and mineral oil to control dust. It is bound into batt form by the use of a phenolic resin. These materials can be bothersome to some people, hence, they are not recommended.

Fiberglass

Fiberglass insulation is manufactured in a similar manner, by melting inorganic materials, often sand, and spinning it into glass fibers. Usually the fibers are held together in batt form by a phenol-formaldehyde resin binder. It is generally not contaminated with the same impurities as rock wool and its cost is somewhat less.

Most of the fiberglass insulation manufactured today is either pink or yellow in color. All brands contain approximately 5 percent of the resin binder. The pink variety contains, in addition, less than 1 percent dye to give it the pink color. The yellow insulation has been recommended for individuals with chemical hypersensitivity syndrome[8], apparently because of the intolerance to the coloring dye. This seems to be a reasonable precaution, avoiding as many unnecessary pollutants as possible. The phenol-formaldehyde binder in all of the fiberglass insulation, both yellow and pink, can, however, elicit symptoms. With age, the outgassing from the binder will diminish, and if the insulation is sealed from the living space, the odors should not reach the occupants.

Pink fiberglass insulation is manufactured by **Owens-Corning Fiberglas Corporation** (not recommended because of the dye used). The yellow variety is manufactured by several companies, including: **Certainteed Corporation, Manville Building Materials Corporation, Knauf Fiber Glass GmbH**, and **Georgia-Pacific Corporation**. At least one manufacturer (**Manville Building Products Corporation**) uses a more odorous urea-extended phenol-formaldehyde binder.

Manville also produces a fiberglass batt insulation without a binder, called "unbonded B fiber" for use primarily in the space program. This material is generally not available for residential applications but can be specially ordered at a cost estimated to be seven or eight times that of the conventional product with the binder. It seems to be one of the most inert insulations available from a chemically contaminated point of view, and may be worth the extra cost for certain applications. It is available in rolls of different thicknesses and must be cut to size for use in residential wall construction.

During a fire, the fiberglass itself is fairly inert, giving off little in the way of toxic gases. The resin, however, can decompose in a fire and produce small traces of hydrogen cyanide. The facing material can produce oxides of sulphur, carbon, and nitrogen.[9] If a plastic facing is used, it too can give off toxic vapors in a fire.

The importance of keeping fiberglass insulation separated from the living space can be seen in a report of nearly all of 13 office workers reporting various symptoms related to glass fibers entering the air due to improper construction methods. Symptoms included itchy rash, burning eyes, sore throats, coughing, and malaise. Eye complaints made it impossible to wear contact lenses. After the insulation was sealed with plastic foil, the health complaints ceased.[10]

Board Insulations

There is a wide variety of materials used in manufacturing insulating boards. Many are specialized industrial products. Those commonly used in residential applications include polystyrene, polyurethane, isocyanurate, cellular glass, rock wool, and glass fiber. Cork, phenolic foam, and rubber foam may also be occasionally encountered.

Most board-type insulations are available in a variety of thicknesses and sizes. Four foot by eight foot sheets are common. They are often used as sheathings, underneath the siding of a house, or as foundation insulation.

Polystyrene

Polystyrene foam insulation is made in two types, expanded and extruded. The expanded type consists of small beads that are fused together inside a mold. It is often called "beadboard." The extruded variety consists of mixture of polystyrene, solvent, and a pressurized gas that is pushed through a rectangular die. Upon cooling it is cut into sheets. Both varieties will deteriorate when exposed to ultraviolet light, so they must be protected from sunlight.

All types of polystyrene insulation can emit noxious fumes when exposed to flames in a house fire.

The polystyrene beads in beadboard are usually expanded with a hydrocarbon such as pentane. Beadboard's R-value is slightly lower than the other variety and it is not as sturdy. Extruded polystyrene is foamed by the use of the pressurized gas, which is usually a fluorocarbon such as Freon. After foaming, it will contain, within its pores, both air and the fluorocarbon gas.

Extruded polystyrene will function very well around a foundation but beadboard will deteriorate when exposed to ground moisture. Only extruded polystyrene and cellular glass foam can be used successfully in damp locations. All other insulations will tend to deteriorate when exposed to continuous ground moisture. Damp locations, around a foundation or under a concrete slab, are areas where a potentially toxic insulation can be used in a healthy house without eliciting symptoms.

Both types of polystyrene insulation are commonly available at lumberyards. "Styrofoam" is a particular brand of extruded polystyrene that is manufactured by **Dow Chemical Corporation**.

Polyurethane and Polyisocyanurate Foam

The basic ingredients of polyurethane foam are isocyanates, polyol resins, and an amine catalyst. Other additives can be used. A blowing agent is used to cause the mixture to expand, creating a foam. The blowing agent is a gas, such as a halocarbon. Polyurethane can be made into a flexible foam as used in upholstery, or a rigid foam as used in insulation, depending on the type of isocyanate used.

Health effects in factories that produce polyurethane include blurred vision, skin, eye, and respiratory tract irritation, asthma, chest discomfort, etc. Some of the chemicals causing these symptoms outgas rather quickly, while others do not. At least one, toluene diisocyanate (TDI), has been shown to be a sensitizer, with a sensitized individual reacting to only trace exposures with attacks of asthma.[11] A group of fireman, who experienced a large exposure to TDI, reported numerous neurological symptoms such as euphoria, headache, difficulty concentrating, poor memory, and confusion.[12]

Polyrethane insluations have higher R-values than other insulations because of the blowing agent that is trapped in its pores. Most other insulations used trapped air to retard the flow of heat, but the halocarbon gas used in polyurethane functions is a much better insulator. However, as the material ages, the gas slowly escapes and is replaced with air. This results in a lower R-value as the insulation gets older. The escape of gas can be largely prevented by coating the polyurethane with a dense skin, or a layer of foil. Polyurethane used, for example, inside a sealed steel entrance door probably would allow little gas to escape.

Polyurethane will degrade and fall apart in sunlight unless ultraviolet inhibitors are used in its manufacture. It will also take on water when in a damp environment or used underground, so it must be adequately protected with a suitable vapor barrier.

Polyurethane is flammable and must be isolated from living spaces. It burns rapidly and releases carbon monoxide, oxides of nitrogen, and hydrogen cyanide. Hydrogen cyanide is indeed lethal but so much carbon monoxide is released that it is probably of more concern.[13]

Polyisocyanurate foam insulations are very similar to polyurethanes, but are slightly more stable. They too must be protected from sunlight and moisture and they have similar characteristics when burned. Like polyurethanes, they are often supplied with a foil facing to protect them from degradation.

"Thermax" and "Tuff-R" are both polyisocyanurate insulations manufactured by **Celotex Corp.**

Cellular Glass Insulation

Cellular glass insulation is usually confined to commercial applications because of its increased cost. It is mentioned here because it will not burn and it is moisture resistant. It can be used in roof and wall systems as well as underground. Various thicknesses are available. This insulation is a foamed glass product that contains no fillers or binders; however, it is not 100 percent safe. During the foaming process, carbon monoxide and hydrogen sulfide gases are trapped in each cell of the foam. Theoretically, they will not be released to the atmosphere because each cell is totally surrounded by glass. Whenever the surface is scratched, or the material is flexed sufficiently, the characteristic "rotten egg" odor of hydrogen sulfide is released; however, once incorporated into a structure, it is doubtful that this will ever become a problem. When installed, it will generally be in a location that is not subjected to abrasion, and most buildings do not flex enough to allow the release of gas. Cellular glass and extruded polystyrene are the only two insulations that function well underground when in contact with damp soil. Cellular glass will cost approximately two to three times more for a comparable thickness that will have a lower R-value. Cellular glass insulation is manufactured under the name of "Foamglas" by **Pittsburgh Corning Corporation**.

Rock Wool and Glassfiber Boards

These products have the same basic advantages and disadvantages as their batt counterparts. They are dense, rigid products made of the same basic materials as rock wool and fiberglass batts and may contain more resin binder.

Loose Fill and Blow-In Insulation

These types of insulations come in several forms; some can be simply poured out of a bag while others are better applied by blowing them through a specially designed machine and out of an applicator hose. Cellulose and chopped fiberglass are generally blown in place, but they can be placed by hand.

Often the only way to insulate an existing house is to drill holes in the wall and blow some type of insulation into the cavity. Blow-in insulations are often used in attics because they can be installed much more quickly than batt insulation and, hence, are cheaper. Some lumberyards will rent blowing machines to do-it-yourselfers. Cellulose and chopped fiberglass are generally used in wood frame construction. Vermiculite, perlite, and polystyrene beads will be often found in masonry construction, because they can simply be poured into the inside of a concrete block wall as it is being built. Shredded tree bark, sawdust, and cork have also been used in the past, but these materials should be treated with chemicals to reduce insect attack or flammability and therefore are to be avoided in a healthful house.

Cellulose

Cellulose insulation is a very popular product today. It is made by chopping old newspapers into a fine, fluffy material. Since newspapers are very combustible and can be eaten by insects, fungi, or bacteria and can be used for nesting material by rodents, the insulation must be treated chemically. Usually approximately 20 percent of the final product will consist of such things as borax, boric acid, ammonium sulfate, aluminum sulfate, lime, ammonium phosphate, mono- and di-ammonium phosphate, aluminum hydrate, aluminum trihydrate, and zinc chloride.[14] If used in improper amounts, these chemicals may not adequately control flammability, and they can cause corrosion of any metal that they come in contact with. In attic areas, roof trusses are often held together with metal plates. Corrosion of these plates could eventually lead to a collapse of the roof system. Cellulose insulation standards today take these problems into consideration, but many older installations could contain flammable or corrosive insulation. A sample of the material can often be obtained from the attic and placed near a flame to test flammability, and an examination of any exposed metal will reveal a corrosion problem.

From a health standpoint, the various chemical additives can cause reactions in sensitive occupants.[15] Symptoms reported after installation of cellulose insulation include severe rashes, hair loss, digestive and respiratory disorders.[16] Some individuals report an intolerance to newspapers, presumably to both the ink and the paper. They can easily be bothered by this insulation. Since cellulose insulation is so finely ground, it can filter through very small openings into the living space, resulting in symptoms requiring removal.[17] It is usually installed in wall cavities through small holes drilled in the exterior siding, which are plugged after the cavity is filled. There are some real horror stories of applicators working their way around the outside of the house without realizing that they were blowing large amounts of insulation into the interior of the home. In older houses, remodeling over the years may have left openings in the walls of closets or behind kitchen cabinets. As a result, a house can have clouds of insulation floating around inside, unknown to applicators. Electrical outlets can also allow insulation to enter the interior of the house. It is always a good idea for someone to be inside the house while the material is being installed. Any problem will be noticed immediately, before an extremely difficult cleaning job is necessary.

There are many manufacturers of cellulose insulation, and it can be purchased through most lumberyards or insulation contractors.

Chopped Fiberglass

This material can be installed in a manner similar to cellulose. It is composed of small fibers of glass, similar to fiberglass batt insulation, but in a loose form, so it can be blown into wall cavities or attic spaces. Glass is inherently noncombustible and is not subject to being eaten, so it does not need to be chemically treated like cellulose.

Certainteed Corporation manufactures a chopped fiberglass blowing insulation, called "Insulsafe," that is widely used. It contains approximately 1 percent mineral oil and silicone sprayed on to control dust. This is the least chemically contaminated glass-fiber insulation available today for the residential market. For many sensitive people, this is a positive point, but it must be weighed against the possible long-term cancer risks. If it is adequately sealed from the living space, the risk will be minimal for the occupants. Since much of the concern over the cancer-causing ability of man-made mineral fibers relates to very small diameter fibers, "Insulsafe" may be more problematic than batt products because of its small fiber size.

Rock Wool

Many older homes are insulated with loose rock wool, primarily in their attics. Installed by simply pouring it in place, it is used today in the residential market less than in the past. It will be contaminated with the same materials that rock wool batts will contain, with the exception of the binding resin. Sensitive people should be concerned about its presence, but should keep in mind that with an old installation it will have outgassed over the years and may no longer be a problem from that standpoint. However, inhalation of the loose fibers may still result in a cancer risk.

Vermiculite and Perlite

These materials are usually poured in place, occasionally in attics, but they are primarily used as a insulation inside concrete blocks. Vermiculite is a mica-like mineral that contains both free and chemically bound water. When it is heated, it expands due to steam being driven off. This puffed-up product is then used for insulation. It is resistant to fire, rot, vermin, and termites. Vermiculite is sometimes treated chemically to make it water repellant.

There is some concern about vermiculite containing small amounts of asbestos[18]; however, the temperatures used in "puffing-up" the vermiculate may cause the asbestos to decompose, yielding a less toxic product.[19]

Perlite is a naturally occurring silicate volcanic rock. When heated it expands, like vermiculite, because of a small amount of water turning to steam. Perlite is also fireproof and resistant to vermin. It is a very dusty material, and is often treated with silicone to control the dust. Its use in attics is often discouraged because the dust can filter down into the living space through light fixtures or other small openings. This dust can be problematic to an asthmatic as can the silicone to other sensitive individuals. There is the possibility of silicosis due to long-term breathing of dust containing silica, but this is a remote possibility outside of a perlite-producing factory.

When these products are used inside masonry walls, there is little chance of them or their contaminants reaching the living space. For someone with unusual sensitivities, extra care should be taken to insure that they stay where they are placed inside the wall cavity.

Polystyrene Beads
The polystyrene beads used to make expanded polystyrene sheet (beadboard) can be used as a loose fill insulation. The beads, when expanded, are approximately 1/8″ in diameter and are often used as stuffing in "bean-bag" chairs. They have the same flammability drawbacks as beadboard. Their use is primarily found in masonry walls, although they can also be used in attics or other installations. Health concerns are similar to polystyrene board products.

Foamed-in-Place Insulation
There are several types of foamed-in-place insulation used in industry, but the best known in the residential market is urea-formaldehyde foam. Another type is known as "Air-Krete." Both have the consistency of shaving cream when applied. They are usually installed through small holes in walls like blow-in insulations, but they can also

be applied to open walls or attic spaces. Polyurethane is sometimes sprayed in place, but its use is primarily in commercial applications. Disadvantages are similar to polyurethane board insulation.

Urea-Formaldehyde Foam

Urea-formaldehyde foam insulation (UFFI) has been installed in thousands of houses in the United States without any noticeable health effects among many of the occupants. There are, however, many instances where negative health effects have been recorded.[20] So many in fact that the **Consumer Product Safety Commission (CPSC)** banned its use in residences and schools in 1982. Even though the ban was overturned by a Court of Appeals, the **CPSC** feels that the decision was based on legal and factual errors, and they continue to warn consumers about its dangers. Even though it is again legal to use UFFI, it is rarely being installed today. It is considered such a liability in houses that some real estate agencies require that its presence be disclosed to prospective buyers.

The primary problem with UFFI is the fact that it can release formaldehyde gas into the living space. This occurs more often in warm weather or in hot attics and can be greatly aggravated if the chemicals were mixed incorrectly during application. Other gases given off by UFFI include benzene, benzaldehyde, acetaldehyde, cresol, methylnaphthalene, acrolein, ammonia, and phenol.[21]

Health effects include eye, nose, and throat irritation, cough, headache, dizziness, bronchopneumonia, pulmonary edema, asthma, dermatitis, rhinitis, conjunctivitis, and allergy. Some people have been sensitized to many other chemicals as a result of formaldehyde exposure, resulting in a wide variety of symptoms.

The story of the Leyda family relates how they were driven from their home after it was insulated with UFFI. Early symptoms included chest problems: colds, bronchitis, and coughs, then proceeded to such things as red, watering, and painful eyes. Mrs. Leyda became very weak and dizzy and she began having irregular heartbeats. Her doctor suspected multiple sclerosis. By the time the problem was related to formaldehyde outgassing, Mrs. Leyda had become hypersensitive to a wide variety of everyday chemicals. They borrowed $15,000 to have the insulation removed, but because of her newly acquired sensitivities, Mrs. Leyda still could not tolerate her home. Mrs. Leyda now is a victim of chemical hypersensitivity syndrome and must avoid many things that the rest of the population takes for granted.[22]

Individuals interested in having UFFI removed from their homes are advised that it is very expensive and time-consuming, involving some major demolition and remodeling. Two publications are available describing the necessary procedures.[23,24]

Air-Krete

"Air-Krete" has been reported in recent articles to be a nontoxic insulating material.[25,26] It is a foamed-in-place product that must be installed by trained technicians. The main ingredients are magnesium oxychloride (a cementitious material), and sodium silicate (water glass). Both are fairly inert. Fluorescent dye is used to give it a pink color. Compressed air is used on the job to cause the liquid material to become a foam having the consistency of shaving cream. Air-Krete contains no formaldehyde or asbestos and has more insulating ability than fiberglass or cellulose.

In new construction, Air-Krete is installed in the walls before the interior drywall or plaster is attached. In existing buildings, it is foamed into the wall cavities through holes in either the exterior siding or the interior wall surface. The holes are then plugged or repaired. Attics and masonry walls can also be easily insulated. After insulation, Air-Krete becomes semirigid within seconds. Final drying takes two to four weeks.

While this material seems to be one of the least toxic insulating products on the market today, a few people report an odor with it even after several weeks. Most people, however, report little or no odor after curing. The odor could be due to the use of the pink dye.

Air-Krete was developed by **Air-Krete Inc.** and there are several licensed manufacturers around the country who distribute the product to various local installers.

Reflective Foil Insulation

Radiant heat can be reflected back where it came from by means of a shiny foil. This foil can be placed inside the wall and still function. Radiant heat can pass through drywall, strike the foil, and be reflected back into the house. The only requirement is that there be an airspace in front of the foil. A layer of reflective aluminum foil inside a wall with a 3/4" airspace in the summer can have an R-value of 3.28 compared to .91 for a 3/4" airspace alone.

Radiant foil insulations are only of minimal value in cold climates, but they can be very useful in hot climates to keep the radiant solar energy out of air-conditioned spaces.

Reflective foils may be made of a variety of shiny metals including aluminum foil, stainless steel, or a foil-coated paper; however, they will not function when covered with dust. The dust factor can be difficult to determine when the foil is inside the structure of the house, where dust can accumulate. Dust is more of a problem in floor systems than in walls or ceiling systems. If reflective foil is well sealed, it can also function as a vapor barrier. Some materials can function both as a sheathing material and a reflective insulation. Reflective foils can be lightly perforated to allow moisture to pass through, if required, while still functioning as a reflecting barrier.

These materials should not pose any health problems if they are metal products. Some reflective foils are made of aluminized Mylar or aluminized polyethylene which could outgas.

Innovative Energy, Inc. manufactures multilayer reflective insulations. These products are rolled out, cut to length, and expanded, then stapled into a wall or ceiling cavity. By being multilayer, they reflect most of the radiant energy and trap different layers of air, thus helping to block other forms of heat loss as well.

Moisture Barriers and Air Barriers

All insulation installations should contain a moisture barrier of some sort. This can be a paint film, a plastic film, or a metal foil. There should also be an air barrier. An air barrier helps to control air transported moisture and reduces the possibility of insulation outgassing into the house. Sometimes the moisture barrier and air barrier can be the same material. The location of the moisture barrier should generally be on the warm side of the wall and the air barrier should be on the inside of the wall. In cold climates, the moisture barrier will be on the inside of the wall (warm side) and the air barrier will be on the inside. Therefore, the same material can perform both functions. In warm climates, the air barrier should be on the inside and the moisture barrier should be on the outside of the wall. For more information on problems associated with air and moisture barrier locations, see Chapter 7.

Polyethylene air and moisture barriers are quite common, but they can be problematic to individuals sensitive to plastics, and they can degrade inside the wall. "Tyvek" is a popular polyethylene air barrier produced by **Du Pont Co.** When polyethylene is degraded by very high heat, it can emit acrolein, formaldehyde, hydrocarbons, carbon monoxide, possible free radicals, and soot.[27] Exposure to sunlight and the lower amount of heat given off by electric baseboard heaters can also cause polyethylene to degrade. For these reasons, foil barriers are recommended. Foil products vary in width, and seams must be taped to be effective. They are not always available in all parts of the country. They can, however, be ordered through the mail. The best tape to use in sealing these products is metal foil tape. Aluminum foil tape can be purchased through some hardware stores and most heating equipment suppliers. Conventional "duct tape" is intolerable to many people because of its synthetic composition.

Stainless steel foil can be used as a vapor barrier, but its cost is quite high. It can be purchased through metal suppliers listed in the telephone book. **Alpine Industries** sells stainless steel foil in 24″ wide rolls and stainless steel tape on a mail order basis.

Aluminum builder's foil usually has a kraft paper backing, sometimes with foil on both sides of the paper. It is available in solid foil for use as a moisture barrier, or with very fine pinprick perforations for use as an air barrier. The perforated foil will allow water vapor to pass through, yet it will prevent wind penetration.

These products were originally designed to be reflective insulations, but function very well as air and moisture barriers. They work especially well for people sensitive to synthetic materials by helping to seal various fumes from the living space. Following is a summary of various manufacturers' products. **Innovative Energy, Inc,** makes an all foil product (R+) with no kraft paper in 24½″ and 49″ wide rolls, both perforated and solid. They also sell aluminum foil tape. **Denny Sales Corporation** sells four different foil/kraft paper sandwich products (Denny foil). They have a solid material with foil on either one or both sides of the kraft paper, and a perforated material with foil on either one or both sides. Some of their distributors will ship material COD. Some of these manufacturers and others also produce foil products that contain polyethylene. They are not listed here because of the problems associated with polyethylene degradation.

Other materials can be used as moisture barriers. Foil-backed drywall is mentioned in Chapter 18. Foil-faced sheathing is also available. It is covered in Chapter 14. Regular drywall, if properly sealed, can easily function as an air barrier.

Air and Moisture Barriers and Outgassing

An air barrier will stop a considerable amount of outgassing from insulation from passing through a wall. However, outgassed chemicals can still slowly diffuse through the surface of the wall like water vapor does. A foil moisture barrier can effectively block this diffusion. Since air is the primary transport mechanism, an air barrier is of greater importance than a moisture barrier, although both are important. See Chapter 7 for a further discussion of air and moisture barriers.

In cold climates where both the air and moisture barrier will be on the inside of the wall, the greatest protection will be provided to protect the occupants from the outgassing. In hot, humid climates, the moisture barrier should be located on the outside of the wall, thus outgassing from insulation can slowly diffuse through the wall to the interior of the house. While the least toxic insulation should be chosen in all climates, it is of even more importance in climates where the moisture barrier is located on the outside of the wall.

Summary

Since there are no 100 percent safe insulations available, care should be taken to insure that they are well sealed from the living space. A barrier of builders foil or well sealed drywall works well. Superinsulated designs or the Airtight Drywall Approach are excellent solutions if they utilize a very well sealed air/moisture barrier.

Of the readily available products, the insulations made from glass or Air-Krete are probably better choices than those of synthetic materials. The use of extruded polystyrene underground would, however, probably be acceptable. For someone with severe sensitivities, all insulations may be bothersome when in direct contact, but can be tolerable when sealed behind an air barrier. If this air barrier is also a foil moisture barrier, additional protection is provided.

Chapter 17

Flooring Systems

Whatever flooring material is chosen, it must be remembered that the square footage of floors is second only to walls and ceilings in the amount of area exposed to the inhabitants. There will be hundreds of square feet of flooring that will be within the living space. If this material is even only slightly unhealthy, the fact that there is so much of it can mean that it easily can be responsible for various illnesses.

Each type of flooring material has certain advantages and disadvantages. No one material will be a perfect choice for all installations, and some choices will not be practical for retrofits in existing houses.

The Structure Under the Floor
The structure of the house may dictate the types of flooring that can be used. A concrete slab will be well suited to using ceramic tile. A wooden subfloor will accept solid hardwood quite well. There are methods of applying ceramic tile to a wooden subfloor but they either involve relatively toxic methods of attaching the tile or they add considerable weight. If the structure isn't designed to support the extra weight, problems will definitely develop. It should also be remembered that some flooring systems will add thickness to an existing floor. This often requires that doors be cut off at the bottom to allow for proper clearances. Wooden doors are easily shortened, but metal doors may involve more work, sometimes requiring the removal of the frame and raising the whole assembly.

Someone designing a new house should consider the finish flooring material prior to selecting a particular subfloor or foundation system. In that way, not only a healthful floor, but a more economical and structurally sound system will result. A complete discussion of foundations will be found in Chapter 10.

It should be remembered that most floor systems require both a subfloor and a finish floor for structural integrity or appearance. Floor systems should also include a moisture barrier, which can prevent odors or radon from penetrating the floor. In a cold climate, floors over crawl spaces should have the moisture barrier as close to the living space as possible. This will usually be under either the subfloor or the finish floor, depending on the particular installation. The purpose is to keep moisture from passing from the living space into the crawl space. For further information about moisture barrier location, see Chapter 7. It will also tend to keep odors from the crawl space from entering the house. Concrete slabs on grade should have the moisture barrier between the concrete and the ground to prevent both ground moisture and radon from migrating up into the house.

Following will be a discussion of various flooring types, installation requirements, advantages, and disadvantages.

The Typical Floor

While no floor can be said to be truly typical, one of the most common installations involves a plywood subfloor on a wooden structure over a crawl space. Particle board is installed over the plywood to add stiffness, and the finish surface is usually carpeting. The use of particleboard subflooring can result in formaldehyde levels in homes that are twice that found in homes insulated with urea-formaldehyde foam insulation and the high levels can last for years.[1] Sometimes adhesives are used to attach the plywood to the floor joists or the carpet to the particle boards. Often, no separate moisture barrier is used.

This common type of flooring system has been developed primarily because it is inexpensive. Health effects have not been considered at all. Both the plywood and the particle board can emit formaldehyde fumes into the house. The adhesives also give off a variety of undesirable odors. While the glue layer in the plywood forms a reasonable moisture barrier, the seams between sheets can allow radon or other pollutants to enter the living area from the crawl space. Finally, the carpeting itself is a terrible choice of flooring material in a healthy house, for a variety of reasons.[2] Since it remains a very popular choice by most consumers, we will discuss it first.

Carpeting

Prior to the introduction of electric vacuum cleaners, when carpets were taken outdoors and cleaned by beating them, it was very apparent just how dirty they could become. Wall-to-wall carpeting simply cannot be removed for the occasional beating, so we do not realize that there are huge quantities of dirt stored there. Their ability to hide dirt is very good, and we are fooled into believing that we have clean houses. Anyone who uses a water/vacuum cleaning machine will be shocked to see how much dirt is removed from their carpet. Even though carpeting is regularly vacuumed by a homeowner, the occasional water/vacuum cleaning results in large quantities of filthy water. If the nozzle on such a machine is transparent, you can watch the dirt being pulled from the carpet. Often it seems as though you can go over the same area again and again, yet there is still more dirt being removed.

The tremendous reservoir capacity of a carpet means that it contains not only large quantities of dirt but food particles and crumbs as well. This results in a breeding ground for dust mites, mold, bacteria, etc. We all shed a certain amount of dead skin every day that contributes to house dust and finds its way to the carpet, providing more food for microbes there. It has been shown that carpeting can contain up to 10,000,000 organisms per square foot.[3] You can imagine that as you walk across carpeting, each footstep creates a small invisible cloud of potentially allergenic materials. This will, of course, be four to six feet from your nose so the symptoms that you immediately experience may not be very severe. Children, however, are much closer to the floor because they are shorter. They are also more likely to be lying or playing on the floor with their noses directly exposed to this reservoir of dust, dirt, and allergens.

Carpeting itself will generate its own dust. As it becomes worn, fibers break off and either become airborne or contribute to the accumulating debris. Today, most carpeting is made from synthetic materials, which generate synthetic house dust. Breathing any kind of dust can be harmful, but synthetic dust has some problems of its own. When synthetic dust is picked up by circulating air and finds its way into a heating system, it can be burned by the high heat inside the furnace. This can result in a variety of toxic vapors being released. Sunlight falling on carpeting can also cause it to disintegrate and release particles or vapors.

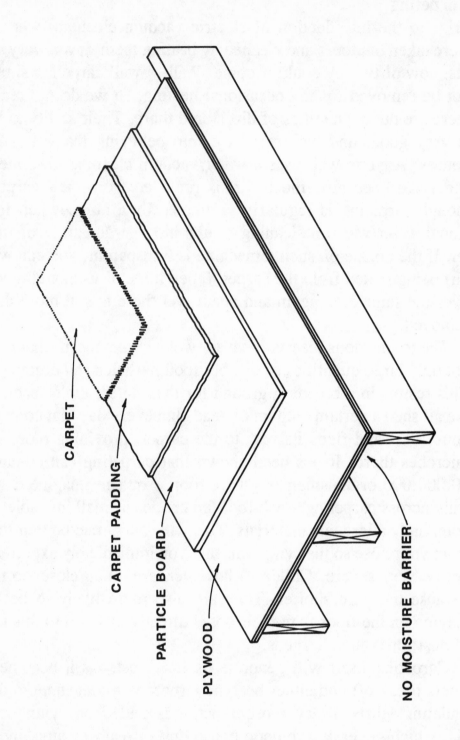

CARPET

CARPET PADDING

PARTICLE BOARD

PLYWOOD

NO MOISTURE BARRIER

An Unhealthy Floor

The carpeting material itself is not the only thing that can be implicated in health problems. The backing that holds the fibers together is generally another type of material with its own problems. The padding, as well, can generate various pollutants as it wears and disintegrates. Carpets are often treated with toxic chemicals such as pesticides, mold retardants, or mothproofing. These will help to keep microorganisms in check, but their effectiveness will be lessened with repeated cleaning. For many people, the chemicals themselves can have a devastating effect.

It is often believed that cleaning a carpet will solve any problems, but it can actually do just the opposite. The shampoo itself has been implicated in health problems of some people because of the toxic cleaning agents involved. Insecticides and fungicides are often added by professional rug cleaners.[4] Cleaning a carpet has also been suspected of causing Kawasaki syndrome, possibly by causing an infectious agent to become airborne during the cleaning process. This is a systemic illness in children, characterized by a high fever. Symptoms have been reported 16–25 days after cleaning.[5] Shampooing will result in a damp carpet which can easily cause any mold spores located there to proliferate. Vacuuming results in much dust becoming airborne, resulting in various symptoms in sensitive persons. Cleaning, therefore, can make a situation worse. Vacuuming with a central vacuum system having an outdoor exhaust will tend to stir up less dust. If a carpet has been cleaned, it should be allowed to dry thoroughly before occupants, especially children, are allowed to return to the house, and cleaners or shampoos should be chosen with care.

New synthetic carpeting can outgas a wide variety of toxic vapors for weeks after installation. This can be due to the carpet itself, chemical additives such as pesticides, fungicides, or soil repellants, the dye, backing, synthetic or treated natural padding, the adhesive, or the subfloor. The outgassing of formaldehyde, toluene, and xylene can cause severe irritations and sensitivities. A complete list of chemicals that can be given off by new carpeting will sound quite frightening and it would take a chemist to fully understand it. Such things as methyl methacrylate, ethylbenzene, hexamethylene triamine, 1-chloronaphthalene, 2-methylnaphthalene, and 1-phenylcyclopentanol can be given off by new carpeting. Many of these vapors will dissipate with time as the carpet ages, but as we have seen, other health problems can result with older carpeting. Untreated 100 percent nylon carpeting with a natural jute backing is reportedly less offensive than other types.[6]

While plywood and particle board are commonly used for floor construction over crawl spaces, older houses are usually built with solid wood. This avoids the fumes given off by the synthetic glues used in man-made wood products, but the use of individual boards means more seams, and a greater chance of the living space being contaminated by odors from the crawl space; also, the cracks provide room for molds and dust mites to flourish.

A "440 Carpet Board" underlayment is being marked for use under a carpet, instead of particle board, by **Homosote Co.** and is advertised as containing "no asbestos or formaldehyde." However, it is made from recycled paper, like cellulose insulation, and is chemically treated to resist moisture absorption, termites, rot, and fungus attack, so it probably outgasses various chemicals as it ages.

Carpets may also be installed over a concrete slab on grade. If the slab has no moisture barrier between it and the ground, dampness can rise up through the concrete and provide just enough moisture for mold and dust mites to thrive. Even with a moisture barrier, if the slab is uninsulated, it can be slightly cooler than the room's temperature. A carpet will act like insulation on top of the slab, causing its temperature to be lower yet. This results in higher relative humidity near the floor and corresponding mold growth in the carpet. This can be especially common in hot muggy weather.[7] Ventilation and air movement will help to keep the temperatures higher near the floor to help dissipate the humidity.

There are several companies that manufacture 100 percent wool or cotton carpeting. This type of material will certainly be an improvement over synthetic carpeting, but individuals with conventional allergies can be bothered by these natural fibers, and they can have certain other drawbacks. Wool carpeting can be treated with toxic mothproofing chemicals. Cotton can have residues of pesticides that were originally sprayed on the cotton crop. Of all the pesticides applied to crops in the United States, almost half are applied to the cotton crop and these are not all removed during processing.[8] Cotton and wool can both can be dyed with intolerable dyes, or have an intolerable backing of latex or another material. **Dellinger, Inc.** makes a quality all-cotton carpeting with cotton backing. It normally comes with an additional latex backing and is dyed, but can be ordered undyed and without the latex. Without the added latex backing, the carpet is less dimensionally stable and should be carefully stretched into place to insure a quality installation. Without dye, the off-white carpeting may be difficult to keep clean. If paddings are intolerable, a carpet can be installed without padding, but it will not wear as well or last as long. A sample should be tested prior to purchasing any carpeting.

Rugs have advantages over wall-to-wall carpeting in that they can be removed easily. Large rugs can be cleaned outdoors by beating or vacuuming, and smaller rugs can be machine washed. Many stores carry natural fiber rugs in a variety of sizes and styles. Untreated Oriental and Navajo Indian rugs are also available.

New synthetic carpeting should be aired out for at least a month to allow major contaminants to outgas. If odors persist, water/vacuum cleaning may help, but most of the chemicals involved are not water soluable. Children should not be allowed to play on carpeting that is suspected of causing symptoms.

A product called "Carpet Guard" is sold by **AFM Enterprises** and is found by some sensitive people to be tolerable. It is used to actually coat the carpeting itself to seal in any outgassing odors. This may help in a few situations, but the best solution for most sensitive individuals is to remove the carpeting.

Resilient Flooring

Resilient flooring is used more often than any material besides carpets, again because of the relatively low cost. The most commonly encountered materials contain vinyl or asphalt, either in individual tiles, or in large sheets that can provide a seamless installation. Sometimes cork, linoleum, and rubber are seen. They can be composed of a wide variety of fillers, pigments, binders, gums, plasticizers, and resins. Some products can contain asbestos. In general, resilient flooring is not well tolerated by very sensitive people because of the outgassing potential; however, it is not as offensive as carpeting. As the materials age, they are better tolerated as the outgassing lessens, so by the time the material is worn out, it may be perfectly tolerable from an outgassing standpoint. Asbestos release can, however, remain problematic for some tiles. Many resilient tiles require the use of a potentially troublesome wax or clear finish. Some "no wax" floors eventually need to be sealed, and sensitive persons may have difficulty finding a tolerated product.

Asbestos is found in some, but not all, vinyl- and asphalt-based flooring. It can be a constituent of the material itself or a part of the backing. If an asbestos containing flooring becomes worn, it can release asbestos fibers into the air.[9] When the floors containing asbestos are removed, the fibers can be released as the flooring is broken, scraped, or sanded. The best solution might be to leave such a material in place and cover it with a more inert product. Testing laboratories can usually determine whether or not asbestos is present in a flooring sample. There is no law currently on the books that forbids the use of asbestos in flooring, but manufacturers should tell you if a certain product contains it.

A plasticizer is used in vinyl flooring to make it easier to clean. Often, this substance is butyl benzyl phthalate, which can emit benzyl chloride and benzal chloride into the air. These chemicals can irritate the eyes and respiratory mucosa and are carcinogenic. The half-lives for these chemicals in vinyl flooring have been estimated to be 100–200 days, meaning that it takes that long for half of the chemicals to dissipate.[10] Obviously, these types of materials should not be used in a healthful house.

Occasionally, a particular brand of sheet flooring is recommended as being tolerable for sensitive people, but since reactions are so individualized, one should test a sample prior to using any synthetic product. Harder materials should be less offensive than softer, cushioned flooring.

Large sheet goods can often be laid without using an adhesive. They are simply cut to fit the shape of a room and held in place with the baseboard molding. All smaller tiles must be installed with a potentially problematic adhesive. If an adhesive is required, it too should be tested, and a water-based product should be used instead of a solvent-based material. Self-stick tiles are sometimes recommended as being less objectionable.[11]

A "natural" material that is occasionally recommended is plain battleship linoleum. This is made from linseed oil, pine resins, and wood flour on a jute backing. It is available in eight solid or several marbleized colors and is advertised as containing "no harmful by-products, toxins, carcinogens, fumes, gases, etc." It does have a slight odor that can bother some people and there are other drawbacks. It is susceptible to moisture and fungus attack and cannot be allowed to be damp for extended periods. If installed on a concrete slab over earth, special installation requirements are needed to prevent moisture damage. It must be installed with an adhesive, and it requires a wax or protective finish that can be problematic. Plain battleship linoleum is distributed by **Forbo North America** and they also have a similar product that uses the same basic materials with the addition of natural cork.

Wood Floors

Wood flooring is available in two basic types: strips and parquet. Strip flooring that is wider than 3¼" is normally referred to as plank flooring. Parquet flooring is available in a wide variety of patterns. All types of wood flooring can be installed over either a wood subfloor or a concrete slab, although installations over concrete require special precautions. The primary health considerations in wood flooring include tolerability of the wood itself, and tolerability of the finishing material or adhesives. From a practical standpoint, wood floors are not recommended in kitchens or bathrooms because of the danger of water damage.

Strip or Plank Flooring

While oak seems to be the most common wood used for strip or plank flooring in the residential market, other species are readily available. Of the hardwoods, maple, beech, birch, and pecan are also manufactured. Occasionally, a local manufacturer will be able to process a batch of another type of wood on special request, but this will obviously result in a higher cost. Of softwood flooring, southern pine is the most common, but Douglas fir, west coast hemlock, spruce, and western red cedar are also seen. All of the species can be found in a number of appearance grades, widths, and thicknesses.

Some wood flooring is seen with squared edges, but most is made in a tongue-and-groove style. This results in a tighter floor, with shallower cracks to collect dirt and dust. Since all wood will expand and contract at different times of the year, depending on the humidity, these cracks will expand and contract as well. There can always be a place to collect debris; however, this is usually not a major consideration.

Strip flooring is easily installed over a wooden subfloor, usually by blind nailing through the tongue. Wider plank flooring is also face nailed to prevent warping. Today, plywood is the preferred subfloor material of the industry because of its strength and lower cost, but for

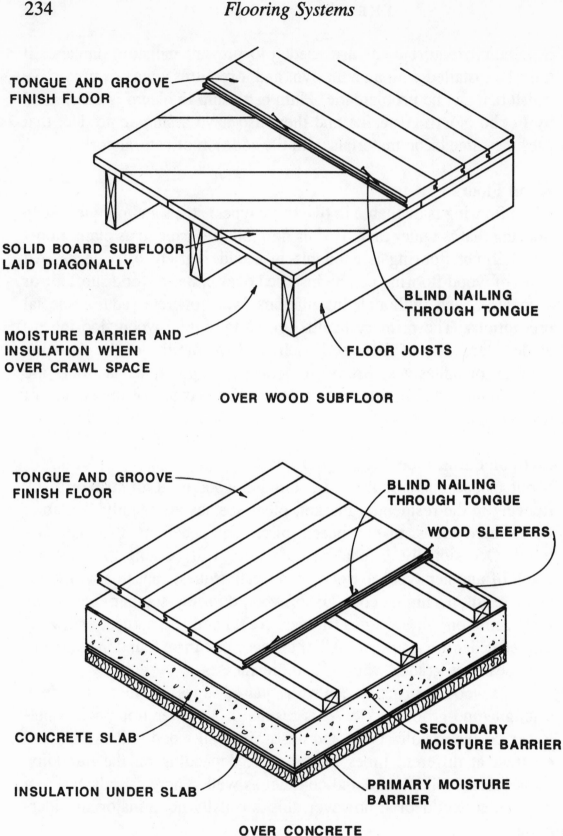

TONGUE AND GROOVE
FINISH FLOOR

SOLID BOARD SUBFLOOR
LAID DIAGONALLY

MOISTURE BARRIER AND
INSULATION WHEN
OVER CRAWL SPACE

BLIND NAILING
THROUGH TONGUE

FLOOR JOISTS

OVER WOOD SUBFLOOR

TONGUE AND GROOVE
FINISH FLOOR

BLIND NAILING
THROUGH TONGUE

WOOD SLEEPERS

CONCRETE SLAB

SECONDARY
MOISTURE BARRIER

INSULATION UNDER SLAB

PRIMARY MOISTURE
BARRIER

OVER CONCRETE

Wood Flooring Installations

a sensitive person, a solid wood subfloor is recommended to avoid formaldehyde fumes. A layer of asphalt-impregnated building paper is installed between the subfloor and the finish floor to protect the home from dust, cold, and moisture that might seep through the floor seams. A sensitive person would be wise to substitute a foil product that will not outgas asphalt fumes. (See Chapter 16.) The foil should be taped at all seams, thus forming a good moisture barrier. Care should be taken during installation because the foil product will not be as sturdy as the asphalt paper.

In an existing house, with a plywood subfloor, the foil will tend to seal any bothersome smells to the outside of the living space. If the plywood is several years old, it may have outgassed sufficiently over the years to be reasonably tolerable. In most cases, any particle board should be removed, because of its more offensive nature.

When installed over concrete, it is extremely important to consider moisture before deciding on a wood floor. Moisture can migrate up from the ground through the slab and cause the flooring to be excessively damp, resulting in expansion of the floor and possible buckling, or a mold problem. A high-quality moisture barrier under the slab, usually polyethylene, is always recommended. In addition, many flooring manufacturers also recommend some type of barrier between the slab and the wood floor because of the possibility of the underslab barrier being damaged. A foil product could be used in this situation as well. In an existing house, where the quality of the underslab barrier is unknown, this additional above-slab barrier is very important. If the concrete slab is uninsulated, the wood floor can be cooler than the rest of the room, resulting in a localized area of higher relative humidity which is not good for the floor. In an existing house with an uninsulated concrete slab, with no underslab moisture barrier, another type of flooring may be a better choice.

The actual installation of a wood strip floor over a concrete slab is relatively easy. Wood sleepers can be attached to the slab with concrete nails or anchors, and strip flooring is blind nailed or face nailed to the sleepers. The sleepers are usually placed on 16″ centers and are ³/₄″ to 1¹/₂″ thick. Another method is to use metal runners rather than wood sleepers. This method is often used in commercial installations. The strip flooring is attached to the runners with metal clips, which fit into a special groove in the flooring itself. The "Permalock" system by **AGA Corporation** is available in several grades of maple or in clear white pine, and the "Lock-tite" system by **Robbins, Inc.** is made in various grades of maple only. These methods of attachment will only work with flooring that has a special groove to accept the mounting clips. Both manufactures recommend a plastic moisture barrier and foam insulation between the slab and the wood floor, but these can be deleted if an adequate foil barrier and underslab insulation is used.

Parquet Flooring

There is a wide variety of patterns of parquet flooring in several different types of wood, such as oak, maple, walnut, cherry, mahogany, and teak. Small individual pieces of wood are held together by either glue or wire into tiles 4" to 12" square and in different thicknesses. Sometimes a glued plywood sandwich is seen, or pieces can be held together with some type of backing material. Tongue and groove edges are common. Most installations today involve the use of an adhesive or mastic to actually glue the material down to either a concrete or wood subfloor. While water-based adhesives are preferable to solvent-based types, both can bother some people, as can self-stick backings. The glue holding the tiles themselves together has also been found to be troublesome because it often emits formaldehyde fumes. Similarly, any backing material should be of concern for those seeking a healthful flooring. When applied over a wood subfloor, blind nailing or face nailing can be used as a method of attachment, but some flooring is too thin to accept the nails. A foil barrier is again recommended instead of an asphalt-impregnated product. The best choice of a parquet flooring would be a type held together by wire and thick enough to be attached to blind nailing. Installations over concrete are less desirable, because they generally will require some type of adhesive.

Finishing a Wood Floor

Some wood flooring can be purchased prefinished. This can be advantageous to someone sensitive to the fumes generated when finishing a floor; however, not all factory-applied finishes will be well tolerated. The baked-on finishes will be the best, but any finish should be tested by a sensitive person prior to purchasing flooring. Open grained woods, such as oak, may require the use of a wood filter. A water-based brand should be selected over a solvent-based product because of lower outgassing potential.

Most strip flooring is sanded after installation to provide a more uniform, smooth surface, and is then finished. The clear finishes and stains can be of a variety of types and are discussed in Chapter 19. If a particular wood is not very tolerable, finishing it can often improve the situation, but it should be remembered that the underneath side of the floor will remain unfinished, so the type of wood chosen should be as inert as possible. In selecting a finish, tolerability is a major consideration, but one should also think about the durability of the finish, so that refinishing does not need to be done very often. When constructing a new house, it can be possible to delay moving in until the finish has outgassed sufficiently, but 15 years down the road when refinishing is necessary, it may be difficult to leave the house for a month during the outgassing period.

Ceramic Tile

Ceramic tile is usually a well tolerated and inert flooring material. The tile itself is a clay product that is fired in a kiln. There are various types, such as mosaic, quarry tile, glazed tiles, etc. All can be installed by similar methods. Glazed or vitreous tiles have an impervious surface and are often recommended because they do not require any additional sealer as do quarry tiles, pavers, and slate. Porous unsealed tiles can harbor bacteria and other microorganisms; however, as a rule, the tile itself will pose no tolerability problems, unless a glaze containing toxic lead has been used. This will be more of a problem with imported tiles than with those produced in the United States. Similarly, foreign tiles may contain asbestos fillers which can release fibers during installation as the tiles are being cut. Reputable manufacturers will be able to tell you if a lead glaze or asbestos filler was used. Lead in a glaze can, for instance, be transferred to foods that are in contact with a tiled countertop. The mortars used to attach the tiles and the grouts used to fill the spaces between the tiles can be sources of symptoms more than the tile itself.

Ceramic tiles are available in a variety of sizes, colors, and surface textures. Larger tiles should be chosen to minimize the number of joints. Skid resistance should also be taken into consideration. Color is generally a matter of personal taste, but darker colors will absorb more warmth from sunlight in solar applications. If used outdoors in cold climates, tiles should be selected to withstand freezing conditions.

Ceramic tile installations can be quite expensive. If you are considering tiling all of the floors in a house, cost will be a definite consideration, and you may want to look into "seconds." The cost savings can be up to 50 percent. These may have a slight color or surface variation. Some may have a small chip or defect on an edge. Since every installation will require cutting along walls, major defects can be cut off and discarded. Tiles with more than usual color variation can be used in closets where they won't be readily noticed.

Although the cost would be even higher, a marble floor would also be inert. It would be installed in a manner similar to ceramic tile. It is, however, more absorbent and softer.

Manufacturers of ceramic tile have instruction sheets available that the do-it-yourselfer can use. There are also several books on the subject for both the homeowner and the professional.[12,13]

Attaching Ceramic Tile

The traditional centuries-old method of attaching ceramic tile is the most inert; however, it is also more expensive than other methods and requires an experienced tile setter. This is known as the thick-bed method and is often referred to as a "mud-job." A 1¼" thick mortar bed of Portland cement, sand, and water is applied to either a wood or concrete subfloor, and while the bed is still plastic, the tile is set in a paste of Portland cement and water. There are no chemicals required with this method, only Portland cement, sand, water, and the ceramic tile itself.

There are many other materials that can be used to attach ceramic tile. Organic mastics or petroleum-based products are commonly used by do-it-yourselfers, but they are usually poorly tolerated by sensitive people. Other choices include epoxies, furans, dry-set mortars, and latex-Portland cement mortar, of which the epoxies and furans will be the more odorous. Latex-Portland cement contains either powdered or liquid latex, and it and the dry-set mortars (sometimes called thin-set mortars) contain a variety of other ingredients that could be bothersome to some people. The actual ingredients are considered trade secrets by manufacturers. They can both be used on a variety of surfaces, depending on the particular manufacturer, such as concrete, exterior plywood, water resistant drywall, cementitious boards, etc. Both are mixed with water and applied with a notched trowel to the floor. The tile is then set into the mortar and allowed to cure. The spaces between the tiles, or joints, will later be filled with grout. These

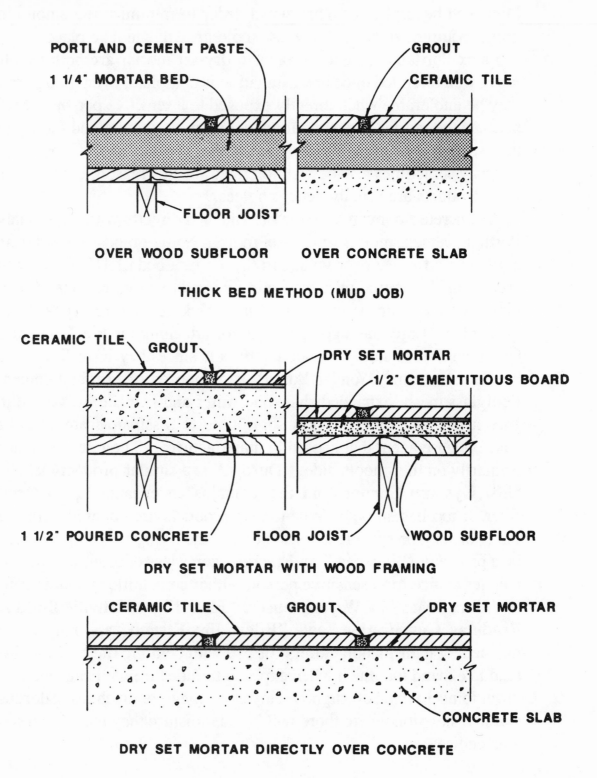

PORTLAND CEMENT PASTE
GROUT
1 1/4" MORTAR BED
CERAMIC TILE
FLOOR JOIST

OVER WOOD SUBFLOOR   OVER CONCRETE SLAB

THICK BED METHOD (MUD JOB)

CERAMIC TILE   GROUT
DRY SET MORTAR
1/2" CEMENTITIOUS BOARD

1 1/2" POURED CONCRETE   FLOOR JOIST   WOOD SUBFLOOR

DRY SET MORTAR WITH WOOD FRAMING

CERAMIC TILE   GROUT   DRY SET MORTAR

CONCRETE SLAB

DRY SET MORTAR DIRECTLY OVER CONCRETE

Ceramic Tile Installations

joints can be kept fairly narrow, in order to minimize the amount of grout required, since this is where mold growth can take place.

Latex-Portland cement mortar and dry-set mortar are both usually fairly well tolerated once the installation is complete, even though they may be intolerable when directly exposed to a sensitive person. This is because the mortar is eventually covered up by the tile and the grout, thus sealing it from the living space. Other types of mortars and mastics may sometimes also be well tolerated for this reason, but the more inert products are usually better choices.

A concrete floor can have the tile attached directly with either latex-Portland cement mortar or dry-set mortar. Some brands of mortar are not suitable for use over wood. In this case, a bed of 1½″ thick concrete could be poured over the floor, allowed to cure, and one of these mortars could then be used. Half-inch thick cementitious boards are available that provide a good surface for attaching the tile. They must be nailed over a sturdy wooden subfloor, since they have little load-bearing strength. "Wonder Board" is composed of Portland cement, fiberglass mesh, expanded shale and water and is made by **Modulars Inc.** It has an odor that takes some time to dissipate from a sulfur-based release agent that is used in manufacturing. The release agent is primarily on the smooth side. "Durock" is a similar product made by **U.S. Gypsum Corporation** that contains an expanded polystyrene filler. It too has an odor. When these products are covered with tile, the odor may be sufficiently sealed from the living space to no longer be a problem. "Eterspan," by **Eternit**, seems less odorous and may be a better choice for a sensitive person. Other cementitious boards, such as "Ultra Board" by **Weyerhaeuser**, "Flex II" by **Manville Building Products Corporation**, and "Eflex" by **Eternit**, are not recommended by their manufacturers for use with ceramic tile because they tend to expand too much when exposed to moisture, and can cause the grout joints to open up slightly. However, they are much less odorous, and in a situation where there will be no moisture they may be reasonable choices.

Grouting Tile Joints

As with mortars, there are several different types of commercial grouts used to fill the joints between tiles. All contain various chemical additives, and the epoxies, furans, and silicones will be the most offensive for sensitive people. Dry-set grouts, latex-Portland cement grouts, commercially prepared Portland cement grouts, and acid resistant grouts will be more tolerable, but unlike mortars the grout will be exposed to the living area. This means that chemical additives in grouts, such as acrylamide or latex, can be more bothersome than those in mortars that are sealed off from the living space.

There can be dozens of different ingredients in these commercially prepared products, so for sensitive persons a more appropriate choice will be to use the traditional Portland cement, sand, and water mixture that is prepared on the job, with no chemical additives. Sometimes lime is added for workability. Marble dust can be added as a filler, but it its softer than sand and can result in a less durable and more absorbent grout. Pure white Portland cement can be used with white sand to achieve a white grout, or tolerable concrete colorants to achieve a bright shade. For joints up to 1/8" wide one part Portland cement is used with one part of fine graded sand; 1:2 for joints up to 1/2" wide; and 1:3 for joints over 1/2" wide. The grout is worked into the joints with a rubber squeegee. The finished joints should be as flush with the surface as possible, rather than concave, so they will be easier to keep clean and dry.

Job-site mixed grouts like this that are made without additives to control setting, must be damp cured for 72 hours in order to have a hard and durable grout. This is done by covering the dampened floor with either a plastic sheet or kraft paper and keeping it moist.

For most people, ceramic tile set on concrete using a dry-set mortar and a sand-Portland cement grout will be quite acceptable. However, if in doubt, test first, by making up a sample using the proposed materials.

Cleaning Ceramic Tile

Glazed ceramic tile is relatively easy to keep clean with a damp mop and a mild cleaner. The grout, however, is somewhat absorbent and susceptible to staining. Commercially prepared grouts contain various additives that make them more resistant to stains. Various commercial sealers are available that can be used to seal the grout (or a porous tile such as quarry tile), but these are usually poorly tolerated by sensitive people. Sodium silicate (see Chapter 9) is, however, often well tolerated. It can be applied to grout with an artist's brush. Beeswax can sometimes be used to seal grout joints, although it may be difficult to apply.

Fuller's earth, a natural clay-like material, can be mixed with water to make a paste for use in absorbing stains from grout. It can be ordered through most pharmacies and is helpful in removing oil stains. The paste is applied to the stain and allowed to remain overnight to absorb the contaminant. It is then simply washed off. Stubborn stains can also be removed with a dilute solution of muriatic acid, but this should not be used as a regular method of cleaning because the acid actually eats away part of the surface of the grout.

Grout joints can often harbor mold if they are allowed to remain damp. Some grout additives such as methyl cellulose can actually encourage mold growth.[14] Most of the allergenic molds live in an acidic environment (low pH) and since Portland cement has a relatively high pH, it will discourage mold growth if kept dry. With narrow joints between tiles and grout flush with the surface of the tile, mold growth should not be a problem unless a lot of water is normally present.

Terrazzo

Like ceramic tile, terrazzo has been around for centuries, and the traditional method is again the best tolerated. It consists of a mixture of marble chips, Portland cement, and water, applied over a variety of surfaces such as concrete or wood. When this mixture has hardened, it is ground and polished smooth. Sometimes metal-divider accent strips are used to separate colors, highlight certain areas, or control cracking. This is becoming a lost art, since newer, faster, cheaper methods have been developed, so a contractor who uses the traditional techniques may be difficult to locate. Traditional terrazzo can be up to $2\frac{1}{2}''$ thick depending on the surface to which is is applied.

Today, latexes, vinyls, rubbers, epoxies, polyesters, or other materials can be used instead of Portland cement and various other minerals can be substituted for marble. This usually results in a less tolerable floor for a sensitive person. Chemical bonding agents can also be used when installing terrazzo over some types of surfaces.

A disadvantage of the traditional terrazzo is the fact that is requires a sealer of some type. Both the marble chips and the cement are porous, so it is not often recommended for use in a kitchen where it could be repeatedly stained. It can also have more of an institutional appearance and it is fairly expensive.

Concrete Floors

Concrete itself has been used as a finish floor and generally it is very inert. The surface can, however, be subject to wearing, which results in a very fine dust. A tolerated sealer such as sodium silicate (see Chapter 9) will help to remedy this. Acrylic, epoxy, or other synthetic sealers will be not as tolerable for sensitive people. A large expanse of gray concrete can be somewhat unattractive, but colored concrete can be much warmer looking. Tooled joints can break up a floor into interesting patterns. While a square, boxlike pattern may not add much to a room, diagonal joints can add a new dimension to the space. The various surface forms discussed in Chapter 9 can also be used. Once furniture and throw rugs are in place, a room takes on a personality that makes the appearance of the floor itself less important.

Concrete floors should be adequately reinforced with steel and poured properly to minimize any cracking which would not only be unsightly, but could allow radon to pass into the living space. If a concrete floor is covered with ceramic tile, a crack in the concrete will result in cracked tile as well.

Existing concrete floors that have had carpets or resilient tile glued down can be cleaned by using a heavy-duty sanding machine, a commercial floor scrubber with an abrasive pad, or a terrazzo grinding machine. TSP can work in some situations. Solvents or strippers should be used with extreme care and never in the presence of a sensitive person.

Gyp-Crete

Gyp-Crete is a farily inert plaster-based product that is mixed with sand and water on the job. Its primary use is as an underlayment for finished floors. Installed as a slurry and quickly leveled by trained workers, it hardens rapidly. Gyp-Crete subfloors can accept a carpet, wood, or resilient tile finish floor if adhesives are used to attach them. Ceramic tile can be attached with thin-set mortar.

Old uneven floors can be easily leveled by pouring a layer of Gyp-Crete, and radiant heating tubes can be cast in place. It is fire and crack resistant and will tend to seal cracks in an existing floor and around the perimeter of ther room. It is the product of **Gyp-Crete Corporation** and is available from a number of installers throughout the country.

Summary

While there are many different types of flooring in use today, the most popular—carpeting and synthetic tile—are the worst from a health standpoint. Ceramic tile and hardwood both make excellent choices if they are installed correctly. The primary problem with ceramic tile is the use of chemical additives in the mortars and grouts. With hardwood, finishing materials should be chosen with care. Terrazzo is a good choice, but its expense and the required sealers can be discouraging. With a little thought, bare concrete can result in a very healthful, attractive, and inexpensive floor.

Chapter 18

Interior Walls and Ceilings

Interior walls and ceilings comprise more surface area than anything else in a house; therefore, they have greater potential to cause indoor pollution than some other components. Not only must the wall or ceiling material itself be considered, but also any required paint or finishing material. The things inside the wall or ceiling structure such as the plumbing lines, electrical wires, and insulation can outgas through the wall into the living space. Moisture and wind barriers inside the wall can have an effect on the quality of the interior air depending on how well they perform their intended function.

In general, plaster or drywall will make for smoother, better sealed surfaces than individual boards or acoustical tiles which can provide crevices for dust to collect. Sometimes these materials can be used for decoration over a plaster or drywalled surface.

Wall Structure
Concrete and masonry can both be fairly inert structural components of walls, and some of the masonry materials discussed in Chapter 9 will be very attractive. However, in climates where high levels of insulation are required, these types of walls will be difficult to insulate properly. Steel framing, as discussed in Chapter 12, is an inert material that can easily be insulated. Yet, wood remains the traditional material to use for the structure of a house. As was discussed in Chapter 11, some woods are better tolerated than others for sensitive people,

but a major drawback to using wood is the fact that sooner or later a potentially toxic termite treatment will probably be required.

In cold climates, the interior of an insulated wall should have a moisture and air barrier (see Chapters 7 and 16). By making the air barrier as tight as possible, any outgassing from materials inside the wall will not be allowed to migrate into the house. Interior partition walls that are uninsulated can also contain a variety of materials that are capable of contaminating the indoor air. Most often it is plastic materials that cause the difficulties: electrical and telephone wires, plumbing or central vacuum lines, etc. While these walls could also be tightly sealed, a simpler solution is to wrap the offending materials with foil prior to applying the interior wall surfacing material.

Plaster

Plaster is a very old building material, and is usually well tolerated by most people. However, as with most other materials, there have been "improvements" over the years that can cause difficulties with those who are very sensitive. Plaster is a gypsum product that is purchased in a powder form, mixed with water, and applied to a wall where it hardens, leaving a very durable surface. Years ago it was applied over wood lath, but in recent years other base materials have been developed. Plastering is a labor intensive process, and can be fairly expensive. As less expensive drywall is becoming more and more common, it can be difficult in some areas to find someone skilled in the art of plastering. Plaster can easily be used to form curved surfaces in order to provide an architectural accent. A major advantage for many people is the fact that it can be finished with a hard surface that doesn't require painting. While the plaster itself is white, it can be tinted slightly to give it some color.

Bases for Plaster

Thin strips of wood lath are no longer used as a base for applying plaster. The most common base for plaster today, a gypsum board product known as gypsum lath, is easily nailed to wood framing or screwed to steel framing. It is a sandwich of gypsum with paper on both sides and can be purchased in different thicknesses. The gypsum core can also contain limestone, glass fibers, perlite, and minor amounts of starch or other additives.

There are several types of gypsum lath for use in different situations, with the standard product being used in most applications. A denser fire-rated material is available where required by certain building codes, and a heat resistant paper is used on sheets in contact with electric heating cables that are sometimes embedded in ceilings. Gypsum lath is also manufactured with a backing of aluminum foil that acts as a moisture barrier. The face paper of all of these products is specially treated for a maximum bond with the plaster. This paper is usually blue in color, hence gypsum lath is often referred to as "blueboard." Although drywall sheets are also gypsum products, they will not accept a plaster surface.

Metal lath is commonly seen in commercial construction, but because of the increased cost of labor and materials, it is not usually encountered in residential construction. It is made from sheet metal that has been perforated with small slits and expanded into several different forms, such as diamond mesh and flat ribbed. Some types have a backing of asphalt-impregnated paper. The metal itself is either painted or galvanized. Metal lath is easily applied to steel- or wood-framing members and generally is quite well tolerated.

Plaster can be applied directly to masonry materials such as clay tile, brick, or concrete block if their surface is sufficiently porous to allow proper bonding. A concrete surface must usually be treated with a bonding agent in order to get the plaster to adhere to it.

Plaster Materials

The main ingredient in gypsum plasters is gypsum rock. When the rock is taken from the earth, it is chemically combined with about 20 percent water. During processing, the gypsum is crushed into a powder and heated to drive off most of the water. When water is added back on the job, the material rehardens back into its original rocklike form. Commercially available plasters are specially formulated to control setting time and provide other characteristics. Fillers include materials such as natural sand, manufactured sand (crushed rock, blast furnace slag, etc.) perlite, vermiculite, or wood fiber. In the past, fillers included animal hair or asbestos. In demolishing older plaster walls, you should first determine if asbestos is present and then take appropriate precautions. Pure gypsum sets very fast and is referred to as plaster of Paris after the huge beds underlying that city. Gypsum plasters are available in a variety of types such as neat plaster, bond plaster, gauging plaster, and finish coat plaster.

When limestone is crushed and heated in the same manner as gypsum, quicklime, often simply called lime, is the result. Quicklime must be mixed with water (slaked) and stored for as long as two weeks before it can be used. Hydrated lime is quicklime that has been slaked before packaging. It is a powdered product that when mixed with water on the job is referred to as lime putty. It cannot be used as a plaster itself because it is subject to shrinkage when drying and lacks a hard finish. Hydrated lime is, however, added to gypsum plaster to control the set, plasticity, early hardness and strength, and to prevent shrinkage cracks.

Keene's cement is gypsum plaster with the addition of alum that, in powder form, has practically all of the water driven off. The resulting material is denser than ordinary gypsum plasters and has greater moisture resistance and hardness. It can be used for surface coats, but is more difficult to work with than other plaster products.

Portland cement may be combined with lime to be used as a plastering material. It is generally only used where very high moisture conditions exist. It cannot be applied to gypsum lath or to smooth, dense surfaces, but is suitable over metal lath. Portland cement plaster must be kept moist by misting water on the surface during the curing period in order to insure a proper set. Its cost will probably be higher than a comparable gypsum plaster installation.

Some plastering materials can contain polyvinyl or other additives to modify the setting time. These may be subject to outgassing. According to **U.S. Gypsum Corporation**, its products only contain plaster of Paris (or Portland cement) and lime. If a filler is used, it is clearly stated on the label.

Application of Plaster

The traditional thick method of applying gypsum plaster involves three coats, but today two-coat methods are also employed. The result is a plastered surface $1/2''$ to $5/8''$ thick. With metal lath, the three-coat system must be used. Over gypsum lath, brick, or masonry, either the two- or three-coat system is acceptable. The first of the three coats is called the scratch coat because it is scratched after application to provide a rough surface. The second coat, the brown coat, is applied after the scratch coat has hardened. It is leveled and left with a rough surface to accept the third, or finish coat. In two-coat work, the first coat is called the basecoat. It is applied in a manner similar to the brown coat above, and is left rough to receive the finish coat. Portland cement plasters are applied in a similar manner: the three-coat method over metal lath, or the two-coat method over masonry.

The finish coat in either the two- or three-coat system can be applied in several textures from a hard, smooth, steel-troweled surface to a more textured finish. Aggregates such as sand can be added to the finish coat to create a rougher finish. The smoother surfaces will be harder and easier to keep clean.

Veneer plastering systems involve very thin layers of plaster over gypsum lath and are more common than the traditional thick method, especially in residential construction. The two-coat veneer system adds less than $1/8''$ thickness of plaster and provides a durable, abrasion-resistant surface. The first coat, or basecoat, is left slightly rough and is allowed to dry before the finish coat is applied. One-coat veneer plaster is not quite as thick, and is lower in cost; however, it may not be finished as true or be quite as durable.

Paints and wallpapers are often problematic for some people, and they can be eliminated entirely when a hard steel-troweled finish is used. Textured surfaces tend to be more absorbent and difficult to clean. For the hardest, densest surface, a lime putty finish coat made of gauging plaster and lime putty is recommended. A minimum amount of water should be used since extra water will render the surface more porous. While this type of surface will be quite hard initially, it will continue to get harder for a couple of years as the lime carbonizes, finally yielding a rocklike finish.

Plaster and Health

There are several components of a plastered wall that can cause problems for some people. However, because the plaster itself is so hard and dense, it usually seals the offensive materials from the living space. An asphalt-impregnated backing on metal lath will certainly outgas some offensive asphalt fumes, and metal lath can have some residual oil from the manufacturing process, but since metal lath is rarely used in residential construction because of increased cost, these are usually not of concern. The paper on the gypsum lath can bother some sensitive persons as can some of the minor additives in the gypsum core, but these are usually not problems because the gypsum lath is totally covered by the layer of hard plaster. Most sensitive people can tolerate plastered walls and ceilings finished with either the tradi-

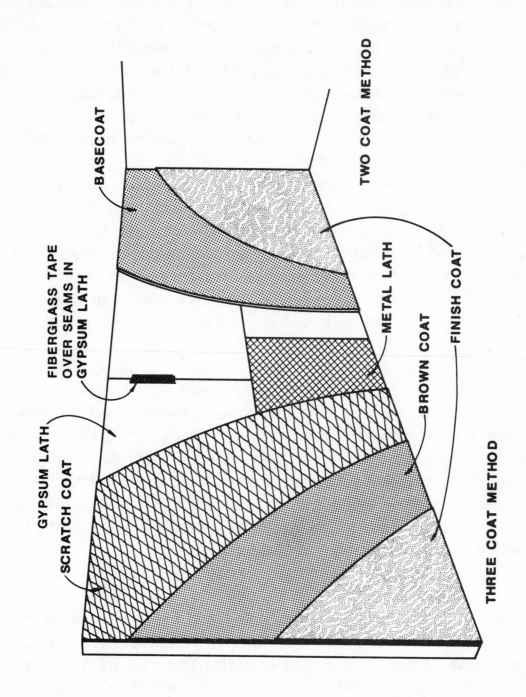

TWO COAT METHOD

BASECOAT

METAL LATH

FINISH COAT

BROWN COAT

FIBERGLASS TAPE OVER SEAMS IN GYPSUM LATH

GYPSUM LATH

SCRATCH COAT

THREE COAT METHOD

Traditional Plaster Application

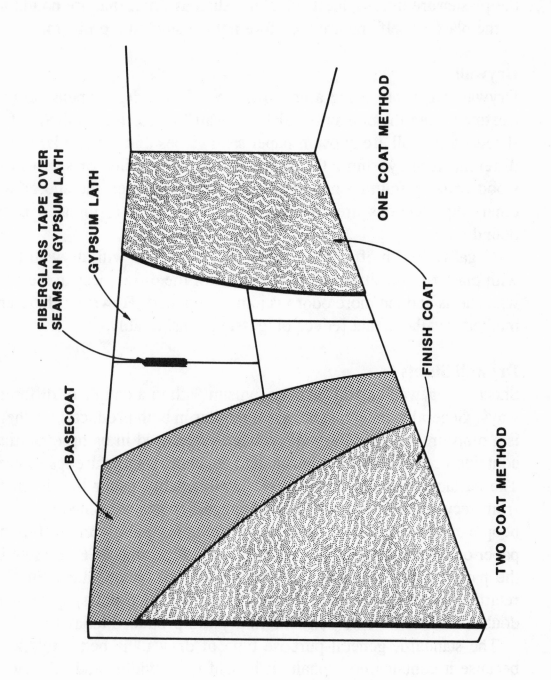

FIBERGLASS TAPE OVER SEAMS IN GYPSUM LATH

GYPSUM LATH

BASECOAT

FINISH COAT

ONE COAT METHOD

TWO COAT METHOD

Veneer Plaster Application

tional thicker methods or the thinner veneering methods. Additives to the plaster are usually inert minerals, such as lime, that are bound up in the plaster itself and are therefore not considered a problem.

Drywall

Drywall came into being after World War II as a less expensive wall treatment than the conventional "wet wall" plastering methods. The sheets of drywall are gypsum/paper sandwiches that are similar to but different from gypsum lath. They can be either nailed or screwed to wood or steel framing members. The joints between the sheets and other imperfections are finished with a specially formulated compound.

Negative health effects are more likely to occur with drywall than with plaster in sensitive persons because of the differences in the drywall sheets and the more odorous joint compound. However, there are methods available that reduce outgassing considerably.

Drywall Sheets

Sheets of drywall can differ from gypsum lath in a couple of different ways. Generally, the gypsum core is similar in both products, but there is a moisture-resistant drywall product, often used in bathrooms, that contains a certain amount of asphalt to enhance its moisture resistance. The surface paper on drywall is a lower quality paper that is made from recycled newspapers, old telephone books, etc. Since sensitive people often react to newspaper and printing ink[1], they can react to the paper on drywall as well. One source, in 1976, found PCBs present in the paper surface and assumed that they were either added for fire retardant purposes or were present in the recycled newspaper.[2] It is doubtful if PCBs would be found in drywall produced today.

The standard, general-purpose type of drywall is better tolerated because it contains no asphalt. It is sold in 4' widths and in various lengths and thicknesses. Like gypsum lath, it can be purchased with aluminum foil backing that acts as a moisture barrier and seals outgassing insulation from the living space. Denser fire-rated drywall panels are also available.

The moisture-resistant type of drywall not only contains a modified core, but the paper is chemically treated to combat water penetration. It is easily recognized because the paper facing is green in color instead of the standard light gray. It should not be used with a moisture

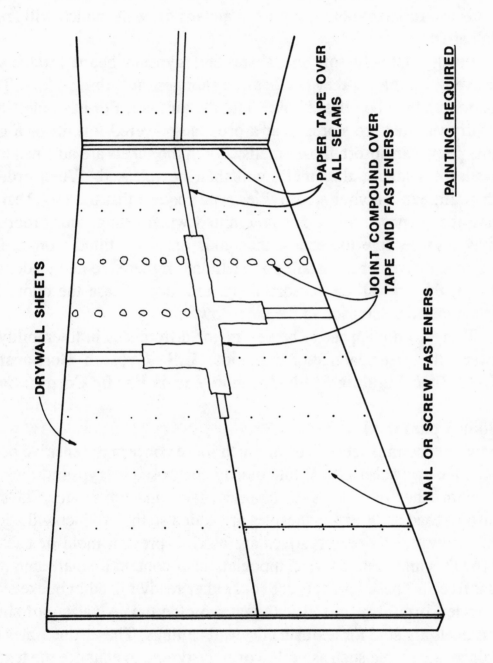

PAPER TAPE OVER ALL SEAMS

JOINT COMPOUND OVER TAPE AND FASTENERS

PAINTING REQUIRED

DRYWALL SHEETS

NAIL OR SCREW FASTENERS

Drywall Application

barrier on the reverse side because of the danger of trapping dampness between the barrier and the face. Ceramic tile can be attached to the moisture-resistant board, but not standard drywall, which will tend to fall apart.

Being relatively soft and absorbent, gypsum board products are scavengers, that is, they can act like sponges, absorbing odors. These odors can then be released back into the air later. For example, sheets of drywall that are stored near a propane-powered forklift or a gasoline pump can absorb those smells. When the sheets are attached to the walls of a house, the smells will then be released. When ordering drywall, explain your sensitivities, and request that the top sheet that has been exposed to the air, be omitted when filling your order. You may also be able to request that your order be filled from a fresh shipment. Even once installed and painted, if there are many odors in a room, the drywall can absorb them and then release the odors later when the concentration in the air is lower.

There do not appear to be any major differences in tolerability between the principal national brands: **U.S. Gypsum Corporation**, **Gold Bond Building Products**, and **Georgia Pacific Corporation**.

Joint Compound

Joint compounds seem to be of much more concern to sensitive people than the drywall itself.[3] While mostly composed of gypsum, they also contain other minerals such as mica, talc, and limestone. Clays can also be used as fillers. Adhesives are added so the product will stick to the drywall, and preservatives are used to prevent mold or bacterial growth while wet. Some compounds also contain a small amount of antifreeze. These products are sold either ready mixed in buckets or in powder form to be mixed with water on the job. A variety of similar products are sold for texturing drywall ceilings. These sometimes contain an aggregate such as perlite or polystyrene to enhance the texture.

Today, the adhesives in joint compounds are usually vinyl products, such as polyvinyl alcohol and polyvinyl acetate. Polyvinyl acetate will probably be better tolerated, since it is the same basic material used in "Elmer's" glue, which is often well tolerated by sensitive people. The preservatives and antifreeze compounds can, however, cause problems. A variety of things can be used as preservatives, such as mercury compounds which have the capacity to release mercury gas into the air during outgassing. Years ago, casein, derived from milk, was commonly used as an adhesive in joint compound, but its use has been discontinued by the major manufacturers because of the limited shelf life of the product once it was mixed with water. It was highly susceptible to mold growth until it was thoroughly dry. Sometimes toxic preservatives were added to extend the shelf life, but eventually the vinyl adhesives became popular. None of the nationally distributed joint compounds seem tolerable to sensitive persons.

Asbestos, once a common ingredient in joint compounds, was banned in 1977 by the **Consumer Products Safety Commission**.[4] Many drywall products manufactured prior to this ban contained asbestos. Some contained as much as 10–15 percent of the chrysotile and 8–12 percent of the tremolite varieties.[5] There is, therefore, a good chance that drywall joint compounds used in houses prior to 1977 contain asbestos. If such materials are loose and flaking, or if they are sanded by the homeowner, they could release asbestos fibers into the air. A solid surface will not release any fibers, and a deteriorating material can be painted to seal in any problems. Any remodeling or demolition should be done with care.

There is a joint compound available from a smaller company that is very well tolerated by sensitive people. "M-100 HiPO Compound" is a powdered material that is mixed with water on the job. It contains "no mildewcides, preservatives, asbestos, formaldehyde or hydrocarbon solvents," and is available from **Murco Wall Products, Inc.** Small samples for testing are sold at a nominal cost. Because of the weight, quantities are usually shipped by truck. While shipping charges can be seem high (up to $100 for enough material to do an entire house), this will certainly not increase the total cost of a house appreciably. This product can be used both for finishing drywall joints or for texturing ceilings.

Painting Drywall

Unlike hard steel-troweled plaster, drywall must be painted to protect it from daily wear and tear. Since the facing paper is made from recycled newsprint and is a potential problem for sensitive people, a paint should be chosen that will seal the paper well. A paint, therefore, should be selected that is not only tolerable by itself, but renders the drywall tolerable. It may be necessary to coat the drywall with one product to seal it and a second product for hiding or coloring ability. Some paints may be quite acceptable when tested on a piece of foil or glass, but may not sufficiently seal the surface of the drywall to render it tolerable.

Since the testing of paints can take some time for outgassing to be complete, they should be tested early in the planning process in conjunction with drywall. If a tolerable painting/drywall system cannot be found, then you will still have time to schedule a plastering job.

Wall Paneling

When most people think of wall paneling, thin 4'×8' sheets will come to mind. These are made with either particle board, plywood, or hardboard and have a decorative face which can be a wood veneer or a printed surface. The products made of hardboard, especially very dense tempered hardboard, will contain the least formaldehyde, but all will be intolerable to many sensitive people. They can also be troublesome because of vinyl surfaces or adhesives used to attach them to the wall.

There are predecorated gypsum panels made with decorative facings that can be used on walls. These do not require any joint compound since the joints are left exposed. The facing materials can be either a plastic film or sheet, a paint, or other liquid material. Textured panels can contain some type of aggregate as well. Since these materials are subject to outgassing, they are not recommended for sensitive people.

Solid wood tongue-and-groove wall paneling is seldom encountered because it is assumed to be higher in cost, and it usually is. However, some 4'×8' paneling with walnut veneer may be high priced as well. In fact, a solid wood poplar paneling might be less expensive than a top-of-the-line walnut veneered product. Solid wood can be used as an accent material on one wall, as wainscotting or as a ceiling treatment. If used on an insulated wall or ceiling, a moisture barrier may be required behind it. Health aspects to consider include tolerance of the wood itself and the finishing material.

Metal Ceilings

Reproduction embossed metal ceilings are being manufactured to resemble those used in the early 1900s. These can be used on walls as well as to provide a striking accent effect. They are attached by tacking the individual tiles of embossed metal to wood furring strips.

Manufacturers include **AA-Abbington Affiliates, Inc.**, and **Pine-**

crest. A drawback to these products is the fact that they must be either painted or coated with a clear finish. Water-based finishes are not suitable since they can cause rusting of the metal. More odorous oil-based paints or lacquers are recommended by the manufacturers.

Contemporary prefinished metal strip ceilings are also available, but their use is generally confined to commercial buildings because of cost. They can, however, be used in homes on walls or ceilings and are available in a variety of colors on an aluminum base. They do not form a continuous barrier so they must be backed up by an appropriate material to seal any offensive smells inside the wall or ceiling. Installed by attaching the strips to special metal tracks, they can be used over most types of surfaces. Manufacturers include **Donn Corporation** and **Levolor Lorentzen, Inc.**

Acoustical Ceiling Tiles

These ceilings are popular with do-it-yourselfers because of their ease of installation. Suspended ceilings consist of individual panels up to two feet by four feet, placed in a metal track system that is suspended from the structure. The panels themselves can be a source of symptoms in some people. They can be made of either mineral fiber, wood fiber, fiberglass, metal, or some other material. Some older products should be handled with care because they contain asbestos; however, a common source of asbestos is in sprayed-in-place ceilings. These are usually only encountered in commercial buildings, schools, etc. They are rarely found in homes.

The panels made of fiberglass tend to emit formaldehyde into the air. Plastic, latex, fabric, or wood finishes can also be used, each having its own outgassing characteristics. Another problem with these materials is the fact that they can be very absorbent. They can soak up any smell in the room, whether it is from a formaldehyde source or fried fish. This can result in a very odorous ceiling.

Individual acoustical tiles, generally one foot square, are made of similar materials. These are attached to wood or metal furring strips with staples, clips, or an odorous mastic glue. They too are fairly absorbent.

The basic manufacturing process used in producing mineral and wood fiber tiles is similar to papermaking and can be contaminated with a variety of materials. It has been reported that 1 to 2 percent of the tiles produced by **Armstrong World Industries** between 1969 and

1970 contained PCBs.[6] At that time, the dangers of PCB were not fully known. These particular tiles were used primarily in commercial buildings and it is unlikely that they would be found in homes. However, it does underscore the fact that materials currently believed to be safe may be found to be dangerous in the years to come.

Ceramic Tile

Ceramic tile or marble can be attached to walls by methods similar to those discussed in Chapter 17. Concrete or masonry walls can be easily covered by using a dry-set or latex-Portland cement mortar, or the thick bed method. In damp areas such as showers, manufacturers usually recommend a cementitious board or water-resistant drywall if a traditional thick bed over metal lath is not used. Since both of these materials are less than desirable for sensitive people, testing of a completed trial assembly should be done.

Course sanded grouts may not be desirable in wall installations. If a commercially prepared wall grout is not tolerable, you should use a Portland cement and water mixture. After filling the joints, the grout will need to be kept damp to allow the Portland cement to cure properly. This can be done by misting or sponging periodically. Grout on walls is more difficult to keep damp for curing than floors.[7]

When using ceramic tile in a shower or bathtub, the joint between the bottom row of tile and the tub or shower base should usually not be grouted. It should instead be sealed with a more flexible caulking. In this location, grout will tend to crack and provide a breeding place for mold.

Porcelain-Enameled Panels

This material is an excellent choice for very sensitive people, but it is also quite expensive. It can, however, be a good alternative to ceramic tile in a bathroom. Porcelain panels can be either steel or aluminum with a glass-like porcelain coating fused to the surface. Ovens and bathtubs often have porcelain coatings. There are several different methods of attaching these panels to the structure of a building, and the details and panel sizes need to be worked out well in advance, since once the panels are manufactured, they cannot be easily trimmed to fit.

Because of the cost and advanced planning required, porcelain panels are seldom seen in residential construction. They are, however, used in commercial applications. Someone interested in this material should remember that for residential applications, the panels will need to be custom made. This can be not only costly, but it can take extra time that will affect other construction schedules. For information about having porcelain panels made, contact the **Porcelain Enamel Institute** for a list of manufacturers. For the designer, standard construction details can be found in a book titled *Basic Building Data*.[8]

Wall Coverings

Wall coverings used to be limited to wallpaper, but now fabric, plastic, and metallic coverings are also available. Not only can the material itself be bothersome to a sensitive person, but also the adhesive that is used to attach it to the wall. When they are to be hung on new unpainted walls, it is usually recommended that the walls be painted with an odorous alkyd paint, to facilitate removal of the covering when remodeling is done in the future.

Many wall coverings are prepasted, either with a glue that must be moistened or an adhesive with a peel-off backing. Other coverings require a paste that is either ready to apply or mixed on the job with water. A wheat flour and water mixture is a popular old wallpaper paste. Water-based pastes and glues are subject to mold growth or insect attack, so they usually have potentially troublesome mold retardants or insecticides added. Without the additives, there is danger of mold growth behind the paper which can eventually attack the old wallpaper. The adhesives that are protected with a peel-off backing, such as "contact" paper, are usually not subject to fungus attack, but they may not be tolerated by sensitive people. Synthetic adhesives can outgas synthetic fumes through porous coverings such as paper or fabric.

Metallic coverings can either be a solid foil type or a metallic/plastic film such as aluminized Mylar. The plastic types should be avoided by sensitive persons, but some of the all-metal products may be acceptable if a tolerated adhesive can be found. All-plastic wall coverings can outgas undesirable odors because of their synthetic nature. Cloth and paper coverings can be troublesome because of chemicals used in their manufacture, such as binders, inks, paints, and dyes. There is also a good possibility that, like the glues, they have been treated with fungicides or pesticides. If very much of this material is used, the home becomes "an insecticide-and-fungicide-lined box."[9] Not a very healthful thought.

In general, wall coverings are not recommended for sensitive persons, although some metal foil products could be acceptable.

Summary

Plaster walls and ceilings are usually the best tolerated for sensitive people; however, in many cases, less expensive drywall can be an acceptable alternative. Solid wood or metal wall covering materials are often reasonable choices, but they do not provide as tightly sealed a surface as plaster or drywall. They can require some type of barrier to adequately seal insulation or to keep moisture from migrating through a wall. Ceramic tile or porcelain panels make good wall materials, but their higher cost makes their use limited to specialized areas like kitchens or baths. Most wall coverings and acoustical ceiling materials make relatively poor choices by comparison.

Chapter 19

Paint, Varnish, and Caulking

The odors of these materials have been shown to cause a wide variety of symptoms in susceptible individuals. The effects can cover the entire range of physical and mental diseases.[1] Since these products often take long periods to outgas completely, they should be the first things tested for tolerability when contemplating a remodeling or construction job. Obviously some products will be better choices than others when deciding what to test, and sometimes painting will not be necessary at all.

Why Paint?

There are several reasons why materials are painted. Decoration is probably the first that comes to mind. Walls are painted to "spruce them up" or add some color. Painting may be necessary to cover up an undesirable color, dirt, or stain. Lighting effects can be improved by the correct choice of color. Washability and cleanliness can often be improved with a coat of paint. Preservation and sealing are other good reasons to consider painting.

For someone sensitive to paint odors, some of these reasons will not be very important. For example, it may be easier to live with an orange bedroom than to risk exposure to fresh paint fumes. If a room simply looks like it needs a fresh coat of paint, it is often possible to wash the walls and ceiling and achieve the same effect, thus avoiding painting. New plaster walls are hard and durable enough to not even require painting, and are often recommended for people with chemical hypersensitivity syndrome for that very reason.

In outdoor applications, paints will not need to be selected with the same care as those to be used indoors, because exposure will be less for sensitive people. Outdoors, the paint's outgassing will constantly be diluted by the surrounding air, while indoors, pollutant concentrations from fresh paint can build up to intolerable levels. Most of the paints and varnishes mentioned in this chapter were developed for indoor use.

If new walls are built with drywall, they may require paint not only to decorate them but also to seal the surface. The paper surface is sometimes intolerable to sensitive individuals, and can be coated with a paint or varnish to keep it from outgassing into the living space. Sometimes one material will be used as a sealer and another used as a decorative coat since not all finishes will effectively act as a sealant.

Hardwood floors, woodwork, and cabinetry should be coated with either a paint or varnish to both seal and protect them. Uncoated wood will usually have a characteristic odor and can be easily stained. Water spilled on a bare wood floor can be a good place for mold to grow.

Composition

Paints and varnishes are made of a wide variety of ingredients. Manufacturers generally consider their formulas to be trade secrets, although some items will be listed on Material Safety Data Sheets. Basically, a paint is composed of a binder, a vehicle, and a pigment. The binder is the glue that holds the paint to the wall. The pigment supplies the color, and the vehicle helps to keep the material dissolved. The vehicle will either evaporate or oxidize into a dried film. A varnish, being clear, contains no pigment. In actuality, there can be dozens of other ingredients, including such things as antiskinning agents, antisettling agents, emulsifying agents, driers, fatty acids, fillers, extenders, fire retardants, flatting agents, plasticizers, preservatives, fungicides, surfactants, thickeners, thixotropic agents, etc.[2] These things can be composed of heavy metal compounds containing lead or arsenic, pine oil, coal tar, kerosene, xylene, alcohols, synthetic oils and resins, mineral spirits, etc.[3] Of course, each manufacturer's product will have different ingredients. While manufacturers are reluctant to release specific information about their complete formulas, if asked whether or not a single ingredient is present, they will often reply.

Even if a paint were composed of only a binder, vehicle, and pigment, it could still be toxic. White lead has been used in the past as a pigment and cadmium compounds are still being used. Biocides containing mercury have been used. Heavy metals such as these tend to accumulate in the body until they reach toxic levels. Vehicles can be water, or they can be composed of various oils or solvents such as linseed oil, tung oil, mineral spirits, lacquer thinner, turpentine, toluene, alcohol, etc. Latex is a popular binder today, with various other natural and synthetic resins also being used. Health effects vary considerably. Tung oil, for example, has immunosupressive effects and has been implicated in reactivation of chronic Epstein-Barr virus.[4]

There are many water-based finishes on the market today that rely on water rather than some other toxic vehicle. These have been developed largely as a result of the potential dangers of exposure to the various solvents; however, some water-based products can also significantly contribute to indoor air pollution. One study found high emissions of alkanes from some water-based adhesives.[5]

Lead is no longer used as a pigment, but children still chew on windowsills that are coated with paint containing lead. Ingestion is not the only method of lead intake. Flaking or peeling paint can result in lead dust being inhaled. A few flakes of lead-based paint can contain over 100 mg. of lead. It has been found that children with elevated lead levels in their blood are most likely to come from deteriorated or dilapidated private housing.[6] Newly painted surfaces will tend to seal a deteriorating paint and minimize the lead dust problem.

Binders can include casein, which might be bothersome to a person with milk allergies. Synthetic latexes, lacquers, and polyurethanes can be bothersome to many sensitive people. Some artists use egg yolks as a binder in tempera paints.

When to Paint
The paint in a typical house covers hundreds of square feet and can overwhelm the system of a sensitive person until it has completely outgassed. Even though a testing sample seemed tolerable, the large, freshly painted surface of an entire house may be intolerable. Therefore, careful testing is only part of the answer. *All* paints and varnishes outgas for a certain period, and during this time should be avoided by sensitive people.

Often, it is a good idea for a paint-sensitive individual to leave the house for a few days while painting is being done. This absence may need to last for several days until most of the outgassing has taken place. It may be desirable to have the painting done while on vacation. By testing various paints, it should be possible to select one that outgasses quickly so any inconvenience will be minimal.

Painting can also be done on a room-by-room basis with window exhaust fans used to keep smells from traveling throughout the house. Painting should be done at a time of year when windows can be left open for several weeks if necessary. It is not a good idea to consider painting when outdoor temperatures are below freezing, or above 100 degrees. Periods of excessively high humidity can cause slow drying of water-based finishes, possibly resulting in mold growth.

Selecting Paints and Varnishes

Of the many nationally distributed paints, several have been recommended in various books, newsletters, etc., as being tolerable. There are other paints especially made without fungicides and there are "100 percent natural" paints available. For someone with sensitivities to paint odors, it must be remembered that everyone's system is different, and a paint that someone else finds tolerable may not be tolerable for you. Testing is always recommended.

Most people assume that all paints or varnishes will outgas completely sooner or later. This may be true, but outgassing that continues for a year could certainly disrupt the life of a sensitive occupant. Therefore, when testing, several finishes should be considered simultaneously, in order to determine which is tolerable the soonest. Outgassing, however, may not be the only problem to consider. The dried finish can possibly cause reactions to someone sensitive to the synthetic resin itself.[7]

Keeping these things in mind, we will consider the various products available, first paints, then varnishes, stains, and caulkings. Most of the paints and varnishes discussed are for interior use. If an outdoor application is planned, check with the manufacturer for suitability.

Off the Shelf Paints

Alkyd-based paints can take up to three months to outgas, yet they have been recommended for sensitive individuals because they leave a hard film that can seal such materials as drywall.[8] Another source states that alkyd paint still has an odor after three years.[9] Obviously, individual testing is necessary, since people's sensitivities vary as well as the products of different manufacturers.

Water-based latex or acrylic paints are recommended much more often than alkyd paints as being tolerated by sensitive people, although they may not seal in odors as well as alkyd-based paints or other sealers. In regard to particular brands, various sources recommend Pittsburgh, Du Pont Lucite, Fuller O'Brien, Benjamin Moore, Sears, and Dutch Boy. Custom-mixed colors are sometimes specified over pre-mixed colors which can contain tetrafluoroethylene. Semigloss paints will dry to a harder film than will flat finishes, and may be better tolerated. Flat finishes will, however, hide imperfections in a wall's surface easier than a semigloss finish.

All water-based latex paints have either fungicides or biocides added to control mold growth and bacterial growth. These can be bothersome to sensitive people.

It is often recommended that baking soda be added to water-based paints to absorb the odor of freshly applied paint.[10] Baking soda can be added in amounts from 1/2 to 1 cup per gallon of paint by using a flour sifter and mixing thoroughly until any bubbling stops. This will tend to thicken the paint and thinning with water may be necessary. It may affect the surface sheen when used with a semigloss paint. In damp areas and especially outdoors it can sometimes bleed to the surface of the dried paint. This can be especially noticeable with darker colors. Occasionally, it will cause the paint to adhere poorly and flake off. In most situations, however, a latex paint with baking soda should adhere well to a new or clean surface.

Many people report that an intolerable paint was made tolerable simply by adding baking soda, but this should be tested by someone with severe sensitivities. Others simply find that by switching brands they have found a tolerable paint, while still others must resort to something that may not be readily available at the local hardware store. Keep in mind that manufacturers are constantly changing their formulas, and that a product that was tolerable last year may no longer be safe for a sensitive person.

Custom-Made Paints

Miller Paint Co. produces what are known as low-biocide paints. The raw materials available to them all have small amounts of biocides and fungicides, but they do not add the large amounts common to other paints which are added primarily to extend the shelf life of the paint while it is still in the can. In order to keep from being contaminated by mold or bacteria in the can, low-biocide paints must be used within four weeks of manufacture. These products are, therefore, made to order and **Miller Paint Co.** requires 30 days' notice in order to supply a fresh product. Orders as small as one gallon can be shipped. They produce both a low-sheen and a flat 100 percent acylic wall paint, and a latex semigloss enamel, all water-based. They also have an alkyd semigloss enamel that is solvent-based and can be used if extra durability is needed.

These products are recommended for use indoors only. The added biocides and fungicides are needed outdoors to adequately resist fungal and mildew attack. Also, in very damp areas indoors, fungus growth on the paint could be a problem. As a rule of thumb, if steam tends to accumulate on a bathroom mirror, there is potential for mildew growing.[11]

Low-Outgassing Paints

These are paints that are claimed by their manufacturers to outgas less than most commercially available paints. They may contain materials that could bother someone sensitive to paint fumes, but generally are fairly well tolerated. Again, testing is recommended for sensitive individuals.

AFM Enterprises, Inc. produces a line of "products for the chemically sensitive." Included in their Safecoat paint line are a primer undercoat, flat finish paint, semigloss enamel, and gloss enamel. These are all water-based products and are advertised as being nontoxic and nonhazardous. The only colors available are white and off-white, but they state that these can be tinted at your local paint store with universal tints. Be sure to test tinting materials if paint sensitive. **Pace Industries Inc.** has a "Crystal Shield" latex base paint that is designed to function as an environmental sealant. It is available in seven colors. These products are sold on a mail order basis from several sources, including **Nigra Enterprises**. Product information sheets are available.

Murco Wall Products, Inc. produces and sells a low odor Hipo flat interior vinyl wall paint and a Hipo gloss latex enamel, as well as a semigloss latex enamel and an alkyd gloss enamel. These products are advertised as not containing "such volatile compounds as ammonia, formaldehyde, ethylene-glycol, or ethylene glycol butyl ether." Eight pastel colors are stocked.

Natural Paints

These paints are made from all natural materials. As a result, they are often assumed to be safer than other paints. Some of the ingredients that are considered natural include oil of turpentine, citrus oil, citrus thinner, pine resin, tung oil, etc. For someone sensitive to hydrocarbons or organic chemicals, these ingredients can be troublesome. The "Livos" and "Auro" brands seem somewhat comparable, but are enough different that someone could be sensitive to one and not the other. Outgassing periods may vary as well. There is the possibility of mold forming in a partially used can after a few weeks, but once on the wall and dried, mold is unlikely except in very wet locations.

Livos Plant Chemistry imports the "Livos" brand of wood finishes from Germany. They have a wide variety of products including a flat water-based interior #7402 Natural Resin Wall Paint in white and an oil-based #4091 Vindo-Enamel Paint in white. They also have a #226 Menos-Primer and a #223 Metal Primer and a #7404 Albion-White Wash Paint. The natural resin wall paint contains a "binder of liquid emulsion of high quality plant resins, plant oils, plant glues and beeswax. Pigments: titan white (Rutin) derived through recycling process, chalk, talcum, and high white powdered wood." Also available are water-based and oil-based earthen and mineral-based stain pastes which can be used to color the paints.

The "Auro" brand, also imported from Germany, is sold by **Sinan Co.** They handle a variety of products, including a water-based #321 Natural Resin Wall Paint (flat, white). They also have some oil-based finishes, #235 White Enamel, #233 Enamel Primer, and #234 Metal Primer. Their earth and mineral tinting pigments can be used for coloring the paints. A complete list of ingredients is available for individuals interested in specifics.

Milk paints are considered natural paints and have been around for centuries. Today, they have been largely replaced with latex and acrylic formulations; however, a powdered milk paint is still manufactured and sold by the **Old-Fashioned Milk Paint Co.** that is easily mixed with water and applied. It contains milk protein, lime, clay, whiting, and earth pigments and is a very low-odor paint. For someone with chemical hypersensitivity syndrome, this paint is often tolerated, but for someone with milk allergies it may be problematic and should certainly be tested before application. It was developed to simulate old milk paint finishes on antique reproduction furniture and comes in eight colors. It is a very thin paint and may not cover well in some applications. It is very durable once applied, but can get moldy while in the liquid state and should be used within a few hours after mixing with water. It will keep indefinitely in powder form if the packages are tightly sealed.

A material that is sometimes recommended as a paint for very sensitive individuals is "B-I-N Primer Sealer," manufactured by **William Zinsser & Co., Inc.** This product is alcohol-based and has a very strong odor when first applied, but tends to outgas relatively quickly as the alcohol evaporates. For some sensitive people this may take several hours, for others, a few days. It is not a true paint because it does not have a great deal of pigment, hence it does not cover very well. In spite of this, it does an excellent job of sealing drywall and will seal water stains that can bleed through other finishes, and it can be used as a vapor barrier. B-I-N contains only denatured ethyl alcohol, regular bleached shellac, titanium dioxide, and silicates. Shellac is a purified resin secreted by an insect, and is one of the few natural ingredients that can still be found in use today. B-I-N can be purchased in many paint and hardware stores. It is sold primarily because of its stain-covering ability. Other synthetic stain-covering products are also on the market, but these are often intolerable to paint-sensitive persons, even when dry. They do not use a rapidly evaporating alcohol solvent and should be avoided.

Varnishes

Varnishes are clear finishes that can be used on wood to let the natural beauty shine through. Polyurethanes and synthetic lacquers are popular today, but they can bother sensitive individuals. Fortunately, there are both natural and low-odor synthetic finishes available to choose from.

Varnishes are usually not recommended to protect outdoor woodwork because ultraviolet light from the sun can pass through the finish and damage the wood. This often results in the varnish peeling. The best outdoor finish for protecting wood is exterior paint.

Shellac is one of the oldest varnishes available. With its alcohol solvent, it is quite odorous when wet, but dries and outgases quickly, usually in a matter of days. The "Bulls Eye" brand is available in many paint and hardware stores and is manufactured by **William Zinsser & Co., Inc.** They have available an excellent booklet titled "How and Where to Use Bulls Eye Shellac" that lists several application and finishing tips. A shellac finish can be dissolved by an alcoholic beverage, and becomes water-spotted if allowed to remain wet for a while. However, shellac finishes are very easy to repair by blending, unlike some synthetic finishes that must be completely removed and then refinished.

"Aqua Fabulon" is one of several Fabulon finishes manufactured by **Pierce & Stevens Chemical Corporation**. It is a low-odor synthetic acrylic water-based product that is available through local Pratt & Lambert paint stores. This is a very durable finish, developed for use on floors and is available in different surface sheens.

Pace Industries, Inc. manufactures and sells "Right-On Crystal Aire I" which is advertised as being an environmental sealant as well as simply a clear finish. It is an acrylic, low-odor, water-based product available in matte, satin, or gloss sheen. To seal particle board or other formaldehyde-containing materials, four coats are recommended to achieve a 94 percent reduction in emissions. Comprehensive descriptive literature is available upon request. They also sell a more durable (and odorous) Crystal Shield for use on floors. Crystal Aire is available on a mail order basis from the manufacturer, **Nigra Enterprises**, and **The Allergy Store**.

"AFM Water Seal" and "Hard Seal" are both produced by **AFM Enterprises, Inc.** and sold through several mail order sources. They are water-based, synthetic, low-odor finishes that can be applied over a variety of surfaces. Hard Seal is more durable and well suited to flooring applications. They both will help to seal in the noxious fumes from outgassing materials. Product information sheets are available.

There is a "Particle Board Sealer" available from **Valspar Corporation** that is effective in sealing formaldehyde emissions. It is a water-based product that is sold in clear, fruitwood, and Italian walnut shades. It is most effective when applied to uncoated particle board.

There are several oil-type finishes that are made for coating woodwork, but these products usually tend to remain odorous for longer periods than do the above-mentioned varnishes and generally are not recommended for sensitive individuals. Oils dry by oxidation and many utilize various additives to speed up the drying process.

Waxes are also occasionally recommended for people with paint sensitivities, but generally these products must contain a solvent such as turpentine in order to render them workable. They may, however, be suitable for some applications after outgassing. Beeswax is often used, but can smell strongly of flowers, the smell having been transferred by the bees that produced the wax. Carnuba wax is harder than beeswax. It is sold by the **Trewax Co.** They also have a "Trewax Beauty Sealer" product that is often well tolerated after outgassing.

Stains

Stains for woodwork have come into regular use for a number of reasons. Most types of wood vary in color from tree to tree, so industry tends to stain everything so that it all looks alike. Inexpensive woods are often stained to resemble more expensive ones. Much fine woodworking is not stained at all, thus allowing the natural beauty of the wood to speak for itself. Many stains are dark, and the resulting wood tends to look gloomy. With "natural living" becoming a popular concept, unstained wood is being accepted more and more. The normal color variations are what give wood its character and do not need to be covered up. For those who prefer to add a little color to their wood, some less toxic stains are available.

Both oil-based and water-based mineral stain pastes are sold by **Livos Plant Chemistry** and **Sinan Co.** under the "Livos" and "Auro" brands respectively. These can be used on wood or stone to highlight the grain or change the appearance. Several colors are produced. Under the "Livos" label, a Bela-Wood Stain is made for use especially on woodwork. Walnut husks can be boiled in water to produce a do-it-yourself stain.

Homemade Paints

Some people may wish to try their hand at making their own paint. If this is considered, one should remember that the end product should be durable and somewhat mold-resistant as well as tolerable to a paint-sensitive person. The basic components of paint, binder, vehicle, and pigment can be from a variety of sources. Probably the easiest vehicle to work with is water. Binders can be milk protein, flour, gum arabic, glycerine, sodium silicate, glue, egg yolk, etc. There are many things that can be used as pigments, but inorganic mineral or clay materials are probably the best to use. Local ceramic shops can often supply powdered potter's clay in various shades that can be used as pigments. These clays can be used in the commercially available paints already mentioned to tint them. It may be advisable to bake the powdered clay in the oven at 225 degrees for 15 minutes to kill any mold spores. Simply measure out the same amount to place in each can, add to the paint with a flour sifter, and stir well with a mixer on an electric drill. Such inexpensive attachments are available at most paint stores.

An excellent place to get ideas for making your own paint is the *Artist's Handbook*.[12] This book gives detailed information on advantages and disadvantages of various materials. Some recipes for whitewash and milk paint are listed in *Nontoxic and Natural*.[13] The brochure describing the milk paint sold by the **Old-Fashioned Milk Paint Co.** has an old basic formula listed.

Other sources for ideas include old formula books. Several of these old books have been reprinted in recent years. Care must be taken in choosing some of the recipes because sometimes very toxic ingredients are specified. Such things as white lead for pigment or gasoline for a vehicle may be recommended, both very dangerous choices. They also often give very imprecise measurements, that will lead to inconsistent results. A typical recipe, for "fireproof paint," says to add as much potash to water as can be dissolved, add a quantity of flour paste the consistency of painter's size, then add pure clay until the mixture is the consistency of cream, then apply with a brush.[14]

Caulking

There is a wide variety of caulking materials available today. They can be similar in composition to some paints. Many require long outgassing periods and are intolerable to those with paint sensitivities. The volatile materials given off vary depending on the particular brand. A test of a clear acrylic latex caulk with silicone found the following products being outgassed: acetone, methyl ethyl ketone, methyl propionate, ethyl propionate, dimethyl pentane, C-6 ester, butanone, toluene, C-8 alkene, dimethyl cyclohexane, butyl propionate, N-octane, dimethyl benzene, and C-8 alcohol.[15] This is certainly not a very healthy-sounding list.

Caulking materials, as well as paints, should be tested early when considering building or remodeling, and plenty of fresh air should be provided until the outgassing period is complete. A few nationally distributed brands have been recommended as outgassing relatively quickly. These materials do have an odor when fresh, and they may not be tolerated by some people.

"DAP Kwik-Seal Tub and Tile Caulk" is manufactured by **Beecham Home Improvement Products, Inc.** and is sold in many paint and hardware stores. It is often tolerated by sensitive people after outgassing. This is a vinyl preparation containing several ingredients, including ethylene glycol and n-butyl acetate. As its name implies, it is for use around bathtubs, but it can be used in other areas as well. The only available color is white.

Contrary to its name, "Phenoseal Adhesive Caulking" does not contain a phenolic resin. It is basically a polyvinyl acetate emulsion, similar to "Elmer's" glue, but it contains other minor ingredients that could bother some people. It is made in ten different colors and seems to be tougher and more flexible than the DAP product. While it is distributed nationally, it can be difficult to find in some areas. Write or telephone the manufacturer, **Gloucester Co., Inc.**, for the nearest supplier.

A 100 percent silicone caulking has been recommended for sensitive people. Although highly odorous when wet, it can be tolerable after extended outgassing. It is a very long-lasting product, so once in place, a repeat application may not be necessary for several years.

Pace Industries, Inc. can supply their Crystal Aire product in a thickened form for use as a caulking material. This is basically the same formula as their clear sealant. It is not available in standard caulking tubes, and must be applied with a putty knife from the can. It can be purchased in various viscosities, depending on the usage.

Summary
Since all paints, varnishes, and caulking materials require an outgassing period, testing should be done ahead of time in order to select a material that will be tolerable in the shortest time. For a few individuals, this can be as long as two or three months, even for low-outgassing materials. Obviously, this can cause some major inconveniences, but it is far better to know about it before beginning a painting project, so proper precautions can be taken.

You should always prepare several testing samples simultaneously and date them. In this way it can be determined which is tolerable the soonest, without having to wait for a fresh sample to air out.

Chapter 20

Kitchens and Bathrooms

Kitchen and bathrooms tend to be the most complicated rooms in the house because of the cabinetry, appliance, electrical, plumbing, and ventilating requirements. All these things combine to make these rooms potential problem areas for sensitive people. A bare, relatively empty bedroom, on the other hand, will usually be better tolerated. We will discuss all of the component parts of these rooms in order to sort out the problems.

Cabinetry

Practically all of the commercially manufactured cabinets, whether for kitchens or bathrooms, utilize plywood or particle board and will out-gas formaldehyde fumes into the house. Even expensive cabinetry will rely on man-made wood products to some degree. The doors and drawer fronts are often solid wood, but the shelves are almost always plywood or particle board. The end panels may appear to be made of solid wood but a close examination will usually reveal that they are veneered, having only a thin layer of expensive hardwood over a particle board core.

Most custom cabinet shops also use these materials because they are easy to work with and their cost is lower than solid wood. They can, however, usually make cabinets out of solid wood on special request. The drawers can be made out of galvanized sheet metal by a shop specializing in furnace ductwork, and have an attractive wood front

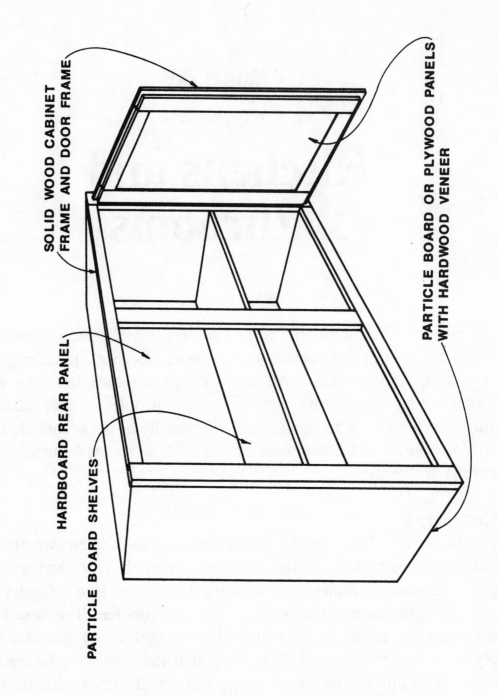

SOLID WOOD CABINET
FRAME AND DOOR FRAME

PARTICLE BOARD OR PLYWOOD PANELS
WITH HARDWOOD VENEER

HARDBOARD REAR PANEL

PARTICLE BOARD SHELVES

Unhealthy Kitchen Cabinet

attached with screws. Wooden drawers can be fitted with sheet metal bottoms, avoiding the usual plywood. If there are no custom cabinetry shops listed in the telephone book, ask the local lumberyard or high school industrial arts teacher for a reference.

Outgassing from existing cabinets can be lessened in a couple of ways, but for very sensitive people, offensive cabinets should be removed. Since the interiors of most cabinets are unfinished, there is nothing to retard the outgassing. They can be simply sealed to reduce the level of formaldehyde release. Four coats of a tolerated finish may reduce the outgassing by over 90 percent. Another method involves covering the inside of the cabinets and the shelves with aluminum foil. This can usually be held in place with tape or staples. While these methods can be somewhat successful in reducing formaldehyde release, they cannot be expected to be 100 percent effective.

When selecting new cabinetry, metal makes a good alternative to wood. Several companies make all-metal cabinets that can be used in kitchens, baths, or utility rooms. **St. Charles Manufacturing Co.** sells a very attractive line of steel cabinets with a baked-on enamel finish in several colors. The surface can be either smooth or textured. The metal doors of these cabinets have a wood core that is held in place with a mastic to give them added rigidity. Even though this core is sealed on the front, back, and all four edges with steel, a sensitive person should test a sample door for tolerability before purchasing a whole kitchen full of cabinets. These cabinets can also be ordered with solid wood doors. **Sears, Roebuck and Co.** also handles an attractive line of steel cabinets in two colors, white and almond. These are somewhat less expensive, and also have a sound-deadening core inside the doors. Other metal cabinet suppliers can be found through local plumbing supply houses or bath shops.

Cabinetry doesn't need to be confined to bathrooms and kitchens. Built-in cabinets in a bedroom closet will eliminate the need for dressers. This can be an important component of a bedroom oasis. For someone sensitive to printing ink, or the moldy smell of old books, bookcases with glass doors will keep those odors from permeating the house. Similarly, glass doors on display cabinets full of collectables will isolate their particular smells from the occupants. A cabinet over the washer and dryer will be a good place to store laundry detergent. Closets are simply large built-in cabinets, and can be used to store other bothersome belongings. Metal shelving and storage systems with baked enamel finishes can make closets much more organized. One manufacturer of such a system is **Leigh Products.**

A problem with storing odorous things in cabinets or closets is the fact that the smells will build up there and be released into the room whenever the doors are opened. This may not be a great problem for a display cabinet that is only opened once a year, but a clothes closet may be opened a couple of times a day. For this reason, a very sensitive person will want to eliminate as many problem articles as possible, or store them outside the house in the garage. Closets and cabinets can be ventilated, so fresh air is always passing through them to the outdoors, carrying with it any offensive odors. While it is a natural moth repellant, cedar should not be used in closet construction if you are sensitive to its aroma.

Countertops

High-pressure laminate is the most often used material today because of its durability and low cost. "Formica" is one popular brand. This material is only about $1/16''$ thick and must be adhered to a heavier base material to produce a sturdy countertop. This base is usually particle board which, of course, emits formaldehyde fumes. The glue gives off a variety of undesirable odors as well. The plastic laminate itself is very hard and dense and many sensitive people can tolerate but not the glue or the particle board. By covering both the top and bottom and all edges of the particle board with laminate, the emissions will be lessened considerably. Also, if a good grade of plywood is substituted for the particle board, there will be less outgassing. Foil taped or stapled to the underside of the counter or several coats of a sealer will also help, but for very sensitive people, another countertop material is recommended.

"Corian," a product of **Du Pont Co.**, is an artificial marble that is tolerated by many sensitive people even through it is composed of marble dust and a plastic resin (methyl acrylate), apparently because it is so hard. It is somewhat more expensive than using a plastic laminate, but can be very attractive. Premolded sinks are available as well as flat sheets in different thicknesses. Other manufacturers make similar products.

Ceramic tile is a popular material for use on countertops. The most tolerable method of installing it involves a thick mortar bed, as discussed in Chapter 17, over a solid wood base. A double layer of $1/2''$

thick cementitious boards will provide a sturdy enough base to use with a dry set mortar. If the cementitious boards are odorous, foil can be taped to the back side prior to installation to help seal in any outgassing. Disadvantages to using ceramic tile on countertops include the fact that foods or beverages can stain the grout joints, and the working surface will not be perfectly flat. Petroleum-based sealers should never be used because they will contaminate foods placed on the countertop. Because of problems with grout cracking, and providing a place for mold to grow, caulking should be used between a tiled countertop and a tiled backsplash.

Wood chopping-block countertops are quite attractive, but they can eventually age, split, and harbor mold.[1] Being absorbent, they also retain food odors. Even relatively new tops will develop a slightly rough surface that can be a haven for food particles and various microorganisms. Some of these tops come with water-repellent preservatives that can cause problems for sensitive persons. The glue used to laminate them together can also be bothersome.

Marble tops will generally be well tolerated, but marble can be easily stained, so it might not be a good choice unless various heavy-duty cleaners are tolerated. A section of marble set in a countertop of another material might be a good solution for someone who prefers a marble surface for preparing pastry, or only one section of a counter could be made of marble, while the rest of the countertops are another material.

Stainless steel makes an excellent countertop material that is durable, nonstaining, and easy to clean. These tops will need to be custom made for each installation. Restaurant equipment suppliers will be able to either make them locally or direct you to a fabricator. If relatively thin 18 ga. stainless steel is used, it will need a backing of solid wood to provide the necessary rigidity. Most suppliers recommend using plywood rather than solid wood, in order to eliminate the possibility of warping which could cause the top to have a wavy surface. Heavier 14 ga. material will usually only need a couple of stiffening ribs that can be a part of the cabinet. These tops can either be glued down with an adhesive caulking or they can be fabricated with small mounting tabs. Some manufacturers apply a soundproofing material to the back side of the stainless steel. This should generally be eliminated because of its outgassing potential. If a backsplash is desired, it can be extended all the way up to the bottom of the wall cabinets, making the countertop and backsplash all in one easy-to-maintain piece. Sinks can be formed into the top as well, making a completely seamless installation; however, this can add considerably to the cost.

A porcelain countertop could be custom made as well, but the brittleness of the porcelain surface would dictate the use of a very stable backing material such as plywood or a cementitious board to which the porcelain should be glued. Porcelain was used in the past for countertops on various kitchen cupboards. Most of the porcelain tops that are seen in antique stores are badly chipped. This is evidence of the fact that it is not a durable material where heavy pots and pans are used.

Laboratory countertops can be an additional material to consider, although they are comparatively expensive. Many of these tops are made with synthetic resins, so care should be taken in selecting them.

Countertop inserts, such as those made by **Vance Industries**, can be nice to use. They are made of tempered glass in a variety of patterns with a stainless steel rim. The smooth, nonporous surface makes a good work or cutting area on ceramic tile tops. They are scratch, stain, and heat resistant and come in three sizes.

Sinks and Bathtubs

Kitchen sinks are made of a variety of materials. "Corian" has already been mentioned. Stainless steel, porcelain on steel, and porcelain on cast iron are all well tolerated. Some sinks have an odorous soundproofing material added to the back side which should be removed. For someone who prefers a colored sink to stainless steel, porcelain sinks will offer a variety of colors and styles. The porcelain on steel, like porcelain countertops, will not be able to tolerate a great deal of abuse. However, they can be easier to replace than a custom-made countertop if they become damaged. Porcelain on cast iron sinks are much more durable and long lasting. They are also considerably heavier and more expensive. Premium quality sinks are usually porcelain on cast iron.

Bathroom sinks are rarely seen in stainless steel, but porcelain sinks are common, both on steel and cast iron. These are "drop-ins" sinks that must be installed in a countertop, leaving a difficult-to-clean seam. Additionally, cultured marble sinks are popular. They usually combine the countertop, sink, and backslash in a one-piece, easy-to-clean unit. Unlike "Corian" tops, these are made with marble dust, or ground limestone, and a polyester binder and finish. They may also have a wax of some type on the surface. These products may not be tolerated very well by sensitive people. Other types of plastics are used in inexpensive bathroom sinks. Vitreous china sinks are also common. Being a glazed clay product they will be well tolerated. They are available in several different styles and colors from sources such as **Universal-Rundle Corporation** and **Sears, Roebuck and Co.** Vitreous china sinks are made either in "drop-in" styles, pedestal models, or one-piece units combining countertop, sink, and backsplash in one attractive piece.

Bathtubs of either porcelain on steel or on cast iron will be well tolerated. Again, the porcelain on cast iron will be a sturdier, heavier, and more costly choice. Various fiberglass and acrylic tubs and one-piece tub/shower combinations are also on the market. These may not be well tolerated by sensitive people, especially when they are warmed by hot water. They may have foam insulation sprayed on the back as soundproofing or utilize particle board stiffeners on the bottom or sides. A major advantage to these units, however, is the fact that they are easy to clean and have no seams that could harbor mold. Some less expensive shower stalls use enameled steel walls that should cause no outgassing problem.

For shower walls, ceramic tile and porcelain panels were briefly discussed in Chapter 18. Both can result in tolerated walls, but it must be remembered that caulking will be required with these installations. Stainless steel sheets can also be custom made to be used as shower walls, but an adhesive caulking will probably again be required to attach the panels to the existing wall and to seal any seams.

Toilets

Vitreous china toilets are well tolerated and can be found in several different styles. Toilet seats are commonly made of either hard or soft plastic or a painted particle board, all of which should be avoided by sensitive people. In recent years, the nostalgic look of the oak toilet seat has made a comeback. These seats make better choices but the finish can be problematic for some. Toilet tanks are notorious for sweating in warm, humid months. This moisture can eventually lead to a mold problem. **American Standard Inc.** and other manufacturers have toilets with insulated tanks that eliminate the sweating problem. While a foam product is used for the insulating material, it will be inside the tank and under water most of the time, so it should be easly tolerated.

Appliances

Appliances can be major contributors to indoor air pollution. These are discussed more completely in other sources.[2,3] Electric motors in clothes dryers, washing machines, or garbage disposers can give off ozone. Garbage disposers are, however, recommended in order to get rid of food scraps quickly, rather than allowing them to stand in a trash container and get moldy. Refrigerator coils get hot and can be bothersome. Cooking odors from stoves will bother some sensitive people as do odors given off by the heating elements themselves. Continuous cleaning ovens outgas whenever the oven is turned on. Microwave ovens have been shown to cause various health complaints. Trash compactors tend to be sources of mold and dishwashers give off a variety of smells from the plastic parts, insulation, motor, and cleaning products. If you are leery of installing a built-in dishwasher because of potential outgassing, simply design the cabinetry so that there is a 24″ wide cabinet next to the sink. At some future date, the cabinet can be removed and a dishwasher installed in its place.

Appliances are usually clustered in the kitchen, so it will be a good idea to have added ventilation in this room. In addition to the regular ventilation system, there should be a high-powered hood over the stove. Cooking odors often contain grease and should not be ducted through a heat recovery ventilator, since the grease could build up and cause a fire. A powerful range hood should be able to remove smells quickly, so it may need to be several times as powerful as the ventilation system that provides daily fresh air to the kitchen. Ductless range hoods with their small charcoal filters are very ineffective and should be avoided. If a gas range is used, an even more powerful ventilator is required because of the many toxic gases associated with burning gas. Gas appliances should be avoided if at all possible, as should all combustion appliances. When selecting a range hood, it is wise to buy one with the largest capacity available, and a variable speed control. In that way, it can be turned up to high speed whenever excessive cooking smells are generated or when a self-cleaning oven is going through its very odorous cleaning cycle. Under normal cooking conditions the fan can be run at a lower speed. At least one operable window should be located in the kitchen area. It can be opened when the range hood is operating at high speed in order to clear the room quickly of odors. A door between the kitchen and the rest of the house will prevent odors from permeating the entire living space.

Other appliances can also have their own ventilation systems. For instance, in an existing house without a well-planned ventilation system, the smell from the hot refrigerator coils may be a problem for some people. In this case, a small, low-powered exhaust fan could be placed behind the refrigerator not only to carry its particular odors outdoors, but to add to the general ventilation requirements of the rest of the room. The drip pan located under self-defrosting refrigerators should be cleaned regularly to minimize mold growth. If the washing machine and dryer are in a closet or small room adjacent to the kitchen or bathroom, the ventilation system can be designed to pull air through both areas. For example, a stale air register or a ventilation hood over a washer and dryer that is located in a closet, off the bathroom, will pull air from the hall, through the bathroom, and past the washer on its way outdoors. Since these rooms generate more moisture and odors than the other rooms in the house, they have higher general ventilation requirements to minimize any mold problems. As a rule of thumb, if moisture builds up on the bathroom mirror, there is not enough ventilation in that room.

Clothes dryers should always be exhausted outdoors separately from other ventilation systems, because of the large amounts of moisture present in dryer exhaust. It also contains allergenic lint and various fumes from clothing dyes and finishes, so indoor exhausts are not recommended.

The various fixtures used in kitchens and bathrooms should be metal or wood rather than plastic to avoid as much outgassing as possible. This includes toilet paper holders, towel racks, glass and toothbrush holders, and medicine cabinets. Towel racks should be wide enough to hold bath towels without folding them, so that they can dry quickly. Mirrors are often attached to the wall with a mastic glue. This should be avoided in favor of screws and clips.

Summary

Kitchen and bathrooms need to be planned out in several different ways. The layout used to be the main consideration, and for ease of working, layout is certainly important, but ventilation and selection of cabinets, fixtures, and appliances may be of more importance to a sensitive person. All that is required is a little forethought and planning to minimize any potential problems with outgassing, moisture, cooking odors, etc.

Chapter 21

Mechanical Components

The mechanical components discussed in this chapter include the heating, air conditioning, electrical, and plumbing systems. General ventilation systems are covered in Chapter 8 and filters in Chapter 22. These can all contribute to indoor pollution, and while it would certainly be possible to eliminate some of them, it is very unlikely that many people would be willing to do so. Therefore, it will be important in healthful houses to carefully select mechanical components and install them in a manner that their contribution to indoor air pollution will be minimal. The most complex system will be that which maintains a comfortable indoor temperature, namely, the heating and air conditioning system. While there are people who are sensitive to extremes of temperature, the larger problem with these systems involves the pollutants that they actually generate, particularly as a result of the fuel used. Chimneys are supposed to carry these pollutants out of the house, yet they are often found to be backdrafting, actually operating in reverse, preventing the combustion by-products from escaping. Newer heating systems can be insulated with materials such as fiberglass, while older systems can be contaminated with asbestos.

Combustion Fuels

As a rule, no combustion fuel of any type should be used in a healthy house. The major indoor air pollutants are, in fact, by-products of combustion and there is much evidence to indicate that the use of combustion fuels contributes to ill health. According to Dr. Theron Randolph, "Clinical susceptibility to gas, oil and coal—including their combustion products and related derivatives—is a common unsuspected cause of chronic symptoms."[1] Furnaces utilizing combustion fuels operate at fairly high temperatures and some sensitive people report symptoms related to various metals when they are heated.[2] For them, even metal cookware can be problematic, especially if made of aluminum.

Wood and coal are very old sources of heat. The use of coal today is generally confined to industrial situations and power plants, but wood heat has enjoyed a revival in recent years as a residential fuel. As an indoor pollution source, it is responsible for a wide variety of pollutants. The effects of particulates, nitrogen dioxide, sulfur dioxide, and carbon monoxide are well documented, but there are over 200 pollutants in wood smoke that are not as well known to the general public, some of which are carcinogenic, such as benz(a)anthracene, chrysene, benzofluoranthenes, etc.[3] These compounds certainly have a negative effect on health, but they have not been studied sufficiently to determine the extent of the damage. Wood stoves add as much as 200 times more particulate matter to the air than other heating methods.[4]

Children living in homes that are heated with wood have a much greater chance of having respiratory symptoms than children in homes without wood heat. One study found that 84 percent of children in wood-heated homes experienced at least one severe symptom of acute respiratory illness during a heating system, compared to only 3 percent in other homes. Symptoms include a history of coughing at night, coughing on most days, or occasional wheezing apart from colds. Allergies were present in 19.4 percent of the children in wood-heated homes compared to only 3.2. percent in the control group.[5] These symptoms are early manifestations of respiratory tract injury, and since young children are generally confined to the house more than adults or older children, especially in winter, it seems logical that they would be the first to exhibit symptoms. Prolonged exposure could certainly have an effect on all occupants. It is often possible to go into a house in the middle of the summer and smell the wood smoke that all of the furnishings have absorbed, evidence of considerable pollution from the heating season. This lingering odor means that burning wood in the winter can have an effect on health all year long. Although the effect will be less in the summer, it could easily bother sensitive people.

Obviously, the newer, tighter, more energy-efficient wood stoves will produce less pollutants than many older models, but they must all be opened in order to load them with wood. When the door is opened for loading, stoking, or ash removal, pollutants can enter the room. If a wood stove is improperly operated or installed, it can be even more polluting. Open fireplaces introduce considerably more pollutants into the living space than closed stoves. The combustion by-products that go up the chimney can easily reenter the living space through natural or forced ventilation. In moderate temperatures, if a stove is operated intermittently, it will not be as efficient (and more polluting) than one that is operated continuously at a constant temperature.

While they are not recommended, wood stoves should be as airtight and energy-efficient as possible, and they should be fitted with combustion air ducting to provide outdoor air rather than indoor air for burning. This creates a closed pathway from the outdoors to the stove and back to the outdoors, and will prevent the stove from pulling air from the living space. When a stove isn't fitted with such an air supply, it creates a lower air pressure in the house which makes it easier for outdoor air and radon to enter the living space. Since the outdoor air will often be contaminated with the wood smoke from the chimney, this is certainly not desirable. Catalytic converters can reduce chimney emissions, but they are rarely used because of increased cost. Only seasoned hardwoods should be burned, not resinous softwood. Treated lumber and nonwood products such as plastic should never be burned because of the highly toxic gases given off.

Unvented kerosene heaters have become popular for use as space heaters. They have been shown to emit not only the well known pollutants such as carbon monoxide, carbon dioxide, nitrogen dioxide, etc. but also mutagenic pollutants such as polycyclic aromatic hydrocarbons.[6] These types of compounds can cause damage to people at the chromosomal level that will show up in later generations. Emissions also include such things as pentachlorophenol, which is associated with many serious health effects. As a result of the tremendous amount of indoor pollution that these heaters are capable of generating, they have been banned in several states.[7] Simply opening a door to another room will not provide adequate ventilation for an unvented heater. It will only mean that two rooms will be contaminated instead of one.

Vented kerosene heaters are not as dangerous because the pollutants are directed outdoors rather than into the room. These will certainly be an improvement over unvented heaters, but they are still not recommended for use in a healthful house.

The major combustion products from natural gas are nitrogen oxide, nitrogen dioxide, and carbon monoxide. Every year many deaths occur from unvented or improperly vented gas heaters, primarily from carbon monoxide poisoning. Lesser quantities of formaldehyde, particulate matter, volatile organic compounds, and polynuclear aromatic hydrocarbons may also be present.[8] Highly toxic methyl mercaptan is the material used to give most natural gas its disagreeable odor.[9] While unvented gas ranges and space heaters should by all means by avoided, furnaces and water heaters that are vented to the outdoors have been often implicated in symptoms as well. Chimneys do not function very efficiently until they are heated up, so when a gas burner first ignites, a certain time period is required before the flue heats up, allowing the fumes to be drawn out of the house. In the meantime, the fumes filter into the living space. Symptoms of exposure to natural gas are very common among sensitive people, and they can range from a stuffed-up head to asthma, hyperactivity, confusion, and loss of consciousness.[10] These symptoms can occur with exposures that are considered acceptable by the gas industry and government agencies. Even the small amounts of pollutants given off by a pilot light can result in symptoms. Often the only way of providing relief to an occupant sensitive to natural gas is not only to remove the appliances and furnace, but to remove all the gas piping from the house as well.

Fuel oil has been implicated in ill health also. This can be due to the fumes given off by the furnace during the heating season, to residual fumes in the off-season, or due to leaking fuel oil. Old storage tanks are notorious for developing small leaks. If they are located in the basement, this smell can soak into the floor and be almost impossible to remove. It can easily permeate the whole house. Dr. Randolph describes what happened to one woman who walked into an oil heated hunting lodge. "She began to cough and wheeze within a few minutes after entering the building, and became unconscious."[11]

Symptoms of exposure to combustion by-products are quite varied, sometimes minor, and sometimes severe. As with exposures to many pollutants, minor exposures over long periods can result in ill health in later years that has no readily discernable cause. There are so many reports of the negative health effects of combustion products, and so many people are exhibiting hypersensitivity reactions to these products that it is becoming apparent that combustion fuels should not be used in houses at all. A possible exception that might cautiously be acceptable would be to have the furnace housed totally outside the home. In a separate structure or enclosure, it could be used to heat water, which could be used to heat the house via insulated piping. While this would remove all of the combustion products from the house, there would still be the possibility of them getting into the house with ventilation air. Such a remote furnace should, therefore, be located downwind. **Amana Refrigeration, Inc.** manufactures a furnace like this in their "HTM Plus" series. Since combustion fuels are so undesirable, we will limit most of our discussion to more healthful fuels such as electricity and solar.

If an existing house is heated with a combustion fuel, the furnace should be separated as much as possible from the living space. If the furnace is located in a utility room or garage, the door should be kept closed and weather-stripped to prevent fumes from seeping into the house. All ductwork should be taped at the seams to prevent fumes from seeping into it and being dispersed throughout the house. The gas company can check to see if there are any leaks in the furnace that would contaminate the warm air. It may be necessary to keep the window in the furnace room open slightly to provide combustion air to the furnace, so there isn't a negative pressure created in the house that could result in unnecessary infiltration of outside air or radon from the ground.

Heating System Types

Heating systems are made in many different styles and types, with forced air, forced hot water, and individual unit heaters all being popular. Any of these can be operated by electricity, thus avoiding the use of combustion fuels. If converting the heating system of a house from a combustion fuel to electricity, it may be necessary to provide more electrical capacity. An electrician can determine whether or not the existing electric service is sufficient for the additional load imposed by electric heat. It may involve changing the meter, some wiring, and the power panel. Electric heat can be more expensive than using combustion fuels, so it would be important to consider upgrading the insulation in order to make the change-over more cost effective.

Each type of heating system has advantages and disadvantages from a health standpoint. Very sensitive people should select a system with care because, according to one authority, "Cumulative experience has indicated that none of the systems...is tolerable to every chemically susceptible person."[12]

Forced Air Heat

Forced air systems utilize a cabinet with a heating unit, fan, and filter enclosed in a variety of configurations. The fan moves air through the filter, across the heating unit, through a ducting system, and into the house by way of registers. A return duct allows the cooler air from the house to reenter the furnace, completing the cycle. The heating coil can be simply a resistance wire like that found in a toaster, that gets hot when electricity is turned on by the thermostat. While this can certainly provide warmth, it is not economically the most cost-effective method of using electricity. Heat pumps have been developed to do this job more efficiently, but they often have the resistance wires also, as a back-up system. This is necessary because heat pumps lose their efficiency as the outdoor temperature drops. During moderate temperatures, however, they can be several times as efficient as a simple resistance coil, so in milder climates they can be very cost effective. In harshly cold climates, a heat pump may still be desirable, but it may be more cost effective to add additional insulation to a house.

There are several difficulties with forced air systems from a health standpoint. The cabinet of the furnace can contain insulation that will outgas. Sometimes this can be removed and reinstalled on the outside of the cabinet, where it will not contaminate the airstream. The electric motor that runs the fan can emit ozone or give off smells from oil or electrical insulation as it warms up during operation. Sometimes, the motor on the fan can be removed and remounted on the outside of the furnace cabinet, outside the airstream. The filter normally supplied with a furnace can be odorous because of various oils sprayed onto it to increase efficiency. If the furnace contains resistance heating wires, they can be responsible for "fried dust."[13] This occurs when house dust passes through the inefficient furnace filter and comes in contact with the very hot wires and is burned. This burnt dust gives off a variety of combustion products. The fried dust phenomenon also occurs in furnaces that use combustion fuels. For this not to be a problem, the heating unit should get no hotter than 250°F. If the dust contains syn-

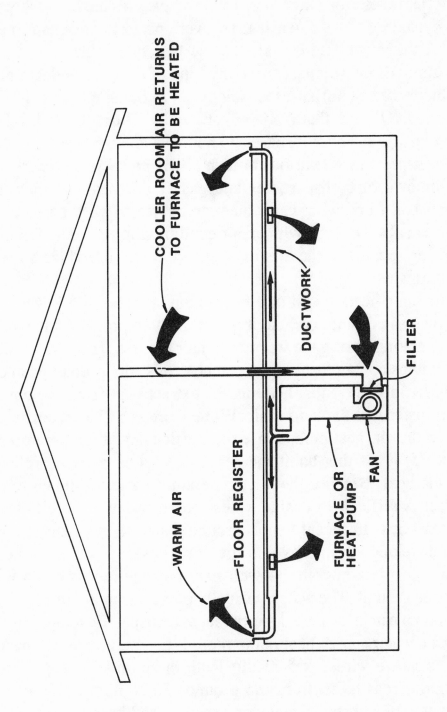

Forced Air Heating System

thetic particles from a carpet, for example, it can produce phosgene and cyanide gases.[14] Even if there were no synthetic materials in the house, the dust could contain a wide variety of "natural" materials. The combustion products from any kind of dust are undesirable.

One forced air furnace that stands out as being more healthful is the "Series IAQ" unit that is manufactured by **Thurmond Development Coroporation**. These furnaces do not have any exposed insulation and can be supplied with various hi-tech HEPA and activated carbon filters for removal of both particles and gases. For heating, they utilize a copper coil filled with water that can be heated with a remote boiler. They can also be fitted with an air conditioning coil. The fan motor is, however, located in the airstream where it can introduce some minor contaminants.

The main heating coil of a heat pump operates at a lower temperature than a resistance coil, so it is less likely to produce fried dust when it is operating during the warmer winter months. However, since most heat pumps contain back-up resistance coils, the problem can develop in colder months. Most heat pumps extract heat from the outdoor air and transfer it to the indoor air. While there is still a certain amount of heat in the air, heat pumps lose their efficiency at temperatures below about 35°F. At this point the resistance wires must be relied on to provide heat. Because the air temperature varies so much during the year, it is difficult to design a heat pump that will be efficient at all temperatures. In recent years, ground water source heat pumps have been developed to improve on the drawbacks of extracting heat from the air. In these systems, a well may be required to bring water up from the ground. The water is usually of a constant temperature, so the heat pump can be designed to operate at that specific temperature. This makes a water source heat pump more efficient, and less dependent on the resistance wires. A difficulty with these units is disposing of the water that was taken from the ground. Some municipalities will not allow it to be returned by way of a second well because of the possibility of contaminating the ground water, and it should not be put into a sanitary sewer. If the water cannot be deposited in a drainage ditch or storm sewer, a very large drainage field will need to be constructed to dispose of it. This field will be in addition to any required septic field, because the amount of water would easily overload a septic system.

Water-source heat pumps are also available that extract heat from the ground by using a closed loop system; thus, the water disposal problem is eliminated. A loop of plastic piping is buried around the house to provide a heat source for the furnace. The depth of the piping is selected to provide a uniform temperature that will allow the heat pump to operate efficiently during the year; however, resistance heating wires may still be required. Manufacturers include **FHP Manufacturing** and **WaterFurnace International, Inc.**

Heat pumps use Freon to transfer the heat from a compressor unit to a heating coil within the furnace cabinet. While this is a closed system, there is still the remote possibility of a leak forming and the house being contaminated with Freon. Freon has been implicated in health problems in sensitive people, and on a larger scale it has been implicated in helping to destroy the ozone layer in the atmosphere. One function of the ozone layer is to protect us from harmful radiation from the sun. Without it, skin cancer rates increase.

Air Conditioning

Air conditioners are mechanically similar to heat pumps. They move heat from the indoor air to the outdoor air (or water). This results in a cooler house. Most heat pumps have a reversing capability that will provide a house with heat in winter and "cool" in summer. The heating coil in the furnace cabinet becomes, in effect, a cooling coil. Some window air conditioning units have this reversing ability as well. Not all air conditioners, however, can supply heat. If it is called an "air conditioner" it can only be used for cooling. If it is called a "heat pump," it should be able to be used for either heating or cooling.

If air conditioning is desired, it will often be necessary to rely on a forced air system, as described above. Drawbacks from a health standpoint include sensitivities to insulation in the cabinet, the filter, and the electric motor. An additional problem with air conditioners concerns mold. The cooling coil can get so cold that the warm humid air passing through it causes moisture to condense, thus air conditioners will remove moisture from the air, resulting in lower humidity. There is a drip pan and a drain line provided to collect this water, but the pan makes a good place for mold to grow. All air conditioners have such a drip pan that should be inspected and cleaned periodically. For very sensitive persons, this cleaning may be required as often as weekly during the cooling season, but generally filters and grilles will need to be cleaned more often than the cooling coil inside the unit or the drip pan. A switch that allows the fan to be run, without the cooling portion of the air conditioner operating, will be helpful. With only the fan running, any residual moisture in the cooling coil or drip pan will be evaporated. However, if mold growth is a continual problem, sprinkling a layer of borax in the pan might help. Another possible solution would be to line the pan with copper, since it will be toxic to many microorganisms. Copper foil can be obtained through craft or hobby stores, and some roofing suppliers may have copper flashing that can be used.

Air conditioners are often recommended for allergy patients. The primary reason for this is the fact that the windows will be closed when the air conditioner is running, thus mold and pollen spores will tend to remain outdoors. Air conditioners usually contain filters, so they will filter out some of the offending particles from the indoor air. These filters, however, are generally not very efficient. Since air conditioners remove moisture from the air, they can make it physically easier to breathe for those with heart or chronic respiratory problems.

When selecting an air conditioner for an oasis, or a superinsulated house, a small capacity unit will be all that is necessary. These will typically contain several plastic parts that can outgas, as can some of the electrical or mechanical components. Small split system units have recently been introduced that utilize an outdoor condenser and a separate indoor unit that are connected only by an electrical wire and two fluid lines. While these still contain plastic parts, they are very quiet, compact, and may be less offensive because much of the equipment is outside the living space. Manufacturers include **Monitor Products Inc.** and **Sanyo.** These can be set up with a single outdoor unit and up to three indoor units located in different rooms, which make them a good alternative to a ducted air conditioning system. Some models are heat pumps that can be used for both heating and cooling.

In some parts of the country, evaporative coolers, also known as "swamp coolers," are used to supply cool air to the house.[15] They operate by pulling the hot air through a water-soaked filter. The water evaporates, resulting in cooler air that is ducted into the house. This can be an economical method of providing cool air, but it can also create a breeding ground for microorganisms such as Legionella bacteria.

Ductwork

Most forced air systems require ductwork to distribute the air around the house. Traditionally this has been made out of metal, which is relatively inert; however, new metal ductwork can contain a thin oil film that will bother sensitive persons. Washing with TSP or a tolerated detergent will easily remove this coating. The joints between straight sections and fittings can allow dust, radon, or microorganisms to enter the airstream and be blown throughout the house. These joints should generally be sealed with tape. The commonly used "duct tape" will not be as tolerable as the slightly more expensive aluminum foil tape, which is available from heating equipment suppliers.

Some older ductwork can be found that is insulated with asbestos. If this material is deteriorating, the easiest solution may be to seal it with a securely taped foil barrier. However, if there are loose-fitting joints between sections of ductwork, the fibers could find their way into the airstream. In this situation, very careful removal may be necessary. (See Chapter 1.) Today, it is often common practice to insulate metal ducts with fiberglass insulation on the inside of the duct. This should never be done because of the danger of contaminating the airstream with fiberglass particles or outgassing products from the insulation's binder. Insulation should only be placed on the outside of the ducting. One household was exposed to so many glass fibers emitted from an air conditioning system that they were forced to abandon their home. A family member and their dog developed cancer, possibly as a result of this exposure.[16]

Some flexible ducting is available that is constructed with a plastic sleeve around fiberglass insulation. It should be avoided for similar reasons since it has no protective inner lining. Some heating systems utilize ductwork that is cast inside the concrete floor slab with the actual duct material being an asbestos cement product. If this is cracked, broken or abraded, it can introduce asbestos fibers into the airstream.

Ductwork used in air conditioning systems will be cool, and when run through unconditioned areas such as attics and crawl spaces, it should be insulated. Without insulation, the humidity in the air can condense on the surface of the duct into liquid water. This can result in a mold problem. If the seams in the ducting are taped, fiberglass can be wrapped around the outside of the duct without contaminating the airstream. This should, in turn, be wrapped with a moisture barrier that is also well sealed. If the moisture barrier is not taped at all seams, moisture will find its way through to the cooler duct and condense there.

Return air lines that allow the room air to return to the furnace or central air conditioning unit are often run through stud spaces or the spaces between floor joists in order to save on the cost of metal ducts. This should not be done because of the possibility of contaminating the airstream with products outgassed from the various building materials.

A general difficulty with all warm air systems that use ductwork is cleaning it. Since the filters used in most systems are somewhat inefficient, they will not trap all of the dust that passes through the furnace. The ductwork, over the years, can become quite dirty as a result, and contribute to reintroducing dust back into the house. If the ducting system isn't very complicated it can sometimes be cleaned with a long vacuum hose, but the cleaning operation itself can stir up accumulated dust that can then be spread throughout the house.

Forced Hot Water Heating

In a forced hot water system, water is heated in a boiler by electricity or another fuel. The hot water is then distributed throughout the house through pipes to radiators, where heat is released into the room. The warm air circulates around the radiators and through the room naturally, without fans. Hot water can also be circulated through tubing that is cast in a concrete slab. As the water cools, it returns to the boiler to be reheated. In a hybrid system, water is heated in a boiler and passed through a heating coil inside a forced air furnace. Some solar systems use a closed loop of water (or another fluid) that is heated by the sun and then piped through the house.

Many older buildings have cast iron radiators that are part of a hot water system. These often operate by gravity. With this method of heating, water is heated in a boiler that is usually located in the basement. The hot water rises through pipes to radiators on upper floors, cools, and falls back to the boiler through another set of pipes. All of this is done without pumps. It is based on the principle that warm fluids rise, and cool fluids fall. The pipes on many of these older systems are insulated with asbestos. This insulation was still being manufactured as recently as 1972.[17] Most modern hot water systems use pumps to distribute the water because they are easier to control and the result is more even and comfortable heat.

Forced hot water systems do not rely on fans to move heated air, so

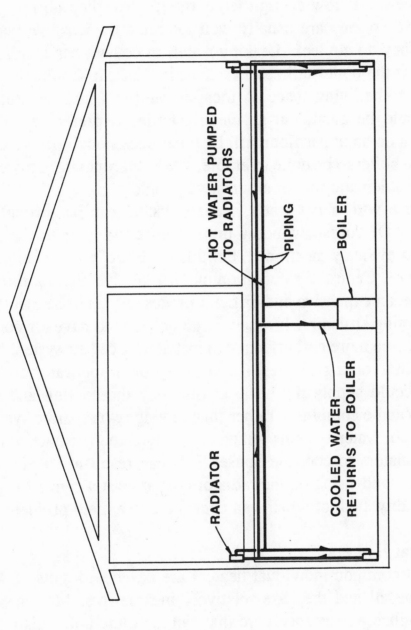

Forced Hot Water Heating System

there is no danger of contamination from fan motors. Nor do they use air filters. If a separate ventilating system is available to filter the air, a filtered heating system may not be necessary. Hot water systems generally operate at low enough temperatures that they do not generate fried dust, so they are usually well tolerated by sensitive people, as long as they do not leak. Leaking water, of course, can result in mold growth. If the boiler utilizes a combustion fuel, it should be well isolated from the living space. A location outdoors, in a separate structure, would be good, but an electric boiler is preferred. Often, an apartment on an upper floor will be separated enough from a combustion-fired boiler to be quite tolerable, while apartments on lower floors can be problematic for some sensitive people.

A house with a hot water heating system can be difficult to air condition. Of course, window units can be used, or the small split systems previously mentioned, but this might be impractical in a very large house. Central air conditioning will involve ducting throughout the house, an expensive and difficult process if it is to be incorporated in an existing structure. If a new large house is to have air conditioning, it may be more cost effective to install a forced air system for both heating and cooling. Either a heat pump or a hot water coil in the furnace could supply the heat. In this way the cooling and heating systems can be combined, rather than having two separate systems.

Some hot water systems utilize a "chiller" to distribute cold water to the radiators to cool the house. This can result in water from the humid air condensing on the radiators, or at least a zone of high relative humidity, both of which can contribute to a mold problem.

Individual Heaters

The most common individual heaters are baseboard units. These are easy to install and they are relatively inexpensive. Most baseboard heaters utilize a resistance wire that can get quite hot. This results in the fried dust problem previously mentioned. Many people notice a disagreeable odor associated with these units.

A less common type of baseboard heater is the hydronic type. These are, in effect, self-contained hot water heaters that operate at approximately 200°F. Outwardly, they look like other baseboard units but they contain a hermetically sealed copper tube that is filled with water (or another fluid). This tube has an internal electric heating wire. The advantage over the more common resistance type heaters is the fact that they operate at a lower temperature. This means no fried dust. They are no less energy efficient than other electric heaters, but are not as efficient as heat pumps. The copper tubes are sometimes fitted with aluminum fins that can gather dust, so they should be cleaned periodically with a vacuum and/or brush. When new, they may contain traces of an oil film that can bother some people. This is easily burned off by leaving the heaters turned on high for three or four days. For sensitive people, this should not be done indoors. Heaters that are "burned off" outdoors should be properly wired by an electrician and protected from the weather to minimize any electrical or fire danger. These individual hydronic heaters are recommended often for sensitive persons; however, a few people do report symptoms with them, so they should be tested prior to use. For individuals sensitive to heated aluminum, it would be wise to avoid heaters with aluminum parts.

Intertherm, Inc. manufactures two basic lines of hydronic baseboards, "Softheat" and "Softheat II," that are available in either models to be permanently attached to the wall, or portable models that can be moved from room to room. The "Softheat" version has a foam plastic strip on the back of the metal case that sensitive persons will want to remove. **Berko Electric** has a similar hydronic baseboard heater in their "EBH series." It is not available in a portable style, only in models to be permanently mounted. All baseboard heaters come in different lengths ranging from two to nine feet. The longer units supply more heat than the shorter ones. An electrician or heating contractor can easily determine the correct size for a particular application.

If a heater is designed to operate at 220 volts, and it is only hooked up to 110 volts, it will not get as hot and as a result may be more tolerable to sensitive people. Of course, there would need to be more heaters installed in a given room to allow for the diminished heating ability.

Many portable heaters of this type are being manufactured and sold through department stores. The oil-filled types should be tolerable as long as they don't leak, but units that have a painted heating element may require an extended outgassing period in order to be tolerated by sensitive persons.

Radiant Heaters

Heat can be transferred from a heater to people by three different methods: conduction, convection, and radiation. Conduction involves

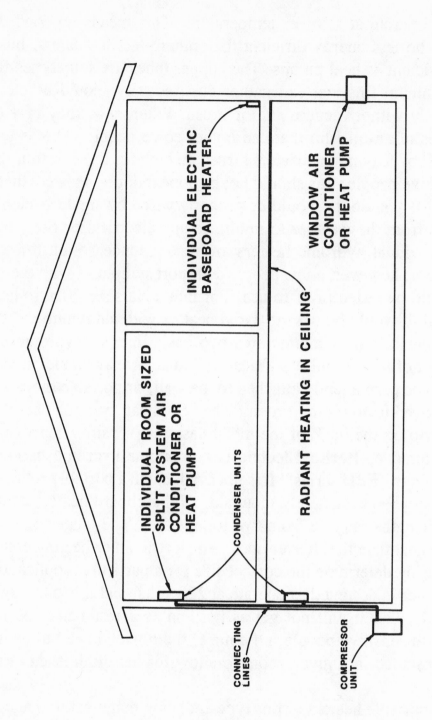

INDIVIDUAL ELECTRIC BASEBOARD HEATER

WINDOW AIR CONDITIONER OR HEAT PUMP

INDIVIDUAL ROOM SIZED SPLIT SYSTEM AIR CONDITIONER OR HEAT PUMP

CONDENSER UNITS

RADIANT HEATING IN CEILING

CONNECTING LINES

COMPRESSOR UNIT

Other Heating and Cooling Systems

the transfer of heat through solid objects. When you actually touch a heater, you will feel its warmth by conduction. This method of heat transfer is important in insulated walls where heat flow is not desired. Convection involves heat transfer by fluids. Air and water are both fluids, so this method of heat transfer is used in forced water and air heating systems. Radiation involves the transfer of energy from a heater to an object. This energy can be in the form of sunlight or infrared waves, and is technically not heat itself. As soon as this energy strikes a surface, it is transformed into heat. The heat that the earth receives from the sun is in the form of radiant energy. The warmth that is felt by someone standing in front of a hot stove is also in the form of radiant energy.

Most heating devices rely on a combination of heat transfer methods to keep the occupants warm. Some are specially designed to create primarily radiant energy. These types of heaters are said to heat "objects, not air." People and other objects will be warmed quickly by these heaters. Radiant energy will not flow around and behind objects, so a piece of furniture could block it from reaching the other items in a room. For this reason, individual radiant heaters are often placed near or on the ceiling, where they are not likely to be blocked. Placement of these heaters is more critical than with other heater types, and when located high on a wall or on the ceiling, they may not be very attractive.

A radiant heater can accelerate the outgassing of objects that are heated by it.[18] This is because the object may get warmer with radiant heat than it would with another form of heat. Most radiant heaters operate at temperatures that can result in fried dust. Residential heaters of this type are available in wall, baseboard, and cove styles, in addition to ceiling, bath, and portable models. They may have either stainless steel, baked enamel, or aluminum parts. One type of radiant heater uses a metal heating element fused to a glass or ceramic plate. These heaters should be chosen with care because they have been implicated in causing symptoms in some sensitive people even after several days of outgassing.[19] This could be due to the synthetic material used to bond the heating element to the plate.

Workers in the glass industry and the iron and steel industry are exposed to a considerable amount of radiant energy, and as a result they can develop cataracts if protective eyewear is not worn.[20] While residential radiant heating systems do not begin to emit the levels of energy that these workers are exposed to, someone with a family history of cataracts might wish to avoid them for this reason.

An advantage to using radiant heaters is the fact that they can usually be operated at a lower cost than heaters that primarily utilize convection to transfer heat. People heated with radiant energy are warmer at lower temperatures, so energy savings can result.

A specialized type of radiant heating system involves heating cables that are embedded in a gypsum ceiling, either plaster or drywall. These operate at a low enough temperature to not result in fried dust and they are totally unobtrusive. Since the ceiling looks no different than any other ceiling, the only evidence of any type of heating in the entire house is the appearance of a thermostat on the wall. A problem that could theoretically occur with very sensitive people living with this type of installation is outgassing from the paper on the gypsum panels when they are warmed by the heating cables. However, since the heat given off is at such a low temperature, it is doubtful that this would be a problem for most people as long as the plaster, drywall joint compound, or paint was not problematic.

Solar Heating

Solar heating is a low temperature method of heating, so it should not result in fried dust. Of the two types of solar heating, passive and active, passive systems are by far the simplest and easiest to maintain. A passive system has no moving parts. It simply involves sunlight passively coming through the windows and warming the house. The design of the house will affect how well it can be heated passively. The size and placement of the windows are very important, as is the shading of the windows in the summer when solar heating is not desired. An improperly designed house that has too many windows can overheat during the day and get too cold at night.

About the only disadvantage of passive solar heating, from a health point of view, is the fact that as the sunlight falls on objects inside the house it can cause accelerated outgassing as it warms them up. This will not be a significant problem if the objects are not synthetic materials that are subject to outgassing, such as artificial fibers in draperies and carpets. Sunlight can, however, degrade natural materials such as cotton or wool rugs and cause them to give off dust particles. Passive solar heating is used in superinsulated house designs because it is an inexpensive way to bring heat into the house and it requires no operat-

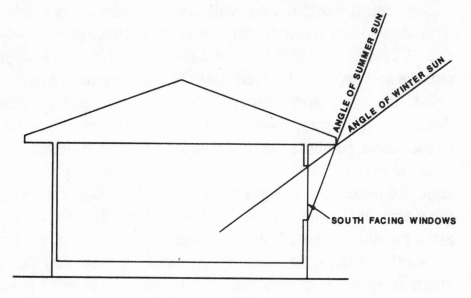

PASSIVE SYSTEM

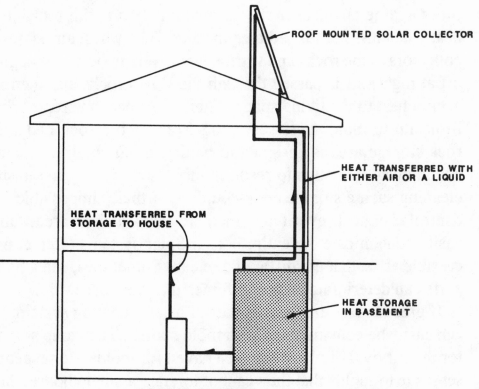

ACTIVE SYSTEM

Solar Heating

ing system. It work automatically and it doesn't break down.

Active solar heating systems involve collecting the sun's energy in one place and transferring it either directly to the living space or to a storage area so it can be used later. These systems can be quite complicated, involving solar collectors on the roof, pumps, fans, piping, ductwork, temperature sensors, storage areas, etc. Many solar-heated houses use a combination of active and passive systems. For example, a greenhouse or sunroom could collect heat passively and store it in a concrete floor, then at night as the house begins to cool off, fans blow the warm air into the rest of the living space. Some active systems use air to transfer the heat from the collector to the house, others use water or another liquid. In freezing climates, precautions must be taken when using water in an outdoor collector, so it doesn't freeze.

There can be several disadvantages to active systems that should be addressed by a sensitive person. If air is used to transfer the heat from the collectors to the house, ducts and fans will be required and the same precautions that pertain to any warm air system apply. Sometimes a large chamber in the basement is filled with rocks to store the heat when it is not immediately needed. The warm air passes from the collectors to the rocks and warms them. When the house begins to cool off at night, air is passed through the warm rocks and then returns to supply heat to the living space. There is at least one report that related ill health to mold spores escaping from such a rock bed.[21] Even if a rock storage area is designed to be dry, a plumbing leak could easily contaminate it enough to result in mold growth. In some installations, cleaning such a storage area would be virtually impossible. If termite control chemicals ever found their way into such an area, fumes could easily contaminate the entire house. Solar systems often contain inaccessible areas that are difficult to clean. Sometimes, sealants or plastic parts can deteriorate and send fumes into the house.

If greenhouses are used as part of a solar heating system, the house can easily be contaminated with mold spores. The damp soil necessary for the survival of plants can be a haven for molds. Some people are so sensitive to molds that they cannot tolerate a single house plant, much less a greenhouse full of plants, pollen, and mold. Commonly used gardening chemicals such as fertilizers and pesticides can also be problematic.

When liquid is used to transfer heat, a large tank may be located in the basement for heat storage. Separate lines may be run from the tank to a furnace or radiators in order to heat the living space. Pumps are used to move the warmed liquid around through a piping system. Plastic pipes are often used that can outgas when warmed by the liquid. If water is used and it freezes, the piping can rupture and water can rain down, usually in an inaccessible place inside a wall. If a leak involves a liquid other than water, such as antifreeze, this will certainly have a negative effect on a sensitive person's health.

There are, of course, many healthful solar heating installations. Since the design of these systems can be quite varied, all of the unhealthy possibilities cannot be adequately covered, but if the designer is aware of the general principles covered in this book, it should be relatively easy to circumvent any potential problem areas. As a rule, passive systems will be less problematic than active systems. It should be remembered that a solar heating system will only work when the sun is shining, and no matter how large the storage system, some form of back-up heating will always be necessary. Therefore, with all systems, insulation is of prime importance, in order to keep the cost of back-up heating low and also to keep the overall heating equipment size small. An uninsulated house needs a large solar system and a large secondary system, but a well insulated house needs only a small solar system and a small secondary system. This is the principle of superinsulated houses: use a lot of insulation, and no matter what kind of heat is used, the requirements will be small.

Electrical Systems

Modern houses have relatively complicated electrical systems compared to houses in the early part of the century, because of the increased use of electrical appliances, electric heating, lighting, etc. Still, there are only a few basic components common to both eras: switches, receptacles, wire, and electrical boxes. Circuit breakers have largely replaced fuses and some plastic materials are being used more and more, but the basic components are the same. The reason for the increased use of plastic is because it is cheaper and it is a good insulator.

There are a couple of things that should be discussed with the electric utility prior to construction. Most healthful houses are "all electric," and they may thus qualify for lower electric rates. If an electrical power pole must be located near the house, request one that is pressure-treated with arsenic salts rather than creosote, to avoid outgassing. Underground electric service may be possible to keep any type of treated poles far from the house.

Receptacles and switches are made of a fairly hard plastic, as are most cover plates. These are subject to very little outgassing, and are often well tolerated by sensitive people. Even less offensive stainless steel cover plates are readily available through electrical supply firms, and ceramic, wood, or brass covers are sold in hardware and department stores or bath shops.

Circuit breakers are also made of a hard plastic that is relatively free of outgassing. They are usually housed in a metal box, or power panel that is painted. While the paint can cause reactions in a few sensitive people, generally it should not be a problem. It can be purchased early in the construction process and allowed to air out before installation.

Some electrical components, such as doorbells, use small transformers to reduce the voltage. These tend to get warm and can give off odors. They should be located where the smell won't migrate into the living space.

The individual electrical boxes that house switches and receptacles have traditionally been metal, but today plastic boxes are often being used because of their lower cost. Metal boxes are still readily available, and they make better choices to someone concerned with outgassing. In superinsulated houses using the airtight drywall approach, where a sealed electrical box is required on some walls to minimize infiltration, most metal boxes can be difficult to make airtight. One solution is to use a cast waterproof box with a plaster extension ring. The ring and the wire entering the box are both caulked, leaving only the front of the box open. A bead of caulking is then used around the plaster ring to seal the box to the rear of the foil-backed drywall. With this type of installation, there should be no infiltration through the switch or receptacle.

A major outgassing component in any electrical installation is the wire itself. Plastic jacketing is used almost exclusively because of its low cost and good insulating ability. Unfortunately, the soft plastic also outgasses considerably. It can be run inside a metal conduit to effectively seal it from the living space. There are several types of conduit available, including plastic which would outgas itself. A lightweight thin-wall conduit, called "EMT," would be the least expensive choice, but a heavier rigid conduit is also available. A flexible metal conduit can be purchased with or without electrical wiring already inside. A flexible steel conduit, or armored cable, without wire inside is commonly called "greenfield," while "BX" is the designation usually given to the prewired product. These flexible products are spiral-wound steel, so they do not form a perfect seal around the wire. While the seal is very good, it is not impervious to water. When electricians pull wire through a conduit, they often use an odorous lubricant that can bother sensitive people. A tolerated liquid soap can be used instead.

There is a type of wire on the market called "metal-clad cable" that is very easy to use. It is encased in a thin layer of aluminum that acts as a protective conduit as well as sealing in any outgassing. It is available in rolls and can be easily bent by hand to snake its way through a house. "Signa/Clad" is one product, manufactured by **Coleman Cable System, Inc.** They also make an aluminum "Corra/Clad" product that resembles the conventional steel armored cable, but is totally sealed, thus forming a better barrier against outgassing.

When upgrading the wiring in an existing house, there are surface-mounted wiring systems that encase the wire in a decorative metal track, thus minimizing any outgassing from the plastic jacketing. One manufacturer is the **Wiremold Co.** These systems are typically painted, so sensitive people should test them for outgassing.

Electric wire that is sealed from the living space by a material like foil-backed drywall should not contaminate the air in the house. Even wiring protected by standard unbacked drywall may be separated enough, but the true test will not come until the house is complete, and a sensitive occupant notices the smell of the wire through the drywall. If using conduit- or metal-clad cable seems too expensive, the plastic wiring can be wrapped with aluminum foil before the drywall or plaster is applied. This will effectively seal in any outgassing. Either builders foil or the grocery store variety can be used. Wire for telephones, TV cable, and doorbells can also be problematic and should be sealed from the living space.

A few people react to the electrical and magnetic fields surrounding electrical wires or appliances. The electric fields can be shielded if the wire is encased in a grounded metal conduit. Foil-backed drywall could possibly be used for this purpose, but would be difficult to ground properly unless it was attached to a grounded steel framing system. Unfortunately, there is no way to shield magnetic fields.

House wiring will generate only very weak fields compared to high-voltage transmission lines, etc.

Light fixtures can be made from a variety of materials such as plastic, ceramic, glass, metal, wood, etc. Since they will become warm from the heat given off by the light bulb, low outgassing materials should be chosen. Plastic fixtures will generally be poor choices and wood will be marginal, depending on the finish and species. Recessed light fixtures will not collect dust, but they can cause interference problems with a continuous vapor barrier when installed in an insulated ceiling.

Lighting

There has been much written about the effects of light on health.[22,23,24] The problem with lighting in houses is that it is artificially created, and is different in composition from sunlight, primarily in that it lacks the beneficial low-frequency ultraviolet portion of the spectrum. Among other effects, it has been shown that the use of full-spectrum light bulbs can improve behavior in hyperactive children and that the children will have less tooth decay.[25] While a certain amount of ultraviolet light is beneficial to health, it can cause a photochemical reaction to take place with some indoor air pollutants, changing them into different types of pollutants.[26]

Full-spectrum "Vita Lite" fluorescent lamps are manufactured and sold by **Duro-Test Corporation** or through various distributors. **Ott Light Systems** sells a complete fixture containing full-spectrum tubes and an auxiliary ultraviolet tube. The fixtures are designed to shield the small amounts of cathode radiation and radio frequency radiation given off by all fluorescent lamps. It should be noted that fluorescent lamp fixtures often contain a ballast that can outgas fumes into living space when it gets warm. Prior to 1978, many of these ballasts contained PCBs.[27]

Full-spectrum lighting has been found to be beneficial in alleviating symptoms of seasonal affective disorder (SAD).[28,29] With this condition, people can experience symptoms of depression, fatigue, weight gain, etc. during winter months because of less exposure to sunlight. Five to six hours of exposure per day to bright full-spectrum lighting can successfully reverse the symptoms.

Whether or not you choose to utilize full-spectrum lighting, it is always recommended that a certain amount of time be spent outdoors in natural sunlight.

Plumbing Systems

Plumbing systems carry water into our houses to be used, and away from our houses when we are done with it. Since most water supplies contain contaminants of some type, it is a good idea to install a water filter or treatment device to insure the quality of the water. For some people, it is not only a good idea, it is mandatory, since many are now finding it difficult to tolerate even the minor contaminants present.

The plumbing lines themselves can be a major contributor to contaminating the water in a house. While lead pipes are no longer used in new construction, they can still be found in some older houses. The lead can leach out into the water causing ill health.[30] Galvanized steel pipes are much more inert, but they are rarely used today in residential construction because of the increased cost. In general, galvanized steel and copper piping are the least toxic materials to use; however, it has been suggested that some galvanizing processes can impart small amounts of cadmium into the water.[31] Copper pipes are believed to be quite safe, but one writer has suggested that people can absorb enough copper from drinking water to result in a zinc deficiency.[32] A larger problem with copper piping is the fact that the joints and fittings are usually soldered together. Solder has typically contained a considerable amount of lead that can leach out into the water, especially if it is soft or acidic. The amount of lead leaching into the water depends on several different factors, and there are many installations where the lead remains in the solder and does not migrate into the water. The best way to determine the lead content of water is to have it tested. Recently, the amount of lead used in solder has been limited to only a trace amount, so it will not be a problem in new installations. Another drawback to soldering copper pipe is the fact that the pipe must be coated with flux before soldering. A certain amount of flux can be transferred to the water where it will bother some sensitive people; however, after a certain time most of the flux should be flushed out of the lines. In order to eliminate soldering completely, flared brass fittings or brass compressions fittings can be used for all connections, but they may be more likely to leak.

Plastic piping is being used more and more because of its low cost; however, there is the danger of it contaminating the water. It can also outgas into the living space and contaminate the air, especially when used for hot water lines. PVC plastic has been shown to outgas diethylphthalate, trimethylhexane, aliphatic hydrocarbons, and aromatic hydrocarbons.[33] The solvents and glues used with plastic lines can also be problematic, contaminating both the water and the air.

Cold water supply lines can allow humidity from the air to condense on them, resulting in "sweating," which can supply the moisture necessary for a mold problem. This can be prevented by using a readily available foam pipe insulation; however, this product can outgas and bother sensitive people. In order to avoid this possibility, the insulation can be wrapped with foil to seal it.

Water heaters should be either electric or solar, instead of relying on combustion fuels. Some water heaters have a plastic lining. This should be avoided in favor of a more inert glass lining. The insulation used in water heaters is usually either fiberglass or a foam product, of which the fiberglass is the slightly better choice. As the unit gets hot, outgassing from the insulation is a possibility, but since it is surrounded by a metal container, it should not be a major problem. Taping all the seams with a foil tape will lessen the effects of outgassing.

Private wells often use a pressurized tank to maintain water pressure in the house. Plastic tanks or those with a rubber bladder should be avoided in favor of galvanized steel tanks. The pipes forming the well casing and the water lines coming from the ground should be metal, not plastic.

Faucets and other plumbing fixtures should contain as few plastic parts as possible to avoid outgassing into the air and contamination of the water. It will be impossible to eliminate all contact with plastic or rubber in a water system. Pumps, valves, dielectric fittings, etc. contain various minor parts that could theoretically contaminate the water. The goal is to eliminate as many contaminants as possible. If the water is still a problem for a sensitive person, a filter or purifying system will be required. Some people must resort to bottled water for drinking and cooking.

The drain lines in the house either take the wastewater to a sewer or to a septic tank. They can be constructed of cast iron, galvanized steel, copper, or plastic. Since drain lines do not carry water to be consumed, the only consideration is contamination of the air from outgassing. Hence, all but plastic are acceptable choices. Because these lines are considerably larger than supply lines (up to 4″ in diameter), the cost difference can be considerable between plastic and the other choices. Plastic drain lines that are underground or within a concrete slab will obviously be well separated from the living space, so plastic in these locations is acceptable. Plastic drain lines within the house can usually be wrapped with foil, like electric wire, to prevent outgassing into the living space. The plastic pipe material can also be purchased early in the construction process and allowed to outgas before installation.

Central Vacuum Systems

While the advantages of central vacuum systems are obvious in houses with wall-to-wall carpeting, they can be very useful even in houses without carpeting. Hardwood and ceramic tile floors do not generate dust like carpeting, but any dust on them is more visible. In other words, there may not be as much dust in a house without carpeting, but you will be able to see it easier. Most portable vacuum cleaners are not only awkward to use, but they tend to blow dust around the house because of inefficient filters.

Central vacuum units should be used in healthful houses only if they have an outdoor exhaust, so that any dust getting past the filter is directed to the outside rather than redistributed throughout the house. Some have an undesirable internal exhaust with a muffler to reduce the noise. All models require the use of plastic tubing within the walls, but this can usually be sealed with aluminum foil to reduce outgassing into the living space. Some manufacturers offer metal wall cover plates rather than plastic. These will be sturdier and aren't subject to outgassing. All units have plastic hoses and plastic tools that can have a very strong odor that will bother some people. When planning an installation, the equipment can be purchased early, and the plastic hose can be allowed to outgas outdoors for a while in a location protected from the weather. If the closets are ventilated, storing such a hose in a closet will not result in minor odors seeping into the house. The vacuum machine itself, when mounted in a ventilated closet, will not allow smells from the hot motor to get into the house where they could bother sensitive occupants. Manufacturers include: **Beam Industries Inc., Filtex, Nutone/Scovill, Thomas Industries**, and **Vacu-Master Corporation**.

Summary

Whenever mechanical systems are used, there is a possibility of indoor air pollution. Heating and air conditioning systems should be selected with care. If you have an existing combustion fired appliance in your house and suspect that it may be causing health problems, the first step would be to have a doctor run a blood test to determine the carbon monoxide content. Hot water heating is one of the more healthful choices, utilizing either a central boiler or individual self-contained hydronic units. Passive solar heating would also be a good choice. Since all air conditioners will have the potential to outgas or grow mold, a model should be selected that is easy to clean and has a minimum of offensive parts. Forced air systems of all types have the potential to contaminate the air with a variety of particles or gases. With electrical, plumbing or vacuuming systems, plastic components should be avoided wherever possible. Electrical wire can be sealed from the living space by enclosing it in a metal conduit or by wrapping it with metal foil. Plastic pipe should be avoided for water supply lines. If plastic drain or vacuum lines are used, they can be wrapped with foil to minimize outgassing. All plastic components should be purchased early in the construction process so that they can outgas before being incorporated into the house.

Chapter 22

Filters and Purifiers

Even after eliminating as many pollution sources as possible from a house, it may be advantageous to install some type of air cleaning system. With a warm air furnace, the standard filter may not be efficient enough to remove the dust generated by the occupants, or the mold or pollen spores that find their way indoors, and these filters are ineffective when it comes to gaseous contaminants. Ventilating systems and heat recovery ventilators can also benefit from an air cleaning system. In an existing house, where it would be difficult to install central air cleaning equipment, individual room-sized units may be more practical.

Besides the air that we breathe, the water that we drink often requires cleaning. Pollutants in water can find their way into our bodies not only when ingested, but some are absorbed through the skin during bathing. Other pollutants are actually dissolved gases that can be released into the air, where they contribute to air pollution. If a whole-house water purifying system is desired, it will be wise to allow extra space in the utility room for it. Adjacent to the water heater is a good location. Sometimes, small "point-of-use" water filters or purifiers will be more practical than a large system.

Air Purifiers

There are many different brands and types of air purifiers available. Some are mounted inside a furnace cabinet or are a part of the general ventilating system. Other models are portable, for use in different rooms, on desktops, or in automobiles. Most will contain at least one component that can bother some people, so it will be important to select a filter or combination of filters with care. Some purifiers are designed to remove particles, others will remove gases, and some combination units will remove a variety of contaminants. Devices that introduce "the pleasing scent of lemons" or other aromas into the air are actually contributing to the pollution because they often use synthetic fragrances. They tend to cover up odors rather than remove them. Unless regular maintenance is performed, microorganisms trapped in a filter can be introduced into the airstream, actually contributing to indoor air pollution.

When considering a whole-house system for use with a furnace or heat recovery ventilator, it will usually be necessary to consult with someone knowledgeable in designing such an installation. Some filter suppliers or local heating contractors may be able to provide this service. All purifiers and filters will restrict the airflow of the system's fan or blower to a certain extent. With several filters or the wrong type of filter, the fan's efficiency can be reduced considerably so that inadequate air is moved through the system. This can result in insufficient hot (or cool) air reaching the registers from the furnace. It can also mean overheating and damage to the fan motor. Sometimes it will be necessary to increase the capacity of the fan or the horsepower of the motor in order to compensate for the resistance of the air cleaning equipment.

Portable units are self-contained and the design work has already been done. All that is necessary with them is to select the correct size or type, and plug it in. As a rule, the very small desktop models are not large enough to remove enough pollutants to be worth the trouble.[1]

It should be remembered that air purifiers are not substitutes for fresh air. They will only remove contaminates from the air, and while this is certainly desirable, they do not create oxygen. In an extremely tight house, it is possible for the occupants to use up the available oxygen, and no amount of filtration will replace it. Some houses have so many internal pollution sources that most methods of air purifying will be impractical. In very polluted houses it would be wise to remove as many sources of air contamination as possible before considering an air cleaning system.

The best way to make use of a filtration system is to design it in conjunction with the structure of the house and the heating/air conditioning equipment. While this is not often done, when designed correctly, the result will be better air exchange rates, filtration of all the air in the house, and less dead air space. A more efficient and cost-effective way of maintaining clean air is achieved by considering the entire house as a system, and designing all of the components so that they work together.

Particle Filters

Particle filters, as their name implies, remove particles from the air. They will not remove gases, like formaldehyde. Mold, pollen, dust, asbestos, viruses, etc. are all particles that can be found floating around inside our houses and they certainly can bother a lot of people. Unfortunately, selecting a particle filter is not an easy matter, because of the wide variety of sizes of the particles that it would be desirable to remove.

The basic unit used in conjunction with filters is the micron (1 micron = 0.000039 inch). A micron is a very small unit. The point of a straight pin is about 75 microns across. Particles smaller than 10 microns are almost impossible to see with the unaided eye. Many of the pollutants in the air, larger than 10 microns in size, are relatively easy to remove. While it is often desirable to remove smaller particles, they are more difficult to trap.

Particulates in smoke may range in size from 0.01 up to 1.0 micron. House dust can be just as small. Animal dander will generally range from 0.5 to 10.0 microns. Pollens, on the other hand, are fairly large in comparison, usually being larger than 10.0 microns. Mold spores can be as small as 1.0 microns and viruses are only 0.01 microns in size.

Mechanical filters remove particles by trapping them on a filter media, somewhat like a very find strainer. The term mechanical does not imply that these filters have any moving parts; it simply means that they are not electronic.

Mechanical particle filters are the most commonly encountered types. The standard furnace filter is a mechanical particle filter that is usually made of fiberglass or polyester in a cardboard frame. Some people are bothered by these types of filters because of the binder used to hold the fibers together, or an oil film sprayed on the filter to increase its dust-grabbing efficiency. Fibers can also be released into the airstream, contributing to air pollution. The conventional furnace filter is usually only capable of removing particles larger than 10 microns. It is, therefore, called a coarse mechanical particle filter. There

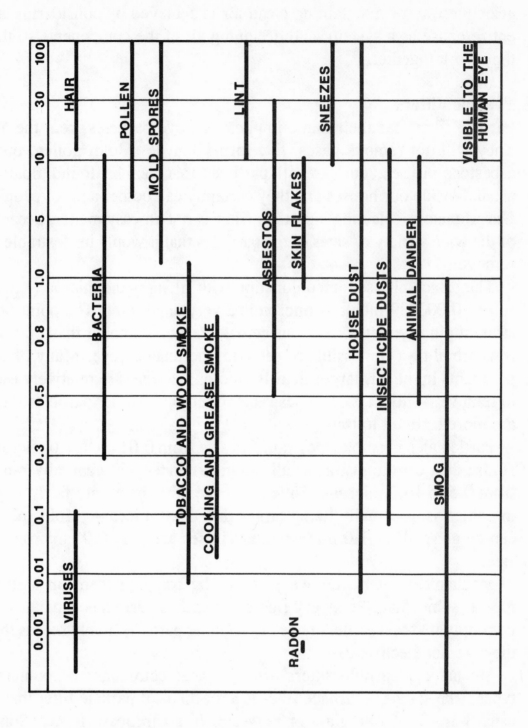

Particle Size in Microns of Air Pollutants

are many different manufacturers of these types of filters and they are available from hardware stores and heating equipment suppliers. One study has found that, although standard furnace filters are somewhat inefficient, dust levels can often be lowered by running the furnace fan continuously.[2] However, some people complain that, although the dust levels are lower, the continually running fan tends to stir up the dust that remains in the air.

For maximum particle filtration, it is desirable to have a coarse particle filter, as a prefilter, in front of a fine particle filter. The prefilter will remove the large particles that quickly clog a finer filter. It should be changed more often than the higher cost fine particle filter.

Fine Particle Filters

Mechanical filters capable of removing the fine, small particles are available in different types from many manufacturers. Since they must be denser in order to capture these very small bits of pollution, they result in more air resistance. For this reason, they are often made in a pleated or "accordion" shape. With all the extra surface area, they have less resistance than a simple flat filter. The very best particle filters are known as HEPA (high efficiency particulate accumulator) filters. These were originally developed during World War II by the Atomic Energy Commission to filter out radioactive dust. HEPA filters typically remove over 95 percent of the contaminants in the air. In fact, some have an efficiency of at least 99.999 percent on particles larger than 0.3 microns. They typically last one to five years before replacement is necessary. Like all filters, their life depends on how dirty the air is. They can, in some cases, be treated with chemicals that will kill molds, viruses, and bacteria.[3] These potentially offensive chemical treatments should be avoided in most cases. HEPA filters are often bonded with some type of adhesive that can outgas unwanted chemicals into the airstream and they may be constructed with frames made of metal, cardboard, plastic, or particle board. While most local heating equipment suppliers have access to HEPA filters, they are not commonly used in residential work. Special ductwork will usually need to be constructed to use them in a ventilating system. There are many manufacturers, including **Airguard Industries, Aluminum Filter Co., American Air Filter, Cambridge Filter Corporation**, and **Farr Co.**

There are readily available medium-efficiency air filters available through **Research Products Corporation** ("Spaceguard") and **Honeywell Inc.** (Model F66A). They are not as efficient as HEPA filters, but they are considerably better than standard furnace filters. While they are relatively easy to adapt to a furnace or ventilating system, they can require some custom ductwork. The "Spaceguard" filters come in two styles: the Model 2250 comes with a grille that can be either mounted in the ceiling or in a wall, the Model 2200 can be installed in a duct run or near the furnace, as can the **Honeywell** filter. Both manufacturers use a small quantity of resin binder to hold the accordion-shaped fiberglass media together. The "Spaceguard" filters use a formaldehyde-based resin and **Honeywell** uses an acrylic resin with a slight amount of silicone. Both types of resin can result in some outgassing into the airstream. This can be minimized by heating the filter media in a low temperature oven prior to installation. These filters also contain some plastic parts that can be coated with foil or an environmental sealant if they prove bothersome. The "Spaceguard" filter cabinets have a small amount of pink fiberglass insulation that can similarly be covered with foil. These filters are generally quite effective with particle sizes down to about 0.5 microns

There are many other manufactures of specialized types of intermediate-range filters that are better than standard furnace filters but not as efficient as HEPA filters. Generally, these will require special ductwork since they aren't often used in residences.

Electrostatic Precipitators

Electronic air cleaners, more correctly called electrostatic precipitators, are typically advertised as being 95–99 percent efficient at removing particles. While this certainly sounds good, it is often misleading. In one test, an electrostatic precipitator was found to have an initial efficiency of 80 percent. The efficiency declined to 50 percent after 20 hours of use and only 20 percent after 40 hours of use.[4] When passing through an electrostatic precipitator, the particles in the airstream are given a negative electrical charge. They are then attracted to a positively charged plate, grid, or screen. When clogged, the screen is simply removed form the cabinet, washed off, and reinserted.

The following disadvantages of electrostatic precipitators have been noted:[5]

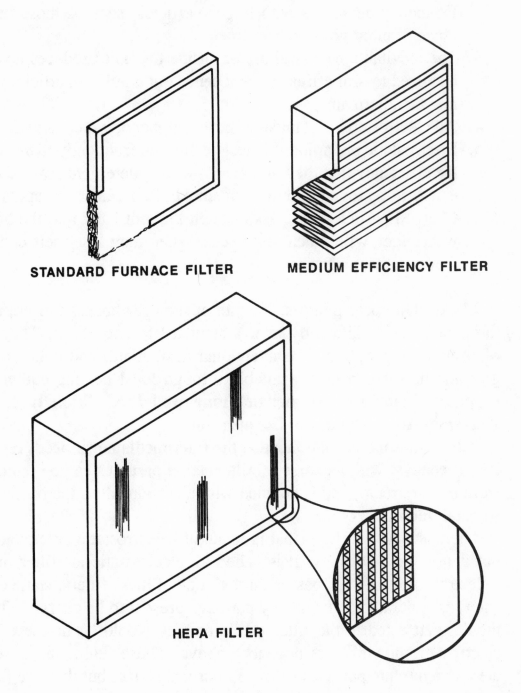

STANDARD FURNACE FILTER   MEDIUM EFFICIENCY FILTER

HEPA FILTER

Mechanical Particle Air Filters

1. Efficiency is low compared to HEPA filters.
2. Efficiency decreases with larger particles, such as those in the range of plant pollens.
3. The inevitable electrical arcing inside the unit produces a small localized loss of efficiency that sends out a puff of particles back into the airstream.
4. All electrostatic precipitators produce ozone, which is toxic.
5. Electrostatic precipitators must be cleaned frequently to preserve the efficiency that they do have. A strong detergent may be necessary to remove buildup from smoke, lubricants, or vapors.
6. Charged particles can pass through the unit back into the house where they will attach to objects. When they lose their charge, they can reenter the air.

Electrostatic precipitators, in spite of the drawbacks, can improve the air quality significantly over a standard furnace filter. They are often used by people with conventional dust, mold, and pollen allergies and they are readily available through local heating equipment suppliers. Manufacturers include **Honeywell Inc.**, **Trion Inc.**, and **Universal Air Precipitator Corporation**.

Advantages include the fact that the filter media never needs replacing. If coupled with a coarse prefilter, large particles can be removed from the airstream, and if coupled with a carbon filter, the ozone can be catalyzed into oxygen.

There is a type of filter that is related to electrostatic precipitators, but it uses no electricity. It is called an electrostatic air filter or an "electret" filter. As air passes through one of these filters, static electricity is generated, causing any particles present to be charged. They then are attracted to the filter media as they would be in one of the electrostatic precipitators described above. These filters are not efficient at removing particles below 6 microns in size, but they are fairly good with larger particles such as ragweed pollen and some mold spores. Since no electricity is used, no toxic ozone is produced. A disadvantage for some people is the fact that they are made of plastic, usually polypropylene and polyester, that can outgas into the airstream. **Air Purification Products Intl.** and **Allergen Air Filter Corporation** sell electrostatic air filters in several standard sizes that can be easily installed as a replacement for conventional furnace filters. They can also be used as a window screen to filter out some of the

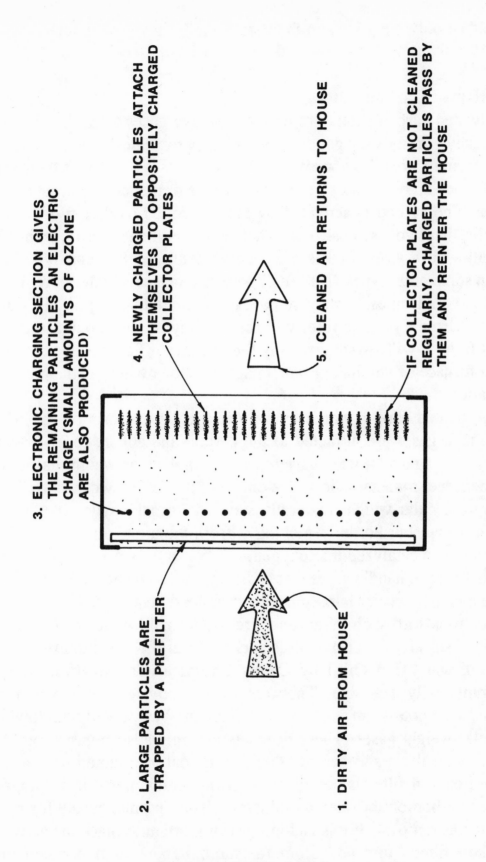

3. ELECTRONIC CHARGING SECTION GIVES THE REMAINING PARTICLES AN ELECTRIC CHARGE (SMALL AMOUNTS OF OZONE ARE ALSO PRODUCED)

4. NEWLY CHARGED PARTICLES ATTACH THEMSELVES TO OPPOSITELY CHARGED COLLECTOR PLATES

5. CLEANED AIR RETURNS TO HOUSE

IF COLLECTOR PLATES ARE NOT CLEANED REGULARLY, CHARGED PARTICLES PASS BY THEM AND REENTER THE HOUSE

2. LARGE PARTICLES ARE TRAPPED BY A PREFILTER

1. DIRTY AIR FROM HOUSE

Electrostatic Precipitator

mold or pollen particles in the "fresh air." They are manufactured by **3M**.

Activated Carbon Filters

Activated carbon filters are used to remove gases from the airstream but they are not very good at removing particulates. The carbon is in the form of granules approximately 1/8" across. In spite of their small size, they are extremely porous and have a tremendously large surface area. The carbon is activated by the controlled oxidation of coconut shells, hardwoods, coal, etc. That which is made from coconut has smaller pore sizes, and is often better tolerated by sensitive people than some other types. The small pore size makes it better at removing smaller molecules. An activated carbon filter that is placed "downwind" from a particle filter will remove any products outgassed from that filter. It will also remove any fumes given off by the electric motor of a furnace or ventilating fan; so again, "downwind" is the preferred location.

Activated carbon works by a process called adsorption, by which pollutant gases are attracted to the carbon and adhere to it. It works very well against a wide variety of high molecular-weight gases such as benzene, toluene, ethers, acetone, etc. It does not work as well with low molecular-weight materials such as formaldehyde. It will deal with ozone, but not by removing it from the airstream. It causes the ozone to be catalyzed into oxygen.

In order to handle gases that ordinary activated carbon is less effective against, special impregnated carbons are available. These can be made to adsorb such things as mercury, formaldehyde, radon, or hydrogen sulfide. Other materials such as "Purafil" by **Purafil Corporation** and "Carusorb" by **Carus Chemical Corporation** are also commercially available. They consist of activated alumina impregnated with potassium permanganate, and they work well with low molecular-weight gases. These products not only adsorb gases, but they react with them and destroy them by oxidation. Sometimes an activated carbon filter is combined with one containing special impregnated carbon or activated alumina/potassium permanganate for maximum gas removal. If this is done, it is important to place the activated carbon filter "upwind" from the alumina/potassium permanganate filter or else hydrochloric acid could be formed if chlorinated hydrocarbons are present in the air.[6]

Since there can be a lot of air resistance with a carbon filter, it is often necessary to increase the surface area so that a powerful fan is not required. The carbon can be placed in trays with a metal screen on the bottom. Several of these trays are inserted in an accordion-shaped cabinet to conserve space. Carbon filters of this type are not often seen in residential situations, but they are available. Manufacturers of multiple-tray carbon filters include **American Air Filter Co., Barnebey-Cheney** (Series FJS and FKS Adsorbers) and **Farr Company** (CF Glide/Pack). These are very efficient, but since they are not often seen in residential installations, many heating contractors will be unfamiliar with them.

E.L. Foust Co., Inc. sells a carbon filter that can be used as a replacement for a standard furnace filter and **Barnebey-Cheney** has a disposable filter of cardboard that is impregnated with carbon. These will help to remove some gases, but will not be nearly as efficient as a multiple-tray filter containing considerably more carbon. The more carbon that is present, the more gases will be absorbed.

Some people are sensitive to activated carbon from one source but not another. For example, coconut carbon may be tolerable, but carbon derived from coal may not. The various carbons all contain dust which can be very irritating to the mucous membranes if it is released into the airstream. In order to minimize this, first place the carbon in one of the trays, then place a vacuum beneath it to pull the small dust particles through. Several passes may be necessary. Some filter manufacturers suggest placing a particle filter after the carbon filter to catch this dust; however, in this location the particle filter could potentially contaminate the airstream.

The life of the carbon will depend on several factors, such as the concentration of pollutants and amount of carbon present. Replacement of the carbon itself after six months is somewhat typical. Various types of carbon are usually available from the different filter manufacturers.

Combination Filters

The ideal filter should be able to remove both particulates and gases. Many readily available portable filters have this capability but, in general, whole house systems must be designed and constructed for each situation. Since many heating contractors are unfamiliar with HEPA filters or activated carbon units, it can be difficult to locate someone

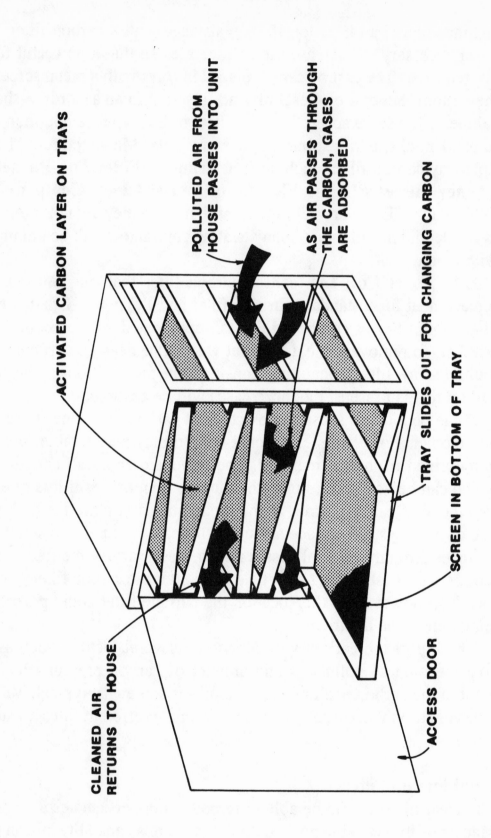

ACTIVATED CARBON LAYER ON TRAYS

POLLUTED AIR FROM HOUSE PASSES INTO UNIT

AS AIR PASSES THROUGH THE CARBON, GASES ARE ADSORBED

TRAY SLIDES OUT FOR CHANGING CARBON

SCREEN IN BOTTOM OF TRAY

CLEANED AIR RETURNS TO HOUSE

ACCESS DOOR

Multiple-Tray Carbon Filter

with the capability to properly design a system.

While the forced air furnaces manufactured by **Thurmond Development** (in Chapter 21) can be fitted with both a HEPA and a carbon filter, most furnaces are simply not designed to accommodate them. There is, however, a package system manufactured by **Control Resource Systems, Inc.** that can be easily added to virtually any warm air furnace system. Their "CRSI 600H" unit consists of a cabinet, motor and blower, prefilter, activated carbon filter, and a HEPA filter. It is a free-standing unit that is attached to the furnace, and wired to operate automatically whenever the furnace fan is running. The carbon filter is located before the HEPA filter and the motor, so there is the possibility of those items outgassing and contaminating the airstream.

Negative Ion Generators

These machines are not true air purifiers or filters, but they can contribute to cleaner indoor air. They operate by sending electrons into the air. The electrons attach themselves to small particulates in the air and cause them to be negatively charged. These charged particles (ions) will then attach themselves to various surfaces. If the negative ion generator has a "downwind" particle filter, the charged particles will attach themselves to that filter. If the ions are simply spewed out into the room, the charged particles will attach to the walls and furnishings. This can result in very dirty walls.

Negative ions themselves have been shown to have positive effects on health, such as increased vigor, friendliness, alertness, and performance. Improved reaction times and diminished anxiety have also been noted. In psychiatric hospitals, negative ions in the air have had a pronounced effect in alleviating symptoms of psychoneurosis, apprehension, and fear.[7] Other researchers have found that high concentrations of both positive and negative ions will inhibit the growth of bacteria.[8] In general, however, it appears from most research that negative ions have a beneficial effect on the health of people, and that positive ions have a detrimental effect.

Portable Air Purifiers

There are many manufacturers now producing portable purifiers of various types. For the best performance, only room-sized models are recommended, so very small desk-sized units are not included in this discussion. The larger, more powerful units will clean the air faster and more thoroughly than moderately sized models. Size, efficiency, appearance, media type, etc. will all have an effect on cost. These air purifiers may contain coarse particle prefilters, fine particle filters, carbon filters, or any combination. It is recommended that the manufacturer's literature of several products be reviewed before deciding on a particular model. For very sensitive persons, it would also be helpful to be able to test a filter before actually purchasing it. Most companies offer a guarantee, whereby a portable filter can be tested in the home and returned if it is intolerable. There are many mail order suppliers of portable room-sized air purifiers, such as **N.E.E.D.S., Nigra Enterprises, Living Source, The Allergy Store**, etc. Manufacturers of portable room-sized air filters include **Air Conditioning Engineers, Aireox Research Corporation, Air Purification Products, Allermed Corporation, Barnebey-Cheney, E.L. Foust Co. Inc., Enviracaire Corporation**, and **King Aire.**

Spider Plants as Filters

There has been some interesting research done through the **National Aeronautics and Space Administration** that involves the use of spider plants (Chlorophytum elatum var. vittatum) to absorb various indoor air contaminants.[9,10] This work was done to find a possible biological method of reducing the concentration of pollutants in the air. In their experiments, known quantities of formaldehyde, carbon monoxide, and nigrogen dioxide were injected into a closed chamber containing spider plants or golden pothos (Scindapsus aureus). Both types of plants absorbed the contaminants, with the spider plant being the most effective. Once the polllutants are absorbed, they are metabolized by soil microbes, rendering them harmless. This research has been widely reported in the media; unfortunately it may not actually help clean the air in a typical house.

NASA's experiments were done in a closed chamber with a specific quantity of pollutants. Houses typically contain pollution sources that continually outgas contaminants. For example, particle board or some other formaldehyde source can outgas for years. With this type of environment, as the plants absorb some pollutants, more are continually added to the air to replace them. Research at Ball State University has shown that for most residential environments, these plants are ineffective at reducing indoor pollution levels.[11] In fact, having plants in a house tends to result in higher relative humidity, and formalde-

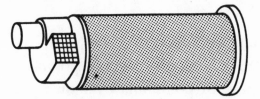

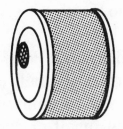

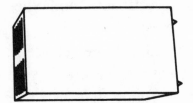

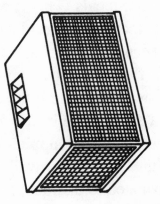

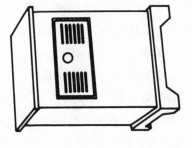

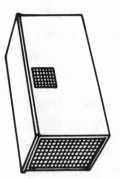

Portable Air Purifiers

hyde emissions increase as the relative humidity rises. Any formaldehyde absorbed by the plants will be quickly replaced by an increased
rate of outgassing. The plants will also release undesirable mold
spores into the air.

Water Filters and Purifiers

Water supplies generally come from rivers, lakes, or wells, all of which
can be easily contaminated. Lakes and rivers become polluted from
agricultural runoff or direct dumping of pollutants by industry, septic
tanks, and sewage treatment plants. Wells that pull water up from underground reservoirs, known as aquifiers, are also often contaminated with
toxic chemicals. This is especially common near landfills or in agricultural areas where herbicides, pesticides, fertilizers, and other chemicals
can seep down through the soil into the aquifier. Water supplies that
come from wells can contain radon, which will be released into the air
as water comes from the tap. Most private water supplies utilize wells,
and a study done by Cornell University found that 63 percent of rural
household water supplies were considered unsafe.[12]

Unless a private well is used, your water will probably have been
chlorinated to disinfect it. Regulations usually require that this be done
routinely, whether the water needs disinfecting or not. It may be
treated with other chemicals as well, such as fluoride. The water
mains buried under the street can be made of iron, galvanized pipe,
copper, asbestos cement, or plastic. Any contaminants from deteriorating mains will be transferred to the water supply where they can
result in ill health. Asbestos fibers released from asbestos cement water pipe can result in an increased risk of developing gastrointestinal
cancer when ingested. Plastic pipes above ground can contaminate
both water and air as they outgas.

Chlorine is the major contaminant that is purposefully added to
drinking water. When it reacts with dissolved organic material in water, it produces, among other things, chloroform, a known carcinogen.
Chloroform is part of a chemical family known as trihalomethanes
(THMs) which are very commonly found in water supplies. Chlorine
can be such a big problem for some people that they cannot even bathe
or wash their faces in water containing it, much less drink it.[13] A major
means of exposure to many of these waterborne chemicals is through
the skin while bathing. One study found that up to 70 percent of the
exposure of adults is through the skin.[14] There are several studies that

have found a link between chlorinated surface water and increased cancer mortality.[15]

If a water filter or purifying system is located on the supply line coming into the house, then the contaminants can be handled before they enter the house piping. This is considered a whole-house system, and while it may be desirable, it is often impractical. Individual units can be used at specific locations. For example, an under-sink unit might be used in the kitchen for water that is to be used for cooking or drinking, or a small carbon filter could be attached to the showerhead. Unfortunately, there is no single type of treatment device that is perfect for all situations. Some work very well with certain contaminants, but poorly with others.

The contaminants routinely found in drinking water supplies fall into four basic categories:[16]

Particulates are small bits of material that do not dissolve in water. They include such things as asbestos, heavy metals, rust, dirt, and sediment.

Dissolved solids are solid materials that dissolve in water. They include fluoride, nitrates, sulfates, and salts.

Volatile chemicals are substances that can be vaporized. Over 700 of these have been identified in drinking water. They include several cancer causing chemicals. Typical examples include chlorine, chloroform, pesticides, and PCBs. When water is exposed to the air, some of these chemicals can be quickly released. This is especially true with hot water.

Microorganisms are microscopic plant and animal life. These include bacteria, viruses, amoeba, molds, etc.

Not all water contaminants are harmful. In fact, some dissolved minerals such as calcium, selenium, etc. can be very desirable. Pure water containing two hydrogen atoms and one oxygen atom is difficult to obtain and would be tasteless, as is distilled water. Water without minerals is said by the **EPA** to be "aggressive," meaning that it will leach out the taste, odor, or substance of whatever it touches. Drinking such water over long periods of time may leach minerals out of the body, creating deficiencies.

Before selecting a filtration or purifying system, you should have your water tested to determine what contaminants are present. If you are part of a large water system, they should be able to supply you with a current water analysis, since this is required by law. Unfortunately, they are not required to test for all possible contaminants, but this is a good place to get some basic information about your water supply. Contact the local or state board of health for a list of laboratories capable of testing a private water supply. This can be quite expensive, up to several hundred dollars, depending on the comprehensiveness of the testing. Equipment manufacturers' specification sheets should also be studied carefully. For some individuals, plastic components in a filter or purifier can result in intolerable water. For them, an all-metal system may be required. Some distillers are made of even more inert glass.

Since this can be quite a complicated subject, it might be a good idea to consult with someone like **Nigra Enterprises** for help in designing a system. They provide a design service to their customers. In this chapter we will only briefly discuss the various types of filtration and purifying equipment available. No particular system will be recommended because it would not be applicable to all situations.

Distillers

Distillation devices boil water into steam. The steam condenses back into water in another chamber, leaving behind dissolved solids and particulates. The heating process will kill any water-based microorganisms. Distillers will allow some volatile chemicals to escape into the air, where they can be problematic, while others remain in the water. Some distillers use a two-stage distillation process, whereby most of the volatile chemicals are driven off first, then the water is boiled to remove other contaminants. With a few people, even triple distillation may not be enough to render water tolerable.[17]

Distillers can potentially remove most of the contaminants found in water, although some have little or no effect on volatile chemicals. When the heating process does drive off the volatile chemicals, they can contaminate the air. Distillers are fairly expensive to purchase and operate, and they are not practical for use as a whole-house method of cleaning up a water supply. Even if used for drinking or cooking water only, they can be inconvenient because they only will produce a limited amount and they need regular cleaning. The distillation process will remove both the oxygen from the water, making it somewhat acidic, and virtually all of the minerals. Stainless steel distillers often

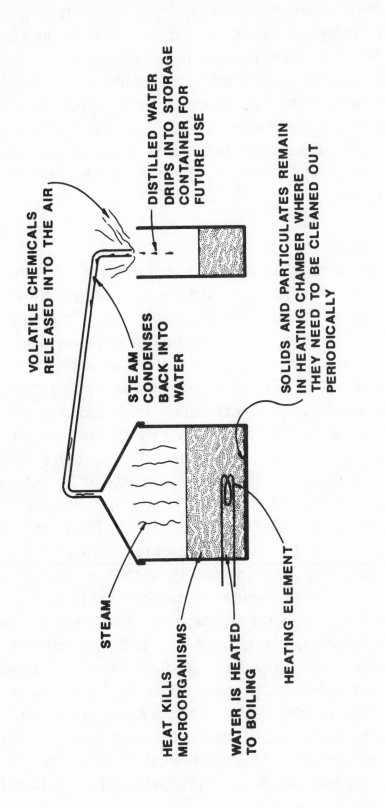

VOLATILE CHEMICALS RELEASED INTO THE AIR

DISTILLED WATER DRIPS INTO STORAGE CONTAINER FOR FUTURE USE

STEAM CONDENSES BACK INTO WATER

SOLIDS AND PARTICULATES REMAIN IN HEATING CHAMBER WHERE THEY NEED TO BE CLEANED OUT PERIODICALLY

STEAM

HEAT KILLS MICROORGANISMS

WATER IS HEATED TO BOILING

HEATING ELEMENT

Distillation

yield water with a metallic taste. This is because the aggressive water can leach chromium out of the stainless steel during the distillation process. Similarly, aluminum can be leached from aluminum parts into the water. Since distillers operate slowly and do not provide water at the turn of a tap, a holding tank or storage jar is required. Typically, several gallons of water a day can be distilled and stored for use. Since distillers will kill bacteria, they can be classified as water *purifiers*. Manufacturers include **Wm. R. Hague Inc., Scientific Glass Co.,** and **Waterwise, Inc.**

Carbon Filters

Filters containing activated carbon are often referred to as taste and odor filters and they are very effective at removing volatile chemicals such as chlorine, chloroform, pesticides, etc. They will not remove dissolved solids, particulates, or destroy microorganisms. In fact, bacteria can grow and multiply inside a granular carbon filter. There will always be some type of bacteria in the water supply even if it has been chlorinated, and a carbon filter can become a breeding ground if it has not had any water run through it for a while. For example, if a family is on vacation for a week, the bacteria in the carbon filter will rapidly multiply. For this reason, it is recommended that the water be run for a few minutes, to flush out the filter, after it has been idle. Some manufacturers recommend that the water be flushed through a carbon filter each morning as a precautionary measure. Carbon filters that utilize a block of carbon rather than granular carbon are much less likely to harbor bacteria. Some manufacturers add silver to the granular carbon to kill the bacteria; however, there has been some concern that the silver can negatively contaminate the water. If a carbon filter is used regularly and changed regularly, generally there is no danger from the small amount of bacteria present. While there is no evidence that bacteria from carbon filters are a common cause of disease, it is a point that must be considered. It should be noted that not all bacteria are harmful, some are very beneficial to human digestion. If a public water supply has been chlorinated, it is doubtful that any harmful bacteria will be present.

Radon can be removed from water with the use of an activated carbon filter; however, most of the smaller filters on the market are not of sufficient size to result in much reduction. To be effective, a

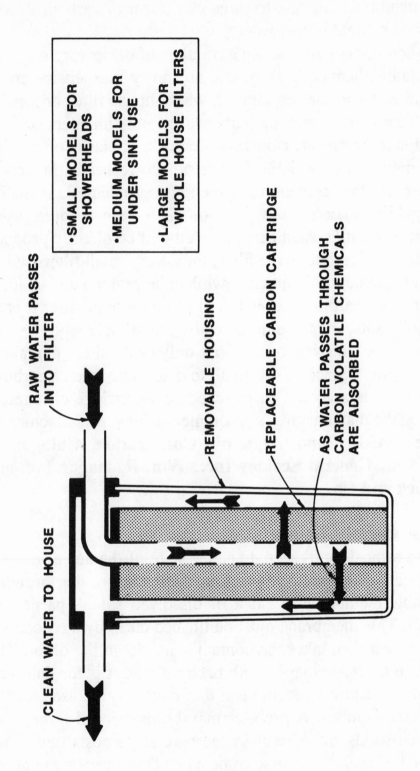

- SMALL MODELS FOR SHOWERHEADS
- MEDIUM MODELS FOR UNDER SINK USE
- LARGE MODELS FOR WHOLE HOUSE FILTERS

RAW WATER PASSES INTO FILTER

REMOVABLE HOUSING

REPLACEABLE CARBON CARTRIDGE

AS WATER PASSES THROUGH CARBON VOLATILE CHEMICALS ARE ADSORBED

CLEAN WATER TO HOUSE

Carbon Water Filter

filter should contain one to three cubic feet of carbon, depending on the radon content of the water.[18]

Carbon filters have the big advantage of being very good at removing volatile chemicals. They also are fairly inexpensive and they are well suited to be used as either a whole-house filter or a point-of-use filter. There are no moving parts and the only maintenance is periodic cartridge replacement. Housings are made of plastic or stainless steel. Small models are available for use on showerheads, faucet, or under the sink. If other contaminants are not a problem, as is the case with most public water supplies, carbon filters can be quite useful. The amount of volatile chemicals removed will be directly proportional to the amount of carbon in the filter; thus, very small filters will have the carbon depleted rather quickly, while a large unit can last for a month or more. If a carbon filter is left in place too long after it is saturated with pollutants, it can begin unloading them back into the water supply; however, this has been noted only with filters containing powdered carbon.[19] Since it is difficult to determine when a carbon filter is saturated, it is a good idea to schedule a cartridge change regularly, based on the manufacturer's recommendations. Manufacturers include **Ametek, AMF/Cuno, Aquathin Corporation, Culligan International Co., General Ecology Inc., Wm. R. Hague Inc.** and **Sears Roebuck and Co.**

Reverse Osmosis Units

Reverse osmosis units seem to be the state-of-the-art in water-cleaning equipment. They operate by forcing a stream of water through a semipermeable membrane to rid it of dissolved solids, particulates, and bacteria. This membrane must be flushed clean by a second stream of water, which then takes the contaminants down the drain. The membrane can become clogged with bacteria, and it is for that reason that some manufacturers recommend that they only be used with chlorinated water supplies. A prefilter may be required if large amounts of dissolved solids are present so the reverse osmosis unit is not overwhelmed. Generally reverse osmosis units are very good at removing all contaminants except volatile chemicals but they are not quite as effective as distillers. They can, however, be easier to use.

These units have the drawback of being inefficient, in that they waste between three and ten gallons of water for each gallon that is processed. This is because the membrane needs constant rinsing.

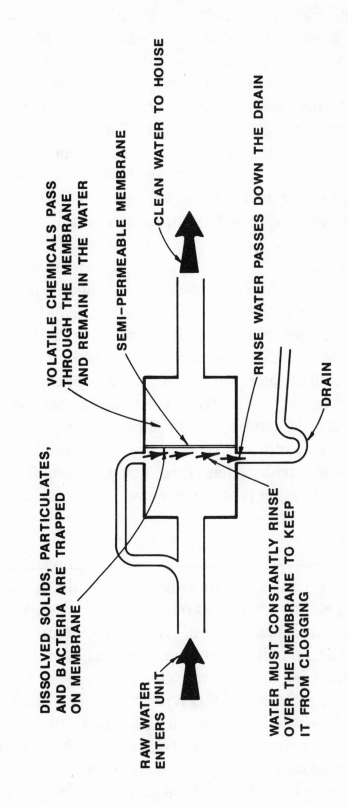

VOLATILE CHEMICALS PASS
THROUGH THE MEMBRANE
AND REMAIN IN THE WATER

SEMI-PERMEABLE MEMBRANE

CLEAN WATER TO HOUSE

RINSE WATER PASSES DOWN THE DRAIN

DRAIN

DISSOLVED SOLIDS, PARTICULATES,
AND BACTERIA ARE TRAPPED
ON MEMBRANE

RAW WATER
ENTERS UNIT

WATER MUST CONSTANTLY RINSE
OVER THE MEMBRANE TO KEEP
IT FROM CLOGGING

Reverse Osmosis System

Their effectiveness is dependent on temperature, pH, and water pressure. Usually at least 30 pounds of water pressure is required. Like distillers, they only produce a limited amount of water each day, so a holding tank or storage jar is needed, and they are not useful as whole-house units. Because they can remove minerals, some produce a slightly aggressive water. They can be relatively expensive and take up a lot of space, and periodic maintenance is required. The operating cost will be less than when using a distiller, but more than with a carbon filter. Manufacturers include: **AFM/Cuno, Ametek, Aquathin Corporation** and **Culligan International Co.**

Other Methods

There are simple dirt and sediment filters available that can be used to clear cloudy water. Others are designed to reduce scale buildup in water heaters, humidifiers, or other appliances. Some are effective at removing iron. None of these are effective for most of the other pollutants found in the water. Many canister-type filters can be fitted with either one of these types of cartridges or a granular carbon cartridge.

Ultraviolet light can be used to kill any microorganisms in water, but it will have no effect on other pollutants. **Ultra Hyd** manufactures several sizes of purifiers that utilize this principle. They can be used for drinking water, hot tubs, spas, or swimming pools.

Water Softeners

Water softeners are usually referred to as conditioners rather than water cleaning devices. They are employed in order to increase the water's sudsing ability. This saves on soap costs and makes cleaning easier. Hard water contains more dissolved minerals than soft water, primarily positively charged calcium and magnesium ions. The most popular residential method of softening water involves the zeolite process. Water softeners of this type utilize salt to cause an exchange to take place between the calcium and magnesium ions in the water and sodium ions from the salt. With this method, hardness can be reduced substantially, and the water takes on a slippery feeling. Unfortunately, it becomes high in sodium content. This can be hazardous to the health of people on sodium-restricted diets.

There is a residential water softener that does not use salt, and hence does not raise the sodium content of the water.[20] The "Stabilizer," manufactured by **Fluid Mechanics Inc.**, is a catalytic water conditioner that works by not adding to the water or removing anything. Nevertheless, it does produce soft water.

Summary

Particle filters and carbon filters are the two primary methods of air filtration that will be applicable to home heating and ventilation systems. There are different approaches to particle filtering that will have advantages and disadvantages in different situations. Coarse particle filters, HEPA filters, and electrostatic precipitators are all possibilities. Usually a combination of carbon and particle filters will provide the best control of airborne contaminants. Since the design of a whole house filtration system can be difficult and may involve some engineering analysis, portable room-sized filters may be better choices for many applications. These vary in the filtration method employed, with some relying only on particle filters and others only a carbon filter. The better models will contain a combination of different types.

Of the water cleaning method, distillation and reverse osmosis are point-of-use units, usually being located in the kitchen. They both work well against a wide variety of water contaminants, except volatile chemicals, which can easily be removed by a carbon filter. A carbon filter can be used either as a whole-house filter or a point-of-use filter. Their main disadvantage is the fact that they can become contaminated with bacteria. By combining a carbon filter with either a distiller or a reverse osmosis unit, the water can be cleaned of all contaminants.

Chapter 23

Putting It All Together

There is no single design that will yield a healthful house. The style will depend on the particular tastes of the occupants; some people will prefer a contemporary house, while others will opt for the country look. The selection of construction materials will also be influenced by personal preference. For example, a brick exterior will be as inert as stucco, but if your tastes lean toward Spanish architecture, stucco will probably be your choice.

Another important consideration will be cost, both for the construction materials and the labor. For most people, cost is a primary factor, since a house is the largest purchase that they will ever make. It will do no good to talk of only exotic and expensive materials, if they are beyond most budgets. Of course, there are some expensive materials mentioned in this book, but there are also lower cost alternatives to most of them.

This chapter will summarize what my wife, Lynn, and I have done in building our own home. Lynn has severe sensitivities to a wide variety of environmental pollutants, primarily formaldehyde, exhaust fumes, pesticides, artificial fragrances, printing ink, and outgassing from most plastic products. Her reactions to hydrocarbons and organic chemicals are so acute that we had no choice but to build with nonpolluting materials, if her health was to be protected. Of course, there were limits to what we could use. Some materials were not available locally, and others were too costly. Although there were some inevitable compromises, the final result has been very successful, and if we ever build another house, there will be few changes made.

Preliminary Considerations

We wanted to remain in the Midwest, yet we ruled out living in a city where exhaust fumes and lawn chemicals proliferate, as well as areas near farm fields where agricultural chemicals were used. We finally selected a location about ten miles from Bloomington, Indiana. For us, it was important to be near a city large enough to have such things as a good hospital, a food cooperative, and the cultural events and library facilities of a large university. Our homesite is in the middle of a hardwood forest and it has been cleared out sufficiently to allow a nice breeze to blow through. During some times of the year there is an abundance of mold spores in the air, but in general, it is quite tolerable. Remember, there is no place that will be 100 percent perfect.

The actual location of the house is 500 ft. from a gravel road, with a deep ravine separating the two. The driveway is crushed stone, running along the eastern side of the five-acre lot. There is a large open area on the west side of the house where the septic field is located, and the detached garage is about 75 ft. east from the house. This allows the prevailing wind from the west to carry away any exhaust fumes near the garage or drive. All of the utilities to the house are underground, so the nearest utility pole is separated from the house by about 500 ft. of wooded land.

Basic House Design

Our particular needs were for a two-bedroom, single-bath house, with an eat-in kitchen. The final design contained 1013 square feet, with an 8′×12′ screen porch. Since this is relatively small by many people's standards, we decided to use sloped ceilings throughout the house to make the rooms seem larger. This, combined with the room sizes and window placement, has yielded an airy home that is more than comfortable for the two of us.

We wanted the house to be very energy efficient, and determined that there were definite advantages to the superinsulated designs being built in very cold climates. The particular construction technique that we chose was the airtight drywall approach utilizing foil-backed drywall. An obvious advantage is energy efficiency. Since the heating requirement is so low, we were able to use nonpolluting hydronic baseboard heaters. Another strong point of superinsulated houses is the fact that they are almost totally airtight and that fresh air must be brought in mechanically. This means that if there happens to be any pollution outdoors, the ventilation system can be temporarily shut off, with the whole house becoming an oasis.

Foundation

An early decision that we made was to use ceramic tile on all of the floors. While this isn't usually seen in residential construction, it has proven to be quite attractive. This decision led to the selection of a concrete slab foundation system. In order to keep the slab from absorbing moisture from the ground, and to keep radon from entering the house, a plastic vapor barrier was used between the concrete and the ground. The slab has three inches of extruded polystyrene insulation around the perimeter and beneath it. Since these materials are separated from the living space by four inches of concrete, they cannot outgas into the house.

A separate masonry foundation wall was used to support the house. It is surrounded by a perforated drainage tile to keep the foundation system dry. This tile can be used in the future to remove radon from the soil if it should ever become a problem. Since the slab was separated from the foundation wall, it was easy to insulate to the requirements of a superinsulated house. This is not only energy efficient, but it also results in a relatively warm floor, one that is not a home for mold.

Framing

We elected to use a light-gauge steel-stud framing system rather than wood for two basic reasons. First, the natural resins in readily available wood framing lumber can contaminate the air in a house. Steel framing is odor free. Secondly, wood framed houses invariably need to be treated for termites, and steel does not. While the cost of steel framing was slightly higher, this was offset by the savings in omitting the toxic termite treatment.

Our superinsulated design required that the walls be 10½″ thick. This was accomplished by actually building two exterior walls. The outer one is load bearing, and it supports the structure. The inner wall is made of less costly nonload-bearing studs. Its purpose is simply to provide a space for more insulation. With sloped ceilings, the wall in the center of the house needed to be constructed of the load-bearing

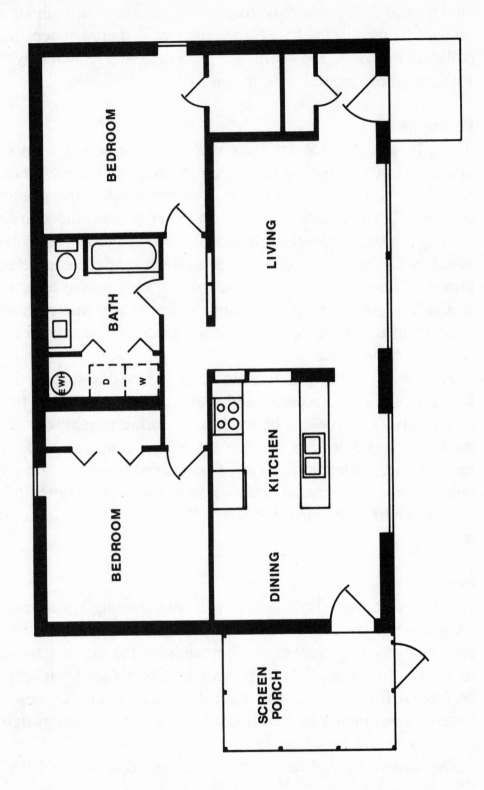

The Author's Home

studs also, but the lighter weight variety was used for all other interior walls. The roof rafters are 13½″ high. This allows for the 12″ of insulation in the ceiling, with a 1½″ airspace above, for roof ventilation.

Exterior

The exterior siding is aluminum, with a baked enamel finish. It is applied over a wind barrier of perforated aluminum builder's foil that has been taped at all seams. The ribbed steel roof is attached to wood purlins. Wood was used in this location in order to maintain the desired roof line. Steel purlins would have needed to be custom made, at a substantial increase in cost. Fir was chosen over pine to minimize outgassing. Since wood in this location is well separated from the living space, the outgassing has not been a problem, and it is far enough from the ground so that subterranean termites cannot reach it. The screen porch is made of aluminum.

Windows are aluminum framed, with thermal breaks to eliminate sweating and be energy efficient. They are triple glazed, having both an insulated unit and an added storm window. In keeping with the superinsulated design, most of the windows are facing south to allow the solar heat to warm the house in the winter. The roof overhang is designed so that they are shaded in the summer. The weather-stripping on the windows does outgas slightly, but since there are so few other components in the house that outgas, this has not been a problem.

The doors are insulated with a foam insulation, but they are sealed on all edges with a steel skin that makes outgassing from the insulation negligible. Again, the small amount of odor from the weather-stripping is minimal. The doors were painted with a latex enamel paint early in the construction process so the paint could have plenty of time to outgas. The windows in the doors are also of insulated glass.

Inside the Walls

We chose yellow fiberglass batt insulation as the lesser of several evils, because of its availability and cost. During installation, a very strong formaldehyde odor was present, but once it was covered with foil-backed drywall, the odor was no longer noticeable. Eventually, all of the smell will have been vented from the walls and ceilings through the ridge vent on the roof. The tightness of the house at this point was becoming quite apparent.

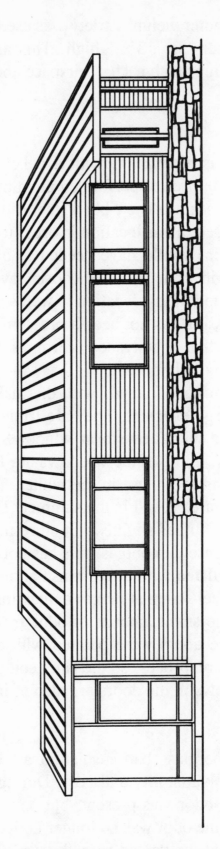

The Author's Home

As a cost-containing measure, plastic sheathed electrical wire and plastic plumbing drain lines were used throughout the house. When these items were well sealed behind the foil-backed drywall in the exterior walls, they could not outgas into the interior of the house. However, we had some reservations about using them within the interior walls, so we wrapped them all individually with aluminum foil. We decided that this was an inexpensive form of insurance, and it has worked quite well in sealing them off from the living space.

Interior

When we elected to use the airtight drywall approach instead of plaster walls, it was both an economic and an energy-related decision. Yet, before we made the final choice, it was necessary to test several samples of paint, in order to determine which would seal the drywall the best. Since Lynn was sensitive to printer's ink, the recycled paper on the drywall was known to be a problem. We found that a white shellac primer worked well in making the paper tolerable, but it did not yield a very attractive finish. For the top coat, we chose a paint that seemed to have only a minimal amount of outgassing after a couple of weeks. Unfortunately, after the interior of the house was painted, the amount of outgassing was quite noticable. It delayed our moving in by three months. This is why testing of several types of paint is always recommended very early in the construction process. Locally available drywall finishing compounds were all quite odorous, but a material made in Texas proved to be very acceptable.

All of the wood used in the interior of the house was tulip poplar, a locally grown hardwood. Like all woods, it has a characteristic odor, but this was reduced by the application of a tolerable, clear finish. All of the interior doors, cabinets, and trim were custom-made of this material. In order to minimize the impact of the smell of the wood, everything was coated on both sides. The trim was all prefinished before it was installed. Tulip poplar was chosen over other hardwoods because of its availability, workability, and relatively low cost.

Kitchen and Bathroom

The kitchen cabinets are all built out of solid wood. The design lent itself to easy assembly, and a minimum of labor. They are finished inside and out. Countertops were also custom-made out of stainless steel. While this was a costly choice, we feel that it was well worth the extra expense. No dishwasher was installed because of the odors associated with them, but the cabinets were designed so that one could be added in the future.

The washer and dryer are located in a closet off the bathroom, so that the major sources of moisture would be in the same room. This closet also contains the electric water heater and the central vacuum unit. The bathtub is a porcelain-on-steel model and the walls around the tub are covered with custom-made porcelain-on-steel panels. The required caulking at the edges of these panels took about three weeks to outgas. The lavatory cabinet matches those in the kitchen and is fitted with a vitreous china top. The toilet has an insulated tank to minimize sweating.

All water supply lines within the house are soldered copper, but since the line outside the house and most of the ten miles of water mains between us and the water plant are plastic, we installed a carbon filter on the incoming line. Plumbing fixtures were chosen from locally available models with a minimum of plastic parts.

Ventilation

The heart of the ventilation system is a heat recovery ventilator that is located above a dropped ceiling in the central hallway. This is the only part of the house that does not have a high sloped ceiling. The model that we chose has a heat pipe core. It was selected because of its compactness and being easy to clean. Fresh air is drawn from the west end of the house and enters the living space through a grille in the center of the house, in the ceiling of the hallway. After the fresh air passes through the heat recovery ventilator, it travels through a fine-particle filter and a bed of activated carbon. The particle filter removes most of the mold spores and pollen that might otherwise enter the house. The activated carbon was added because there was a slight odor from the fan in the heat recovery ventilator and also from the particle filter.

The stale air is pulled from several locations in the house, directed through the heat recovery ventilator and discharged outdoors about 25 ft. downwind of the fresh air intake. The stale air pickup points include the kitchen, the bathroom closet, the entry closet, and the two bedroom closets. In this way, the air in the house is circulated and is constantly being replaced with fresh air. This system is capable of changing the air in the house every hour, but we have found that with so few outgassing sources inside the house, we only need to run it between eight and ten hours a day to keep the air fresh.

The kitchen range hood is a fairly powerful model and is vented outdoors separately, as are the clothes dryer and the central vacuum exhaust. These appliances could contaminate the heat recovery ventilator with dust or cooking grease and cause a fire danger, so it is important to exhaust them separately. The house is so airtight that when one of these items is running, a slight negative pressure is created in the house. As a result, the ventilation air in the heat recovery ventilator is slightly unbalanced. This is not a problem unless all are running simultaneously, when it helps to temporarily crack open a window.

Summary

Our house was designed as a system, rather than a collection of component parts. The superinsulated concept and the ventilation requirements were central to decisions about room placement. Walls were located so that plumbing and ventilation ducting could be easily run without piercing the barrier created by the airtight drywall approach. Room placement was determined by window locations, and vice versa. While there were some less than desirable materials used, they were well separated from the living space. Those materials wholly within the living space were chosen with care to be as minimally polluting as possible. Following the guidelines in Chapter 6, we first *eliminated* everything economically possible that could cause indoor air pollution. Secondly, what couldn't be eliminated, for whatever reason, was *separated* from the living space. Thirdly, the house is thoroughly *ventilated* in order to supply fresh air and to remove any contaminants that do turn up inside the house.

While our house is built somewhat differently than most houses today, it doesn't look unusual. There is little about the exterior to suggest that is was designed to be as healthful as possible. Upon entering, you notice the attractive woodwork, the high sloping ceilings, spacious windows, and deep window sills. The major thing that makes its appearance different from other homes is the fact that there is no carpeting on the floor, but most people comment on the attractiveness of the ceramic tile which is accented with Oriental and cotton throw rugs. In other words, healthful doesn't have to look strange or ugly.

It would be difficult to compute the added cost of healthfulness to our house. Since I built the entire house myself, I can't guess what another builder, with a full crew of workers and more overhead, would charge. Depending on your specific requirements, the added cost of healthfulness may be nothing or it could be as much as 25 percent. Much of the increased cost is due to the fact that many of the materials are not readily available at local lumberyards. While steel framing is easily obtained, it must still be specially ordered, so the cost of handling will be higher than wood. Ordering drywall joint compound or paint from across the country can also be costly. Our house has energy-efficient features that alone would seem to justify the added dollars spent.

The costs of healthfulness go far beyond the construction expense. A house that doesn't result in indoor air pollution means fewer trips to the doctor. Most of the materials used will outlast their unhealthy counterparts, so maintenance and repair in the future will be less. As an example, we have found the routine maintenance of ceramic tile floors to be very minimal.

For very little added effort and money, you too can create a healthful house.

Appendix I

Locating Materials

There are many suppliers and organizations mentioned throughout this book, for whom addresses and telephone numbers are given in Appendix III. The notes and selected bibliography can be helpful if you are interested in further documentation about health effects. However, since sensitivities vary greatly, it may be necessary to locate the producer of an unusual material, or to obtain a more detailed description about a particular product. This Appendix will show you how to contact suppliers in order to obtain health-related information that might not be covered here.

The purpose of this book is to tie together all of the loose ends and to provide a comprehensive guide for healthful housing information. Since new materials and products are constantly being developed, it may be necessary to contact a new supplier directly in order to obtain the necessary information or a small sample to test.

Material Safety Data Sheets
The **Occupational Safety and Health Administration (OSHA)** has issued "right-to-know" regulations for the workplace. Material Safety Data Sheets (MSDS) are a big part of these requirements. The purpose is to insure that hazardous chemicals that are produced, imported, or used within the U.S. manufacturing sector are evaluated, and that that information is then given to the affected employers and employees. An MSDS should be available to all employees for each hazardous chemical that they come into contact with.

The MSDS will provide basic information such as the product name and physical characteristics. It should also list known health effects,

347

for both short-term and long-term exposure. Exposure limits, carcino-genicity, precautionary measures, and emergency procedures are also to be listed.

An MSDS can usually be obtained from the manufacturer by any-one interested in a particular product. They are available for every-thing from paint to insulation to caulking to treated lumber. Anyone interested in learning about the safety of a given product should start by first requesting some general product literature and a current copy of the MSDS.

Unfortunately, the regulations do not require all hazardous sub-stances to be listed. Trade secrets are excluded from the listing re-quirement, although there is a clause requiring that this confidential information be revealed to health professionals in the event of an emergency. If a hazardous ingredient, other than a carcinogen, com-prises less than 1 percent of the product, it need not be listed. Carcino-gens need not be listed if they are present in quantities less than 0.1 percent. This means that there are many hazardous and cancer-causing ingredients that are not required to be listed on the MSDS.

Furthermore, the definition of what is a hazardous chemical further shortens the list of components that must be listed. There needs to be hard scientific data on humans or animals showing that a material is either hazardous or cancer-causing. Since most of the thousands of chemicals have not been subjected to this type of testing, only a rela-tively small number of substances are actually required to be listed on an MSDS.

In spite of these drawbacks, an MSDS is a valuable tool when ana-lyzing a product. It should not be used alone, but in combination with other information and personal testing when determining the safety of a product. As more is learned about the long-term effects of small exposures of various chemicals, the MSDS will become a much more effective tool.

Locating Suppliers

All material manufacturers and organizations shown in this book in **bold type** are to be found in the Appendix III. In general, the manufac-turer is listed rather than the distributor because there may be several regional distributors. These regional distributors may sell to dozens of local retail outlets. Occasionally a manufacturer will be listed as well as a retail or mail order source. If a particular product is not readily available locally, simply write to the manufacturer and ask ask for the nearest supplier.

The public library can be a good source of further information. Several books will prove invaluable when searching for an unusual material. The reference desk personnel will help patrons find information that is not easy to come by. They are usually available by telephone, if you are too sensitive to printing ink to enter the library itself. The *Thomas Register* (Thomas Publishing Co.) and *Blue Book* (MacRaes Publishing) both list manufacturers by what they produce. If you need metal roofing, these will both list several sources. They are like a national industrial yellow pages. Both contain a listing of trademarks, as does the *Trade Names Directory* (Gale Research Co.) This can be helpful if you know the brand name of a product but not the manufacturer.

The *Encyclopedia of Associations* (Gale Research Co.) contains a listing of trade organizations. Names, addresses, and a description of their function are listed, as well as the number of member firms. If you need some general information about marble, it would be a good idea to start with the Marble Institute. If you have a specific question about steel doors, the Steel Door Institute would be a good source.

Different types of *Sweets Catalogs* (Sweets Division, McGraw-Hill Information Services) are kept by engineers, architects, and general contractors. These consist of several volumes of building material information. Unfortunately, the health effects of building materials are poorly publicized, but sometimes these catalogs can be helpful. The catalogs themselves are supplied by various manufacturers and are assembled and distributed by Sweets. While many manufacturers are represented in these catalogs, it is by no means a complete listing. For one reason or another, many building materials companies do not use the service.

There is a growing number of consultants who are interested in healthful housing. As with consultants in any field, there are some who are more knowledgeable and have more experience than others. Selecting a safe building consultant or architect is no different than selecting a television repairman. A competent professional will be happy to provide references that can be contacted. The important thing to remember is that no matter what you are told by a consultant, if you have severe or unusual sensitivities, everything should be personally tested.

Contacting Suppliers

Manufacturers are usually happy to give out information about their products because advertising of any sort is how things are sold, and selling is why they are in business. They can also be receptive to constructive criticism and complaints. However, they may not be receptive to someone who complains about how their product is killing the world and is part of a communist conspiracy. In order to receive an intelligent reply, you must have a specific, well worded request. Later requests can follow as you become better acquainted with their literature. Requests for information can either be made by telephone or mail.

When first contacting a manufacturer, it is best to only ask one simple and straightforward question. Asking ten different and somewhat unrelated questions can cause your letter to be placed in the "crackpot" file. The first things to request are general product literature and, if available, an MSDS. These items may supply you with enough information to determine that you don't want to have anything to do with the product. They may also lead you to ask a question that you haven't thought of. For instance, a brochure might mention a "specially treated" cardboard lining. You may then want to ask what it is treated with. Often, a first inquiry to a company will supply you with the name of a specific individual whom you can contact directly.

After your initial contact, you may have several questions. These should be very specific and written down in front of you, if you are telephoning. In a letter, it may be helpful to number the questions, so that all are more likely to be answered. If you are using the telephone and do not know of a specific individual to speak with, tell the switchboard operator something like: "I have some technical questions about the paint that you manufacture." You will then be put in touch with someone in customer relations or possibly a chemist. It may be helpful to state that you are hypersensitive to hydrocarbons and as a result have some points that need clarifying. You can also ask for a small sample to personally test for tolerability. Such samples are often available but they may be stored in an office area, where they can be contaminated by cigarette smoke. This may not seem an important consideration to them, but if you briefly explain your situation, many companies are happy to comply.

Unfortunately, some companies are much more secretive than is necessary. If a reasonable request has been denied, it may be easier to contact another source than "bucking the system." You may be only one person, but if you don't purchase their product and your friends follow suit, sooner or later they will feel the pressure.

Occasionally, a sales representative will be very interested in your request. Someone concerned with the healthfulness of their product could mean an entirely new market and more sales. "All natural" and "non-toxic" are catch words that can increase profits.

Summary

While this book is filled with sources of less toxic building materials, it will sometimes be necessary to contact a manufacturer directly in order to obtain an unusual product, or further information. Various library reference books can be helpful in obtaining addresses and telephone numbers. When contacting a company, product literature and Material Safety Data Sheets will aid in analyzing the healthfulness of materials.

Appendix II

Testing Materials

Someone with no known sensitivities may not need to test materials. By simply choosing the less toxic products mentioned in this book, they can maintain their good health. However, very sensitive people should test everything because, according to one engineer, "Individual testing is the only known way to guarantee that you will be able to tolerate your home."[1]

In order to accurately test various products, it is advisable to only test one at a time. Otherwise it is difficult to know just what is causing a reaction. With so many possible pollutants floating around in the air of our houses, this can often be difficult. If an oasis has been created, this will be a good place to perform the testing. If the entire house is suspect, testing should be done outdoors, away from pollution sources. This may mean driving some distance away. You should allow your body to "clear" before beginning the testing. This may take a few hours, depending on your particular sensitivities.

Several methods for testing materials are available. It may be necessary to utilize a different method for different materials. It may also be necessary to test some things in combination. For example, the insulation found inside the walls of a house can be a problem, yet it will not ever be directly in contact with the occupants. If required, a small sample wall can be built to see if the assembly itself elicits symptoms.

Some people are delayed reactors. They may not experience symptoms until several hours have elapsed. A diary of exposure methods, materials, and symptoms over several days will usually turn up a pattern if this is the case. Since many people have allergies to foods or pets, the diary should include references to them as well.

Office Procedures

It should be emphasized that with severe sensitivities, all testing should be done under the supervision of a qualified physician, since there could be the possibility of unusual reactions.

There are environmental control units set up for this purpose, but they can be quite expensive, often running into thousands of dollars. For information, contact the **American Academy of Environmental Medicine**. In effect, a person is placed in a sterile environment for several days and given only spring water to drink. In this way, the body becomes totally devoid of symptoms of not only environmental chemicals, but also unrealized food allergies. At this point, if a substance is introduced into the clean environment, a reaction can be noted almost immediately.

There is a variety of office procedures that your doctor may wish to utilize in testing for environmental pollutants. Scratch tests and intradermal tests are very good for determining allergies to such things as mold, and pollen.[2] The provocative-neutralization intradermal test can be used to evaluate sensitivities to pollutants like formaldehyde.[3] By using this procedure, a physician can both cause a reaction to take place, and turn the reaction off.

Preparing a Sample for Testing

Samples can be prepared in several ways. When tesing a single material, it is important to make sure that the sample is not being contaminated by something else. For example, when testing paint, it is important not to coat something that could possibly outgas itself. Painting a piece of cardboard is not recommended, because some people will react to the cardboard. Coating a piece of glass or metal foil would be a better choice. When in doubt, test the material to be coated first, without any paint. If no reaction is noted, then paint it and test again.

Sometimes two or more materials will need to be tested simultaneously. If an individual reacts both to paints and to the paper on drywall, then a paint must be found that will be tolerable itself and will seal the drywall, rendering it tolerable. The best way to handle a situation like this is to prepare several samples using different paints and see which one is the most tolerable the soonest. In the case of drywall, both sides of the sample must be coated so that the paper on the back side is not the source of a reaction.

A small sample is often sufficient for testing purposes. Place the material in a glass jar and screw on the lid. This is then placed out-doors in the sun. The sun warms up the sample and causes it to outgas at an accelerated rate. When the jar is then opened, the amount of outgassing will be comparable to a much larger sample that might be found in a house. Sometimes it is recommended that the jar be placed in a 300° oven for 20 minutes, allowed to cool, then opened and tested. In either case, the purpose is to cause an accelerated rate of outgassing to take place, thus simulating a large sample. In the case of paint, there are hundreds of square feet to which occupants are ex-posed in a house, and while a small sample may be tolerable, 20 gal-lons spread out over all the walls and ceilings may be devastating.

Larger samples can be prepared with a large section of the product itself or, as with paint, on a piece of glass or metal foil. This sample can then be placed indoors, near a sensitive person, to determine toler-ability. Sometimes, it can be placed in an oasis, near the bed. If sleep comes naturally with such a sample present, it is probably tolerable.

Most materials outgas to some degree and they must be allowed to air out before they should be brought near a sensitive individual. When using a glass jar for testing, leave it open for a certain number of days before sealing it and placing it in the sun. Some products, such as paints, may require several weeks of drying before they will be aired out enough for testing. For this reason, preparing several large sam-ples may be a better way to test. They can outgas naturally and can be tested on a regular basis until they are determined to be safe.

It is important to date all samples to be tested. For instance, when several paints are to be tested, they may all outgas sufficiently to be tolerable eventually. If you are going to be living in a house while it is being painted, it will be important to select the paint that outgasses the fastest.

Sniff Testing

Sniff testing is perhaps the easiest method. Simply sniff the sample with your nose. A short sniff is recommended initially. If no reaction is noted, it should be followed by a longer sniff. Immediate reactions can include such things as clogged sinuses, inflamed sinuses, headache, dizziness, feeling "spacey," etc. Symptoms are highly individualistic so your symptoms will likely be quite different from someone else's. If you are testing in a very relaxed place, free of pollution, it should be fairly easy to sense any minor changes in your system. If the testing is done in a noisy, polluted area, there may be so many other background factors that symptoms will not be noticeable. If you have already rid your life-style of the major pollutants, testing should be easier. The fewer the number of background problems, the sharper will be your ability to read your body's reaction.

A variation of this method involves sleeping with the sample. A piece of metal foil that has been painted can be placed inside your pillowcase. A sleepless night or nightmares will indicate intolerance.

While it has been noted that the human nose is very sensitive to odorous pollutants, this method of testing can also be used to test materials that have no apparent odor because the outgassed molecules will still come in contact with the soft sinus tissues and be absorbed.

Touch Testing

It will be possible for some people to simply touch a sample and determine whether or not it is tolerable. For example, many people report that when wearing synthetic clothing, they experience a tingly, "crawly," or burning feeling on their skin. This is simply a reaction to the synthetic material, indicating an intolerance. Occasionally a red spot or hives will develop when performing this type of testing. The method is simple: place a sample on the back of your hand for a while. Sometimes a reaction will be noted immediately, occasionally it will develop within an hour or so. Again, it is important to do the testing in a clean, relaxed atmosphere.

Pulse Testing

This involves learning to take your own pulse. A physician or other health-care worker can assist in teaching you this fairly simple procedure, or you can purchase an electronic instrument to assist you. Begin by determining your pulse every two hours and recording it. Normal may be anywhere from in the mid-50s to the mid-80s. The pulse is taken five minutes before testing and 20, 40, and 60 minutes after exposure. It should be taken for a full minute each time in order to obtain maximum accuracy, and then written down. The testing can be either sniff or touch testing, whichever seems to give the best results. Any form of physical activity will invalidate the test, even something as simple as going to the bathroom. Eating a food to which one is allergic can also invalidate the test, since it will also result in an increase in the pulse rate. A noticeable change in the pulse rate will indicate that your body is reacting to the sample. Usually an increase of 10 beats is considered significant enough to indicate a reaction.

Combustion Appliances

Combustion appliances are often implicated in illness. As a rule, the healthy house will not have any of them, whether they are furnaces, water heaters, or ranges. However, these appliances are quite common and many times are not suspected of causing symptoms. Ideally, in order to test for tolerability, an individual should be isolated from exposure for 72 hours. This may involve staying in an all-electric house for a few days or some time spent in a tent or camper. After this waiting period, the individual can simply breathe the gases escaping from the kitchen range, or the warm air register of the furnace. Furnace fumes will be more noticeable immediately upon start-up. Symptoms can be quite varied and may be immediately noticeable or may be delayed for some time. The best way to test a house in general is to leave it for a few days in this manner. Your system then tends to forget that it was used to the daily exposure. For this reason, people may experience reactions to their house upon returning from a vacation. The constant daily exposure takes it toll, but a sudden return causes the symptoms to be immediately noticeable.

Radon Testing

There is a number of inexpensive radon testing devices on the market, but, as with any product of technology, they are constantly being outdated. Radon is in the news a great deal today and as a result many companies are selling testing devices. Since many of these will be out of business as soon as this book is in print, it was decided not to list any here. Instead, the reader is directed to his local Board of Health. Your local Board of Health will be listed in the telephone book in the yellow pages under Governmental Agencies, and will be able to give you the most up-to-date information about finding a testing device. Sometimes they will be able to provide the service themselves. If your local agency does not have the information, ask for the address or telephone number of the appropriate state agency. Occasionally, local offices are not large enough to have the latest information, but the State Board of Health will be able to help.

Commercial Water and Air Testing

Commercial testing of the air inside your home or your drinking water can be done by many laboratories. It is important, however, to know just what to test for, since the possible list of pollutants could number in the hundreds. Testing for all of them could run into thousands of dollars.

Local and state Boards of Health can often provide some of this testing either at no charge or at a reasonable cost if it is apparent that your health is at risk. Usually, they will do screening tests of the most likely pollutants, such as formaldehyde, by-products of combustion, chlordane, or organic compounds. With these results, it can then be determined whether or not additional testing is required. Unfortunately, commercial air testing may not be able to detect the very low pollutant levels to which many people react.

Commericial testing labs can be found in major cities in the telephone book under Laboratories, or your Board of Health may be able to provide a list.

Summary

There are several different methods of testing various materials. Each material must be evaluated to determine which method will work best. There is no single preferred method and reactions can be varied. There has been at least one case of someone hypersensitive to natural gas returning home after an absence and falling into a coma; however, most reactions will not be this severe. In fact, they will often be fairly minor. Therefore, an individual who has extreme sensitivities should always do the testing under a doctor's supervision. Minor reactions should not, however, be ignored. It is these minor reactions that add up to produce disease.

Appendix III

Organizations and Suppliers

3M
3M Center
St. Paul, MN 55144
(612) 733-1110

AA-Abbington Affiliates, Inc.
2149–51 Utica Avenue
Brooklyn, NY 11234
(718) 258-8333

AFM Enterprises, Inc.
1140 Stacy Court
Riverside, CA 92507
(714) 781-6860

AGA Corporation
P.O. Box 246
Amasa, MI 49903
(906) 822-7311

AMF/Cuno
400 Research Parkway
Meriden, CT 06450
(203) 237-5541
(800) 238-8660

ASC Pacific Inc.
2141 Milwaukee Way
P.O. Box 2075   5256
Tacoma, WA 98401
(206) 383-4955

Air Conditioning Engineers
211 Railroad Ave.
Blue Mound, IL 62513
(217) 692-2812
(217) 422-0311

Air Krete, Inc.
P.O. Box 380
Weedsport, NY 13166
(315) 834-6609

Air Purification Products
P.O. Box 519
Royce City, TX 75089
(214) 635-9565

Aireox Research Corp.
P.O. Box 8523
Riverside, CA 92515
(714) 689-2781

Airguard Industries
P.O. Box 32578
Louisville, KY 40232
(502) 969-2304

Alcan Aluminum Corp.
100 Erieview Plaza
Cleveland, OH 44114
(216) 523-6800

Alcoa Building Products
P.O. Box 716
Sidney, OH 45365
(513) 492-1111

Allergen Air Filter Corp.
5205 Ashbrook
Houston, TX 77081
(713) 668-2371
(800) 333-8880

Allermed Corp.
31 Steel Rd.
Wylie, TX 75098
(214) 442-4898

Alpine Industries
P.O. Box 944
Mt. Shasta, CA 96067
(916) 926-2460

Alside
P.O. Box 2010
Akron, OH 44309
(216) 929-1811

Alumark Corporation
P.O. Box 61
Roxboro, NC 27573
(919) 599-2151

Aluminum Filter Co.
1000 Cindy Lane
Carpinteria, CA 93013
(805) 684-7651

Amana Refrigeration Inc.
Amana, IA 52204
(319) 622-5511

American Academy of Environmental
Medicine
P.O. Box 16106
Denver, CO 80216
(303) 622-9755

American Air Filter Co.
P.O. Box 35690
Louisville, KY 40232
(502) 637-0011

American Architectural Manufacturers
Assoc.
2700 River Road, Suite 118
Des Plaines, IL 60018
(312) 699-7310

American Cyanamid
1 Cyanamid Plaza
Wayne, NJ 07470
(201) 831-2000

American Standard Inc.
40 W. 40th St.
New York, NY 10018
(212) 840-5100

Ametek
502 Indiana Ave.
Sheboygan, WI 53081
(414) 457-9435

Amico/MAS, Inc.
Clark-Cincinnati
5210 Duff Drive
Cincinnati, OH 45246
(513) 874-9631
(800) 543-7140

Ampax Aluminum Co.
350 Fifth Ave.
Empire State Bldg., Suite 3902
New York, NY 10001
(212) 564-6600

Angeles Metal Systems
4817 East Shiela St.
Los Angeles, CA 90040
(213) 268-1777

Aquathin Corp.
2800 West Cypress Creek Road
Ft. Lauderdale, FL 33309
(305) 977-7997

Armstrong World Industries, Inc.
P.O. Box 3001
Lancaster, PA 17604
(800) 233-3823

Asbestos Information Center
Center for Environmental Management
Tufts University
Curtis Hall
Medford, MA 02155
(617) 381-3486

Ashland Chemical Corp.
Div. Ashland Oil Co.
Box 2219
Columbus, OH 43216
(614) 889-3333

Automated Controls & Systems
935 N. Lively Blvd.
Wood Dale, Il 60191
(708) 860-6860

BASF Corp.
Fibers Division
P.O. Drawer D
Williamsburg, VA 23187
(804) 887-6000

Barnebey Cheney
835 N. Cassedy Ave.
P.O. Box 2526
Columbus, OH 43216
(614) 258-9501

Beam Industries Inc.
1607 E. Second St.
P.O. Box 189
Webster City, IA 50595
(515) 832-4620

Beecham Home Improvement Products,
Inc.
8707 Millegrove Dr.
Santa Fe Springs, CA 90670
(213) 692-0911

Benchmark Windows
P.O. Box 2351
Prescott, AZ 86302
(602) 778-2795

Berko Electric
P.O. Box 188
Highway 19 North
Peru, IN 46970
(317) 472-3921

Berridge Manufacturing Co.
1720 Maury St.
Houston, TX 77026
(713) 223-4971
(800) 231-8127

Bilco Company
Box 1203
New Haven, CT 06505
(203) 934-6363

Bio Integral Resource Center (BIRC)
P.O. Box 7414
Berkeley, CA 94707
(415) 524-2567

Boise Cascade
1600 S.W. 4th Ave.
Portland, OR 97201
(503) 224-7250

Boss Aire
2901 SE Fourth St.
Minneapolis, MN 55414
(612) 278-0049

Brookstone Co.
5 Vose Farm Road
Petersborough, NH 03458
(603) 924-9541

Buckingham Virginia Slate Corp.
Box 11002
4110 Fitzhugh Ave.
Richmond, VA 23230
(804) 355-4351

Burns and Russell Co.
506 S. Central Ave.
Box 6063
Baltimore, MD 21231
(301) 837-0720

Cambridge Filter Corp.
P.O. Box 4906
Syracuse, NY 13221
(315) 457-1000

Carus Chemical Corp.
P.O. Box 1500
LaSalle, IL 61310
(815) 223-1500

Celotex Corp.
P.O. Box 22602Z
Tampa, FL 33622
(813) 871-4811

Certainteed Corp.
P.O. Box 860
Valley Forge, PA 19482
(215) 341-7000

Chicago Metallic Corp.
4849 S. Austin Ave.
Chicago, IL 60638
(312) 563-4600

Clopay Corp.
101 East 4th St.
Cincinnati, OH 45202
(513) 381-4800
(800) 225-6729

Coleman Cable Systems Inc.
2500 Commonwealth Ave.
North Chicago, IL 60064
(708) 689-9090

Combustion Engineering Inc.
Q-Dot Corp.
701 N. First St.
Garland, TX 75040
(214) 487-1130

Consumer Product Safety Commission
1111 18th St. NW
Washington, DC 20207
(800) 638-2772

Control Resource Systems Inc.
670 Mariner Dr.
Michigan City, IN 46360
(219) 872-5519
(800) 272-3786

Culligan International Co.
One Culligan Parkway
Northbrook, IL 60062
(312) 498-2000
(800) 451-3260

Dale Industries, Inc.
1001 NW 58th Court
Ft. Lauderdale, FL 33309
(305) 772-6300
or
6455 Kingsley Ave.
Dearborn, MI 48126
(313) 846-3400

Davis Colors
Mineral Pigments Corp.
7011 Muirkirk Road
Beltsville, MD 20705
(301) 792-7700

Dellinger, Inc.
P.O. Drawer 273
1943 North Broad Street
Rome, GA 30161
(404) 291-4447

Denny Sales Corporation
3500 Gateway Dr.
Pompano Beach, FL 33069
(305) 971-3100
(800) 327-6616

Des Champs Laboratories, Inc.
P.O. Box 440
17 Farinella Dr.
East Hanover, NJ 07936
(201) 884-1460

Diamond Shamrock Corp.
Diamond Shamrock Tower
717 N. Harwood St.
Dallas, TX 75201
(214) 922-2000

Donn Corporation
1000 Crocker Rd.
Westlake, OH 44145
(216) 871-1000

Dow Chemical Corp.
2020 Dow Center
Midland, MI 48674
(517) 636-1000
(800) 232-CHEM

Drakenfeld Colors
P.O. Box 519
Washington, PA 15301
(412) 223-5900

Du Pont Co.
1000 Market St.
Wilmington, DE 19898
(302) 774-9096
(800) 527-2601

Duro-Test Corp.
2321 Kennedy Blvd.
North Bergen, NJ 07047
(201) 867-7000

Ecologically Safe Homes
7471 N. Shiloh Rd.
Unionville, IN 47468
(812) 332-5073

Ecology Ministries
Jane Harmon
14232 Marsh Ln.
Dallas, TX 75234

Eljen Corp.
15 Westwood Rd.
Storrs, CT 06268
(203) 429-9486

Enviracare Corp.
747 Bowman Ave.
Hagerstown, MD 21740
(301) 797-9700
(800) 332-1110

Environmental Construction Network
Ed Lowans
R.R. 1
Caledon East
Ontario, Canada LOH 1EO
(519) 941-6499

Environmental Protection Agency
Public Information Center
201 M St. SW
Washington, DC 20460
(202) 382-2090

Eternit
P.O. Box 679
Excelsior In. Pk.
Blandon, PA 19510
(215) 926-0100
(800) 233-3155

FHP Manufacturing
601 N.W. 65th Ct.
Ft. Lauderdale, FL 33309
(305) 776-5471

Fairfield American Corp.
238 Wilson Ave.
Newark, NJ 07105
(201) 589-0263

Farr Co.
P.O. Box 92187
El Segundo, CA 90245
(213) 772-5221

Fenestra Corp.
4040 West 20th St.
P.O. Box 8189
Erie, PA 16505
(814) 838-2001

Filtex
900 Palomares Ave.
Suite F
Laverne, CA 91750

Fluid Mechanics
345 Burnette Rd.
W. Lafayette, IN 47906
(317) 742-2338

Forbo North America
P.O. Box 32155
Richmond, VA 23294
(800) 233-0475
(804) 747-3714

E.L. Foust Co. Inc
P.O. Box 105
Elmhurst, IL 60126
(312) 834-4952
(800) 225-9549

General Ecology Inc.
151 Sheree Blvd.
Lionville, PA 19353
(215) 363-7900
(800) 441-8166

General Products Co., Inc.
P.O. Box 7387
Fredericksburg, VA 22404
(703) 898-5700

Georgia-Pacific Corp.
133 Peachtree Street N.E.
Atlanta, GA 30303
(404) 521-4000
(800) 447-2882

Glidden Paint
925 Euclid Ave.
Cleveland, OH 44115
(216) 344-8206

Gloucester Co., Inc.
P.O. Box 428
Franklin, MA 02038
(508) 528-2200
(800) 343-4963

Gold Bond Building Products
A Natural Gypsum Division
Gold Bond Building
2001 Rexford Road
Charlotte, NC 28211
(704) 365-7300

Gyp-Crete Corp.
P.O. Box 253
Hamel, MN 55340
(612) 478-6072

Gladding, McBean & Co.
P.O. Box 97
Lincoln, CA 95648
(916) 645-3341

Wm. R. Hague, Inc.
4343 S. Hamilton Rd.
Groveport, OH 43125
(614) 836-2195

Harrison Manufacturing Co.
415 E. Brooks Rd.
Memphis, TN 38109
(901) 332-4030

Homasote Co.
Box 7240
W. Trenton, NJ 08628
(609) 883-3300
(800) 257-9491

Honeywell Inc.
Honeywell Plaza
Minneapolis, MN 55408
(612) 870-2142
(800) 328-5111

Human Ecology Action League (HEAL)
P.O. Box 49125
Atlanta, GA 30359
(404) 248-1898

Hydrex of San Diego
Raymond Stansbury
P.O. Box 2611227
San Diego, CA 92196
(619) 695-0455

InCor, Inc.
4601 North Point Blvd.
Baltimore, MD 21219
(301) 477-4000
(800) 345-STUD

Innovative Energy, Inc.
1119 West 145th Ave.
Crown Point, IN 46307
(219) 662-0737

Intertherm Inc.
10820 Sunset Office Drive
St. Louis, MO 63127
(314) 822-9600

J-DRain Enterprises Inc.
725 Branch Drive
Alpharetta, GA 30201
(404) 442-1461
(800) 843-7569

King Aire
126th St. & S.R. 37 N.
Noblesville, IN 46060
(317) 845-1170
(800) 999-KING

Knauf Fiber Glass GmbH
240 Elizabeth Street
Shelbyville, IN 46176
(317) 398-4434

Leigh Products
411 64th Ave.
Coopersville, MI 49404
(616) 837-8141
(800) 253-0361

Levolor Lorentzen, Inc.
One Upper Pond Road
Parsippany, NJ 07054
(201) 299-1190
(800) 223-0193

Living Source
3500 MacArthur Dr.
Waco, TX 76708
(817) 756-6341

Livos Plantchemistry
1365 Rufina Circle
Santa Fe, NM 87501
(505) 438-3448
(800) 621-2591

Lomanco Inc.
P.O. Box 519
Jacksonville, AR 72076
(800) 643-5596

Ludowici Celadon Co.
415 W. Golf Rd.
Ste. 19
Arlington Hts., IL 60005
(708) 228-1808

May Aire
Standex Energy Systems
P.O. Box 1168
Detroit Lakes, MN 56501

Manville Building Products Corp.
Ken Caryl Ranch
P.O. Box 5108
Denver, CO 80217
(800) 654-3103

Marino Industries Corp.
Montrose Road
Westbury, NY 11590
(516) 333-6810

McElroy Metal, Inc.
1500 Hamilton Road
Bossier, LA 71111
(318) 747-8000

Metal Building Components, Inc.
14031 West Hardy
Houston, TX 77060
(713) 461-0505

Metal Lath/Steel Framing Assoc.
600 S. Federal St.
Suite 400
Chicago, Il 60605
(312) 922-6222

Metal Sales Manufacturing Corp.
10300 Linn Station Rd.
Louisville, KY 40223
(502) 426-5215

Met-Tile, Inc.
P.O. Box 11677
Spokane, WA 99211-1677
(509) 534-6612

Michelin Canvas
Sanford Burger
7254 N.W. 34th St.
Miami, FL 33122
(305) 594-2091

Mirati Inc.
P.O. Box 240967
Charlotte, NC 28224
(704) 523-7477
(800) 438-1855

Modulars, Inc.
P.O. Box 216
Hamilton, OH 45012
(513) 868-7300

Monitor Products Inc.
Box 3408
Princeton, NJ 08543
(201) 329-0900
(800) 524-1102

Moultrie Manufacturing Co.
P.O. Box 1179
Moultrie, GA 31776
(912) 985-1312
(800) 841-8674

Mountain Energy Resources Inc.
15800 West Sixth Ave.
Golden, CO 80410
(303) 279-4971

Murco Wall Products, Inc.
300 N.E. 21st Street
Fort Worth, TX 76106
(817) 626-1987

N.E.E.D.S.
120 Julian Place
Syracuse, NY 13210
(315) 446-1122
(800) 634-1380

N-Viro Products Ltd.
610 Walnut Ave.
Bohemia, NY 11716
(516) 567-2628

National Aeronautics and Space
Administration (NASA)
Life Sciences Branch
Washington, DC 20546
(202) 453-1000

National Bugmobiles
Lester Meis
2305 N. Laurent St.
Victoria, TX 77901
(512) 575-6401

National Center for Appropriate
Technology (NCAT)
3040 Continental Drive
P.O. Box 3838
Butte, MT 59702
(406) 494-4572
(800) 428-2525

National Foundation for the Chemically
Hypersensitive
P.O. Box 9
Wrightsville Beach, NC 28480
(919) 256-5391

National Institute for Occupational
Safety and Health (NIOSH)
Health and Human Services Department
200 Independence Ave. SW
Washington, DC 20201
(202) 472-7134

National Institutes of Health and Safety
9000 Rockville Pike
Bethesda, MD 20814
(301) 496-4000

National Wood Window & Door
Association
1400 East Touhy Ave.
Des Plaines, IL 60018
(312) 299-5200

Nigra Enterprises
5699 Kanan Road
Agoura Hills, CA 91301
(818) 889-6877

Nor-An
3509 Silverside Rd.
P.O. Box 7895
Wilmington, DE 19803
(302) 575-2000

Norton Performance Plastics
P.O. Box 3660
Akron, OH 44309
(216) 798-9508

Nutech Energy Systems
124 Newbold Ct.
London, Ont., Canada N6E 127
(519) 686-0797

Nutone/Scovill
Madison and Red Bank Roads
Cincinnati, OH 45227
(513) 527-5100

Miller Paint Co. Inc.
317 SE Grand Arc
Portland, OR 97214
(503) 233-4491

Occupational Safety and Health
Administration (OSHA)
Department of Labor
200 Constitution Ave. NW
Washington, DC 20001
(202) 523-6091

Old-Fashioned Milk Paint Co.
Box 222
Groton, MA 01450
(508) 448-6336

Owens Corning Fiberglas Corp.
Fiberglas Tower
Toledo, OH 43659
(419) 248-8000
(800) 342-3754

Ott Light Systems
306 E. Cota St.
Santa Barbara, CA 93101
(800) 234-3724
(805) 564-3467

Pace Industries, Inc.
779 S. LaGrange Ave.
Newbury Park, CA 91320
(805) 499-2911

Pemko, Inc.
4226 Transport St.
Ventura, CA 93003
(805) 642-2600

Pierce & Stevens Chemical Corp.
710 Ohio Street
P.O. Box 1092
Buffalo, NY 14240
(716) 856-4910

Pinecrest
2118 Blaisdell Ave.
Minneapolis, MN 55404
(612) 871-7071

Pittsburgh Corning Corp.
800 Presque Isle Drive
Pittsburgh, PA 15239
(412) 327-6100

Porcelain Enamel Institute
1101 Connecticut Ave.
Suite 700
Washington, DC, 30036
(202) 857-1134

Purafil Corp.
2654 Weaver Way
Dovaville, GA 30340
(404) 662-8546

Research Products Corp.
P.O. Box 1467
Madison, WI 53701
(608) 257-8801
(800) 356-9652

Reynolds Metals Co.
Construction Products Division
Ashville, OH 43103
(614) 983-2571

Rib-Roof Industries, Inc.
2745 Locust Dr.
Rialto, CA 92376
(714) 875-8529

Rising and Nelson Slate Co.
West Pawlet, VT 05775
(802) 645-0150

Robbins, Inc.
3626 Round Bottom Rd.
Cincinnati, OH 45244
(513) 321-1837

Rohm and Haas Co.
Independence Mall West
Philadelphia, PA 19105
(215) 592-3000

St. Charles Manufacturing Co.
525 Dunham Rd.
St. Charles, IL 60174
(708) 584-3800

Sanyo Electric Inc.
200 Riser Road
Little Ferry, NJ 07643
(201) 641-2333

Scientific Glass Co.
113 Phoenix NW
Albuquerque, NM 8710
(505) 345-7321

Sears, Roebuck and Co.
Sears Tower
Chicago, IL 60684
(312) 875-2500

Shepherd Products Co.
P.O. Box 427
Kalamazoo, MI 49005
(616) 382-4995

Simplex Products Div.
P.O. Box 10
Adrian, MI 49221
(517) 263-8881

Sinan Co.
P.O. Box 181
Suisun City, CA 94585
(707) 427-2325

Stanley Door Systems
1225 E. Maple
Troy, MI 48084
(313) 528-1400

Stark Ceramics, Inc.
P.O. Box 8880
Canton, OH 44711
(800) 321-0662
(216) 488-1211

Steelcraft
9017 Blue Ash Road
Cincinnati, OH 45242
(513) 745-6400

Steeltile Company
40457 Ave. 10
Suite A
Madera, CA 93638
(209) 431-5820

Steel Window Institute
1230 Kieth Building
Cleveland, OH 44115-2180
(216) 241-7333

Structural Slate Co.
222 E. Main St.
Pen Argyl, PA 18072
(215) 863-4141

Taylor Building Products
631 N. First St.
West Branch, MI 48661
(517) 345-5110
(800) 248-3600

The Allergy Store
7345 Healdsburg Ave.
P.O. Box 2555
Sebastopol, CA 95473
(800) 824-7163
(800) 950-6202

Thomas Industries
4360 Brownsboro Rd.
Suite 300
Louisville, KY 40232
(502) 893-4600

Thoro System Products Inc.
7800 NW 38th St.
Miami, FL 33166
(305) 592-2081

Thurmond Development Corp.
P.O. Box 23037
Little Rock, AR 72211
(501) 227-8888
(800) AIR-PURE

Torrence Steel Window Co.
1814 Abalone St.
Torrance, CA 90501
(213) 328-9181

Trewax Co.
11641 Pike St.
Santa Fe Springs, CA 90670
(213) 695-0761

Trion Inc.
101 McNeill Rd.
P.O. Box 760
Sanford, NC 27331
(919) 775-2201

Tri-Steel Structures
5800 Campus Circle
Las Colinas
Irving, TX 75063
(800) TRI-STEEL

Ultra-Hyd
361 Easton Rd.
Horsham, PA 19044
(215) 674-5511

U.S. Geological Survey
507 National Center
Reston, VA 22092
(703) 860-6045

U.S. Gypsum Corp.
101 South Wacker Drive
Chicago, IL 60606
(312) 321-4000

Universal Air Precipitator Corp.
1510 McCully Rd.
Monroeville, PA 15146
(412) 372-0706
(800) 255-8406

Universal-Rundle Corporation
North & East Streets
New Castle, PA 16103
(412) 658-6631

Vacu-Master Corp.
North St.
Saugerties, NY 12477
(914) 246-3408

Valspar Corp.
P.O. Box 1461
Minneapolis, MN 55440
(612) 332-7371

Vance Industries, Inc.
7401 W. Wilson Ave.
Chicago, IL 60656
(708) 867-6000

Vermont Structural Slate Co., Inc.
Box 98
Fair Haven, VT 05743
(802) 265-4933

Victims of Fiberglass
P.O. Box 440
Meadow Vista, CA 95722

Water Furnace International
4307 Arden Lane
Ft. Wayne, IN 46804
(219) 432-5667

Waterwise Inc.
26200 U.S. Highway 275 South
Leesburg, FL 34748
(800) 874-9028
(800) 321-5141 in Florida

Western Metal Lath
15220 Canary Ave.
La Mirada, CA 90638
(714) 523-2160

Weyerhaeuser
Box B
Tacoma, WA 98477
(206) 924-2345

William Zinsser & Co., Inc.
39 Belmont Drive
Somerset, NJ 08873
(201) 469-8100

Winthrop Pharmaceuticals
90 Park Ave.
New York, NY 10016
(212) 907-2000

Wiremold Co.
Wiremold Place
West Hartford, CT 06110
(203)233-6251

World Health Organization
(American Association)
2001 'S' Street NW, Suite 530
Washington, DC 20009
(202) 265-0286

Wrisco Industries Inc.
4039 S. Peoria St.
Chicago, IL 60609
(312) 847-8036

Xetex Inc.
3536 E. 28th St.
Minneapolis, MN 55406
(612) 724-3101

Notes

Chapter 1. Indoor Air Quality

1. M. De Bortoli and others, "Concentrations of Selected Organic Pollutants in Indoor and Outdoor Air in Northern Italy," *Environment International* 12 (1986): 343–350.

2. A.R. Hawthorne, R.B. Gammage and C.S. Dudney, "An Indoor Air Quality Study of 40 East Tennessee Homes," *Environment International* 12 (1986): 221–239.

3. Theodor D. Sterling and Diana M. Kobayashi, "Exposure to Pollutants in Enclosed 'Living Spaces'," *Environmental Research* 13 (1977): 1–35.

4. Charles C. Ossler, "Men's Work Environment and Health Risks," *Nursing Clinics of North America* 21 (March 1986): 25–36.

5. MDAC-Houston Materials Testing Data Base, Report # 85-19534 Ol, (Tra Bond F113/F117-STEX), NASA computerized database.

6. Jane M. Crum, "Indoor Air Pollution Source Database," Paper 86-52.6 presented at the 79th Annual Meeting of the Air Pollution Control Association in Minneapolis, MN on June 22–27, 1986.

7. E.R. Kashdan, J.E. Sickles and M.B. Ranade, *Review of Recent Research in Indoor Air Quality* (Washington, DC: EPA, May 1984), EPA-600/2-84-099.

8. R.L. Chessin, J.E. Sickles II and Y.S. Crume, *Update of Indoor Air Quality Bibliography* (Research Triangle Park, NC: Research Triangle Institute, n.d.) RTI/3065/05-03F, 68-02-3992-005.

9. Environmental Protection Agency, *Bibliography on Indoor Air Pollution* (Washington, DC: EPA, June 1985), #EPA/IMSD-85-002.

10. "Dust to Dust," *USA Today*, October 28, 1986, D1.

11. Environmental Protection Agency, *Asbestos Fact Book* (Washington, D.C.: EPA, August, 1985).

12. Consumer Product Safey Commission, *Asbestos in the Home* (Washington, D.C.: CPSC, August 1982): 10.

13. Environmental Protection Agency, *Guidance for Controlling Asbestos-Containing Materials in Buildings* (Washington, D.C.:EPA, 1985), EPA 560/5-85-024.

14. John G. Ingersoll, "A Survey of Radionuclide Contents and Emanation Rates in Building Materials Used in the United States," *Health Physics* 45 (August 1983): 363–368.

15. L. Morawska, "Influence of Sealants on Radon Emanation Rate from Building Materials," *Health Physics* 44 (April 1983): 416–418.

16. Rena Corman, *Air Pollution Primer* (American Long Association, 1969):44.

17. Judith A. Douville, "The Chemical Nature of Indoor Air Pollution," *Dangerous Properties of Industrial Materials Report*, May/June 1984, 2–8.

18. Thad Godish, *Indoor Air Quality Notes: Formaldehyde—Our Homes and Health #1* (Muncie, IN: Ball State University Department of Natural Resources, Summer 1986).

19. Phil Gunby, "Fact or Fiction about Formaldehyde?," *JAMA* 243 (May 2, 1980): 1697.

20. National Institute for Occupational Safety and Health, *Formaldehyde: Evidence of Carcinogenicity* (Cincinnati, OH: Department of Health and Human Services, Centers for Disease Control, April 15, 1981), *Current Intelligence Bulletin* 34, DHHS (NIOSH) Publication #81-111.

21. Godish, *Indoor Air Notes #1*.

22. Peter Fossel, "Sick House Blues," *Harrowsmith* (U.S.), September/October 1987, 46–55.

23. Godish, *Indoor Air Notes #1*.

24. Thad Godish, *Indoor Air Quality Notes: Residential Formaldehyde Control #2* (Muncie, IN: Ball State University Department of Natural Resources, Summer 1986).

25. Richard A. Wadden and Peter A. Scheff, *Indoor Air Pollution, Characterization, Prediction and Control* (New York: John Wiley and Sons, 1983): 73.

Chapter 2. Building-Related Illness

1. Gary L. Lattimer and Richard A. Ormsbee, *Legionnaires' Disease* (New York: Marcel Dekker, Inc., 1981).

2. David E. Root and Joan Anderson, "Reducing Toxic Body Burdens Advancing in Innovative Technique," *Occupational Health and Safety News Digest* 2 (April 1986).

3. L. Molhave, B. Bach and O.F. Pedersen, "Human Reactions to Low Concentrations of Volative Organic Compounds" *Environment International* 12 (1986): 167–175.

4. Martin L. Pernoll, "Abortion Induced by Chemicals Encountered in the Environment," *Clinical Obstetrics and Gynecology* 29 (December 1986): 953–958.

5. Alan Scott Levin and Merla Zellerbach, *The Type 1/Type 2 Allergy Relief System* (Los Angeles: Jeremy P. Tarcher, 1983): 25.

6. Ibid., 25–26.

7. Andrew Nikiforuk and Barbara Binczyk, "The Pariah Syndrome," *Harrowsmith* (U.S), August/September 1982, 51–61.

8. Charles T. McGee, *How to Survive Modern Technology* (New Canaan, CT: Keats Publishing, 1979).

9. Rene Dubos, "Adapting to Pollution," *Scientist and Citizen* 10 (January/February 1968): 1–8.

10. Anthony V. Colucci and others, "Pollutant Burdens and Biological Responses," *Archives of Environmental Health* 27 (September 1973): 151–154.

11. Irene Ruth Wilkenfeld, "Is Your Home Hospitable?," *Heal Prints #8* (May 1987), Newsletter published by HEAL of Louisiana, Baton Rouge, LA, 1–5.

12. E.J. Calabrese, *Pollutants and High Risk Groups* (New York: John Wiley and Sons, 1978): 187.

13. Bruce Small, *Indoor Air Pollution and Housing Technology* (Ottawa, Ontario: Canada Mortgage and Housing Corporation, 1983): 91.

14. Theron G. Randolph and Ralph W. Moss, *An Alternative Approach to Allergies* (New York: Harper and Row, 1980; New York: Bantam Books, 1982).

15. Robert T. Edgar, Ervin J. Fenyves and William J. Rea, "Air Pollution Analysis Used in Operating an Environmental Control Unit," *Annals of Allergy* 42 (March 1979): 166–173.

Chapter 4. Location, Location, Location

1. A.P. Krueger, "Preliminary Consideration of the Biological Significance of Air Ions," *Scientia* 104 (September/October 1969): 460–476.

2. Alayne Yates and others, "Air Ions: Past Problems and Future Directions," *Environment International* 12 (1986): 99–108.

3. P.F. Scalon, "Heavy Metals in Small Mammals in Roadside Environments: Implications for Food Chains," *The Science of the Total Environment* 59 (1987): 317–323.

4. "Pesticides May Alter Brain Function," *Science News* 129 (February 8, 1986): 88.

5. Thomas H. Maugh II, "Acid Rain's Effects on People Assessed," *Science* 226 (December 1984): 1408–1410.

6. Nancy Wertheimer and Ed Leeper, "Electrical Wiring Configurations and Childhood Cancer," *American Journal of Epidemiology* 109 (1979): 273–284.

7. Nancy Wertheimer and Ed Leeper, "Adult Cancer Related to Electrical Wires Near the Home," *International Journal of Epidemiology* 11 (1982): 345–355.

8. Andrew A. Marino and Robert O. Becker, "Hazard at a Distance: Effects of Exposure to the Electric and Magnetic Fields of High Voltage Transmission Lines," *Medical Research and Engineering* 31 Ref. (November 1977): 6–9.

9. Susan Molloy, "Electromagnetic Field Reactions," *The Reactor*, March/April 1987, Newsletter published by Environmental Health Association of San Francisco, 6–7.

10. E.E. Ketchen, W.E. Porter and N.E. Bolton, "The Biological Effects of Magnetic Fields on Man," *American Industrial Hygiene Association Journal* 39 (January 1978): 1–11.

11. Paul Brodeur, *The Zapping of America* (New York: W.W. Norton & Co., 1977): 36.

12. Ibid., 55.

13. Nancy Shute, "The Other Kind of Radiation," *American Health*, July/August 1986, 54–59.

14. M.A. Persinger, "Geophysical Variables and Behavior: XXII. The Tectonogenic Strain Continuum of Unusual Events," *Perceptual Motor Skills* 60 (1985): 59–65.

Chapter 7. Mold and Moisture

1. Lawrence D. Dickey, ed., *Clinical Ecology* (Springfield IL: Charles C. Thomas, 1976): 259.

2. Phillip R. Morey and others, "Environmental Studies in Moldy Office Buildings: Biological Agents, Sources and Preventative Measures," *Ann. Am. Conf. Gov. Ind. Hyg.* 10 (1984): 21–35.

3. Rodney C. De Groot, "Wood Decay Ecosystem in Residental Construction," in *Trees and Forests for Human Settlements*, Proceedings of papers presented during P1.05-00 Symposia in Vancouver, BC on 11–12 June 1976 and in Oslo, Norway on 22 June 1976 at the XVIth IUFRO World Congress, 345.

4. Peter P. Kozak and others, "Factors of Importance in Determining the Prevalence of Indoor Molds," *Annals of Allergy* 43 (August 1979): 93.

5. Peter P. Kozak and others, "Currently Available Methods of Home Mold Surveys. II. Examples of Homes Surveyed," *Annals of Allergy* 45 (September 1980): 167–176.

6. Anton Tenwolde and Jane Charlton Suleski, "Controlling Moisture in Houses," *Solar Age* 9 (January 1984): 34–37.

7. A.V. Assendfelt and others, "Humidifier-Associated Extrinsic Allergic Alveolitis," *Scandinavian Journal of the Work Environment* 5 (1979): 35–41.

8. "Ultrasonic Humidifiers," *Consumer Reports*, November 1985, 679–683.

9. Kozak, "Factors of Importance," 91.

10. Small, *Indoor Pollution*, 149.

11. Ib Andersen and Jens Korsgaard, "Asthma and the Indoor Environment: Assessment of the Health Implications of High Indoor Air Humidity," *Environment International* 12 (1986): 121–127.

12. R.P. Bowen, C.J. Shirtcliffe and G.A. Chown, *Urea Formaldehyde Foam Insulation: Problem Identification and Remedial Measures for Wood Frame Construction* (Ottawa, Ontario: Division of Building Research, National Research Council of Canada, August 1981), Building Practice Note #23, C1.

13. T.A. Oxley and E.G. Gobert, *Dampness in Buildings* (Kent, England: Butterworths, 1983).

14. National Center for Appropriate Technology, *Moisture and Home Energy Conservation*, (Butte, MT: NCAT, n.d.), GPO 061-000-00615-0.

15. D. Eyre and D. Jennings, *Air-Vapour Barriers* (Ottawa, Ontario: Energy, Mines and Resources Canada, 1983).

16. G.E. Sherwood, *Condensation Potential in High Thermal Performance Walls—Cold Winter Climate* (Madison, WI: U.S. Forest Products Laboratory, May 1983), Research Paper FPL 433.

17. "The Vapor Barrier Goes on the Outside???," *Energy Design Update*, February 1986, 3–5.

Chapter 8. Airtightness and Ventilation

1. Mark Alvarez, "Healthy Buliding," *Practical Homeowner*, February 1987, 30–35.

2. Peter A. Breysse, "The Health Costs of 'Tight' Homes," *JAMA* 245 (January 16, 1981): 267.

3. "Heat Recovery Ventilators," *Consumer Reports*, October 1985, 596–599.

4. Ibid.

5. William A. Shurcliff, *Air-to-Air Heat Exchangers* (Andover, MA: Brick House Publishing, 1982).

6. National Center for Appropriate Technology, *Heat Recovery Ventilation for Housing* (Butte, MT: NCAT, n.d.), GPO-061-000-00631-1.

7. Ibid., 6.

8. Ibid., 11.

9. Bruce M. Small, "Creating Your Own Safe Environment," *Environ #4* (Spring/Summer 1986): 8–11.

10. R.W. Besant, R.S.Dumont and D. Van Ee, "An Air to Air Heat Exchanger for Residences," *Engineering Bulletin* (Saskatoon, Saskatchewan: Extension Division, University of Saskatchewan, June 1980), Pub. #387.

11. Michael B. Schell and others, *The Complete Heat Exchanger Book* (Regina, Saskatchewan: Northern Scientific, Inc., 1985).

12. NCAT, *Heat Recovery Ventilation*, 28–29.

13. John R. Hughes, "Heat Recovery Ventilators," *Fine Homebuilding #34* (August/September 1986): 34.

14. William A. Surcliff, *Super-Insulated Houses and Double Envelope Houses* (Andover, MA: Brick House Publishing Company, 1981).

15. Ed McGrath, *The Superinsulated House* (Fairbanks, AK: That New Publishing Company, 1981), Chapter IX.

16. John R. Hughes, "Retrofit Superinsulation," *Fine Homebuliding #20* (April-/May 1984): 35–37.

17. J.D. Ned Nisson and Gautam Dutt, *The Superinsulated Home Book* (New York: John Wiley & Sons, 1985).

18. John R. Hughes, "The Superinsulated House," *Fine Homebuilding #9* (June/July 1982): 56–59.

19. Robert Corbett, Wally Hansen and Jon Sesso, *Superinsulation: A Housing Trend for the Eighties* (Butte, MT: NCAT, 1980).

20. *Super-Insulation Primer* (Langley, WA: Homestead Designs, 1983).

21. McGrath, *The Superinsulated House*.

22. G.E. Sherwood, *Condensation Potential in High Thermal Performance Walls—Cold Winter Climate* (Madison, WI: Forest Products Laboratory, May 1983), Research Paper FPL 433.

23. G.O. Handegord, *A System for Tighter Wood-Frame Construction* (Ottawa, Ontario: Division of Building Research, National Research Council Canada, January 1984), Building Research Note #207.

24. Joseph W. Lstiburek, *The Drywall Approach to Airtightness* (Toronto, Ontario: Center for Building Science, University of Toronto, n.d.).

25. "Feature, The Airtight Drywall Approach," *Energy Design Update*, September 1984, 5–10.

26. Rich Slayton, "The Airtight Drywall Approach," *Fine Homebuilding #9* (February/March 1987): 62–65.

Chapter 9. Concrete and Masonry

1. Susan H. Early and Roger L. Simpson, "Caustic Burns From Contact With Wet Cement," *JAMA* 254 (July 26, 1985): 528–529.

2. Ibid.

3. Peter R. Lane and Daniel J. Hogan, "Chronic Pain and Scarring From Cement Burns," *Archives of Dermatology* 121 (March 1985): 368–369.

4. S.H. Zaidi, *Experimental Pneumoconiosis* (Baltimore, MD: Johns Hopkins Press, 1969).

5. A.J.R. Curtis, "Cement Dermatitis" (letter), *Journal of the American Concrete Institute*, November 1943, 175–176.

6. *Standard Specification for Blended Hydraulic Cements* (Philadelphia, PA: American Standard for Testing Materials, 1986), ASTM C-595-86.

7. Frederick S. Merritt, *Building Construction Handbook* (New York: McGraw-Hill, 1965, 2nd ed.): 5.12–5.16.

8. Sybil P. Parker, ed., *Encyclopedia of Science and Technology* (New York: McGraw-Hill, 1987), s.v. "Air Entraining Portland Cement," by J.H. Walker.

Chapter 10. Foundation Systems

1. Phillip J. Walsh, Charles S. Dudney and Emily D. Copenhauer, *Indoor Air Quality* (Boca Raton, FL: CRC Press, 1984): 146.

2. Ronald C. Bruno, "Sources of Indoor Radon in Houses," *Air Pollution Control Association Journal* 33 (February 1983): 105.

3. *All Weather Wood Foundation System* (Tacoma, WA, American Plywood Association, 1979), Publication #A400.

4. Oxley, *Dampness*.

5. Jennifer A. Adams, "Down the Drain," *New Shelter*, March 1986, 12–13.

6. Environmental Protection Agency, *Radon Reduction in New Construction: An Interim Guide* (Washington, D.C.: EPA, August 1987), Publication #OPA-87-009.

7. Environmental Protection Agency, *Radon Reducation Methods: A Homeowner's Guide* (Washington, DC: EPA, August 1986), Publication #OPA-86-005.

8. Environmental Protection Agency, *Radon Techniques for Detached Houses: Technical Guidance* (Washington, DC: EPA, June 1986), Publication #EPA/625/5-86/019.

9. NCAT, *Moisture*, 20.

Chapter 11. Wood and Wood Products

1. Raymond R. Suskind, "Dermatitis in the Forest Product Industry," *Archives of Environmental Health* 15 (September 1967): 322–326.

2. Carey P. McCord, "The Toxic Properties of Some Timber Woods," *Industrial Medicine and Surgery* 27 (1958): 202–204.

3. B. Woods and C.D. Calnan, "Toxic Woods," *British Journal of Dermatology* 94 (13 Supplement, June 1976): 1–97.

4. Bjorn M. Hausen, *Woods Injurious to Human Health: A Manual*, (New York: Walter de Gruyter, 1981): 158.

5. Ibid., 22.

6. FPL, *How to Protect Logs from Decay and Stain While Drying* (Madison WI: Forest Products Laboratory, April 1984), #84-010.

7. Edmund Frederick Rasmussen, "Dry Kiln Operators Manual," *Agricultural Handbook #188*, (U.S. Dept. of Agriculture, Forest Service, March 1961): 142.

8. Don Graf, *Basic Building Data*, 3rd ed., (New York: Van Nostrand Reinhold, 1985): 23.

9. Harry Ulrey, *Questions and Answers for Carpenters and Builders* (Indianapolis: Theodore Audel, 1966): 76.

10. Charles Thom and Kenneth P. Raper, "The Arsenic Fungi of Gosio," *Science* 76 (December 9, 1932): 548–550.

11. Guy O. Pfeiffer and Casimir M. Nikel, *The Household Environment and Chronic Illness* (Springfield, IL: Charles C. Thomas, 1980): 33.

12. T.G. Matthews and others, "Surface Emission Monitoring of Pressed-Wood Products Containing Urea-Formaldehyde Resins," *Environment International* 12 (1986): 301.

13. G.K. Sangha, M. Matijak and Y. Alarie, "Comparison of Some Mono- and Diisocyanates as Sensory Irritants," *Toxicology and Applied Pharmacology* 57 (1981): 241–246.

14. Roger M. Rowell, "Nontoxic Wood Preservative Treatments," *Wood & Wood Products* 83 (February 1978): 81–82.

15. Larry Stains, "EPA Gives Wood Preservatives a Cautious Okay," *The Family Handyman*, July/August 1986, 86.

16. H. Levin and J. Hahn, "Pentachlorophenol in Indoor Air: Methods to Reduce Airborne Concentrations," *Environment International* 12 (1986): 333–341.

17. R.T. Johnson (letter), *Fine Homebuilding* #1 (February/March 1981): 6.

18. Nisson, *The Superinsulated House*, 122.

19. Paul Cooke, "Wood," *Nontoxic and Natural Newsletter* #1, (May/June 1985): 6.

20. William Olkowski, Helga Olkowski and Shiela Daar, "Termites—New, Less Toxic Controls," *Common Sense Pest Control Quarterly* #1 (Fall 1984): 7–19.

21. Ibid., 16.

22. Daniel Zwordling, "All Things Considered," on National Public Radio, WFIU Bloomington, IN, January 22, 1987.

23. Michael J. Hodgson, Geoffrey D. Block and David K. Parkinson, "Organophosphate Poisoning in Office Workers," *Journal of Occupational Medicine* 28 (June 1986): 434–437.

24. Rodney C. Degroot, "Alternatives to Termiticides in Building Protection," in: Khasawinah, Abdallah M., ed., *Termiticides in Building Protection*: Proceedings of a Workshop; September 22–23, 1982, Washington, DC (Chicago: Velsicol Chemical Corp., 1983): 91–94.

Chapter 12. Steel Framing
1. Don Ellis, "Safe Homes with Safe Materials," *Environ* #3 (Winter 1985–86): 4.

2. M.F. Marti, "On Screw Guns and Screws," *Fine Homebuilding* #34 (August /September 1986): 42–45.

3. Metal Lath/Steel Framing Association, *Lightweight Steel Framing Systems Manual*, 2nd ed. (Chicago: ML/SFA, 1984).

4. Metal Lath/Steel Framing Association, *Introduction to Steel Framing*, Technical Bulletin #131 (Chicago: ML/SFA, 1978).

5. "Galvanized Steel Framing for Homes," *Construction Dimensions*, June 1984, 21.

6. Carl & Barbara Giles, *Steel Homes* (Blue Ridge Summit, PA: Tab Books, 1984).

7. United States Gypsum Corporation, *Load-Bearing USG Steel Framing Systems* (Chicago: USGC, 1986), #SA-510.

8. Gold Bond Building Products, *Gold Bond Gypsum Wallboard Construction* (Charlotte, NC: GBBP, 1985), Technical Bulletin #9-2171.

9. Steve Mead, "Light-Gauge Steel Framing," *Fine Homebuilding* #32 (April /May 1986): 67–71.

Chapter 13. Roofing Systems
1. Red Cedar Shingle & Handsplit Shake Bureau, *Recommended Care and Treatment of Red Cedar Shake and Shingle Roofs* (Belleview, WA: RCS&HSB, n.d.).

2. Brian Buchanan and Dewayne Weldon, *Southern Yellow Pine, An Alternative Roofing Material* (Lufkin, TX: Texas Forest Products Laboratory, Texas A&M University, May 1981), Publication 123.

3. David Heim, "Roofing With Slate," *Fine Homebuilding* #20 (April/May 1984): 38–43.

4. J. Azevedo, "Metal Roofing," *Fine Homebuilding* #24 (December 1984/January 1985): 42–46.

5. "Metal Roofing Finds Good Home in Multi-Family Dwelling Market," *Metal Construction News* 6 (August 1986): 1.

6. I.C. MacSwan and M.G. Huber, *Controlling Moss on Roofs* (Corvallis, OR: Oregon State University, Reprinted January 1966), Fact Sheet #FS10.

7. Giles, *Steel Homes*, 182.

Chapter 14. Exterior Siding

1. The Aluminum Association, *Specifications for Aluminum Sheet Metal Work* (Washington, DC: TAA, n.d.).

2. Zamm, *Why Your House*, 75–76.

3. Dana Miller, "Electromagnetic Bodies," *The Human Ecologist* #34 (Spring 1987): 7–10.

Chapter 15. Windows and Doors

1. John Ott, *Light, Radiation and You* (Old Greenwich, CT: Devin-Adair, 1982).

2. Mary Oetzel, "Selecting Windows," *The Human Ecologist* #34 (Spring 1987): 29.

3. James C. Benney, Manager of Technical Services of the National Wood Window & Door Association, personal correspondence, February 4, 1987.

4. *Product Data* sheet #SWC 1407 ROO 8407 for "Tribucide P-75," (St. Louis, MO: Koppers Company, Inc.).

5. *Product Data* sheet #PPD 1257 8602 for "Woodtreat MB," (St. Louis, MO: Koppers Company, Inc.).

6. American Architectural Manufacturers Association, *Certified Products Directory* (Des Plaines, IL: AAMA, 1986).

7. Anita & Seymour Isenberg, *How to Work with Stained Glass* (Radnor, PA: Chilton Book Co, 1972): 14–15.

8. William K. Langdon, *Movable Insulation* (Emmaus, PA: Rodale Press, 1980): 57–59.

9. Debra Lynn Dadd, *Nontoxic and Natural* (Los Angeles: Jeremy P. Tarcher, 1984): 150–151.

Chatper 16. Insulation Products

1. CPSC, *Asbestos in the Home*, 8.

2. Georg Kimmerle, "Toxicity of Combustion Products with Particular Reference to Polyurethane," *Annals of Occupational Hygiene* 19 (1976): 269.

3. Consumer Product Safety Commission, *Home Insulation Safety* (Washington, DC: CPSC, July 1980), Product Safety Fact Sheet #91.

4. Cynthia F. Robinson, J.M. Dement, G.O. Ness, R.J. Waxweiler, "Mortality Patterns of Rock and Slag Mineral Wool Production Workers: an Epidemiological and Environmental Study," *British Journal of Industrial Medicine* 39 (1982): 45–53.

5. Jean J. Moulin and others, "Oral Cavity and Laryngeal Cancers among Man-Made Mineral Fiber Production Workers," *Scandinavian Journal of Work and Environmental Health* 12 (1986): 27–31.

6. Mearl F. Stanton, and others, "Carcinogenicity of Fibrous Glass: Pleural Response in the Rat in Relation to Fiber Dimension," *Journal of the National Cancer Institute* 58 (1977): 587–603.

7. John R. Goldsmith, "Comparative Epidemiology of Men Exposed to Asbestos and Man-Made Mineral Fibers," *American Journal of Industrial Medicine* 10 (1986): 543–552.

8. "Label This Building Very Healthy," *The Human Ecologist* #31 (Winter 1985–86): 8.

9. Knauf Fiber Glass GmbH, *Material Safety Data Sheet, Kraft Faced Fibrous Glass Insulation* (Shelbyville, IN: Knauf Fiberglass GmbH, 1985): 2.

10. S.J.A. Verbeck, E.M.M. Buise-van Unnik and K.E. Malten, "Itching in Office Workers From Glass Fibers," *Contact Dermatitis* 7 (November 1981): 354.

11. Carl U. Dernehl, "Health Hazards Associated with Polyurethane Foams," *Journal of Occupational Medicine* 8 (February 1966): 59–62.

12. Pamela M. LeQuesne and others, "Neurological Complications after a Single Severe Exposure to Toluene Di-isocyanate," *British Journal of Industrial Medicine* 33 (1976): 72–78.

13. A.R.D. Lambert, "Foamed Polyurethane Insulation," in *Energy Conservation and Thermal Insulation*, ed. R. Derricott and S.S. Chissick (New York: John Wiley and Sons, 1981): 445.

14. Brookhaven National Laboratory and Dynatech R/D Co., *An Assessment of Thermal Insulation Systems for Building Applications* (Washington, DC: U.S. Department of Energy, June 1978), # BNL-50862, 84.

15. David Buscher, "Problems with Cellulose Insulation," Presentation given to the 16th Advanced Seminar in Clinical Ecology at Banff, Alberta, Canada on October 5, 1982.

16. "Insulation Attacks Woman, Son, Dog," *The Reactor*, November/December 1987, Newsletter published by the Environmental Health Association of San Francisco, 4.

17. Zamm, *Why Your House*, 148.

18. H.E. Amandus and others, "The Morbidity and Mortality of Vermiculite Miners and Millers Exposed to Tremolite-Actinolite, Part 1, Exposure Estimates," *American Journal of Industrial Medicine* 11 (1987): 1–14.

19. Stephen B. Hayward and Glenn R. Smith, "Asbestos Contamination of Vermiculite" (letter), *American Journal of Public Health* 74 (1984): 519–520.

20. Lester Levin and P. Walton Purdom, "A Review of the Health Effects of Energy Conserving Materials," *American Journal of Public Health* 73 (June 1983): 683–690.

21. Bruce M. Small, *The Susceptibility Report* (Cornwall, Ontario, Canada: Deco Books, 1982).

22. Nancy Pappas, "The House on Pickerel Lake Road," *Northeast/Hartford Courant*, December 8, 1985, 14.

23. G.A. Chown, R.P. Bowen, and C.J. Shirtcliffe, *Urea-Formaldehyde Foam Insulation: Building Practice Note No. 19* (Ottawa, Ontario: Division of Building Research, National Research Council of Canada, April 1981).

24. Bowen, *Urea-Formaldehyde Foam Insulation: Problem Identification.*

25. Peter Fossel, "Sick Home Blues," *Harrowsmith* (U.S.) #11 (September/October 1987): 46.

26. "The All-Natural House," *Everything Natural*, September/October 1986, 10–13.

27. Helen E. Robinson and others, "The Effects of Fumes from the Thermal Degradation of Polyethylene on Health," *Annals of Occupational Hygiene* 25 (1982): 291.

Chapter 17. Flooring Systems

1. Fossel, "Sick Home."

2. Francis V. Silver, "On the Carpet," *The Human Ecologist* #20 (Winter 1982–83): 2–3.

3. Roger L. Anderson, "Biological Evaluation of Carpeting," *Applied Microbiology* 18 (August 1969): 180–187.

4. June Larson, "Pesticides in New Nylon Carpets and in Carpet Cleaning Services," *The Human Ecologist* #31 (Winter 1985–86): 31.

5. Peter A. Patriarca, "Kawasaki Syndrome: Association with the Application of Rug Shampoo," *The Lancet*, September 11, 1982, 578–580.

6. Mary Oetzel, "Build for Health," *The Human Ecologist* #21 (Spring 1983): 2–7.

7. Harry F. Ulrey, *Questions and Answers for Carpenters and Builders* (Indianapolis, IN: Theodore Audel & Co., 1966): 184.

8. Gene Bruce, "The Bedroom Goes Natural," *East West*, March 1987, 56–59.

9. P. Sebastien, J. Bignon and M. Martin, "Indoor Airborne Asbestos Pollution From the Ceiling and the Floor," *Science* 216 (June 1982): 1410–1413.

10. Lars Rittfeldt, Maria Sandberg and Mats S. Ahlberg, "Indoor Air Pollutants Due to Vinyl Floor Tiles," (Stockholm, Sweden: Proceedings of the 3rd International Conference on Indoor Air Quality & Climate, Vol. 3, Sensory and Hypersensitivity Reactions to Sick Buildings, 1984): 297–302.

11. Oetzel, "Build for Health."

12. Michael Byrne, *Setting Ceramic Tile* (Newton, CT: Taunton Press, 1987).

13. Tile Council of America, *Ceramic Tile Installation Handbook* (Princeton, NJ: TCA, 1986).

14. John Bower, "Safe Ceramic Tile," *Environ* #5 (Fall/Winter 1986–1987): 21–22.

Chapter 18. Interior Walls and Ceilings

1. Natalie Golos, Frances Golos Golbitz and Frances Spatz Leighton, *Coping With Your Allergies* (New York: Simon and Schuster, 1979): 47.

2. F. Silver, "The Wallboard, Flexible Plastic, and Polyester Problem," Presented to the 10th Advanced Seminar in Clinical Ecology, Dallas, TX on December 7, 1976.

3. Mary Oetzel, "New Wall Treatment," *The Human Ecologist* #29 (Summer 1985): 20.

4. CPSC, *Asbestos in the Home.*

5. Alf Fischbein and others, "Drywall Construction and Asbestos Exposure," *American Industrial Hygiene Association Journal* 40 (May 1979): 402–407.

6. J. Fagliano and others, "PCB Contamination of Ceiling Tiles in Public Buildings—New Jersey," *JAMA* 257 (March 13, 1987): 1297.

7. E.W. Carles and L.G. Wines, *The Art of Tilesetting* (Peoria, IL: Charles Bennett Co., 1954): 114–117.

8. Graf, *Basic Building Data*, 565–580.

9. Zamm, *Why Your House*, 58.

Chapter 19. Paint, Varnish, and Caulking

1. Randolph, *An Alternative Approach*, 89.

2. Ernest W. Flick, *Handbook of Paint Raw Materials* (Park Ridge, NJ: Noyes Publishing, 1982): 1–2.

3. Robert E. Gosselin, Roger P. Smith and Harold C. Hodge, *Clinical Toxicology of Commercial Products* (Baltimore, MD: Williams and Watkins, 1984): V1.82-V1.84.

4. Dana Miller, "Chronic Epstein Barr Virus—What is it?," *The Human Ecologist* #33 (1986): 7.

5. J.R. Girman, A.T. Hodgson and A.S. Newton, "Emissions of Volatile Organic Compounds From Adhesives with Indoor Applications," *Environment International* 12 (1986): 317–321.

6. C.S. Clark and others, "Condition and Type of Housing as an Indicator of Potential Lead Exposure and Pediatric Blood Lead Levels," *Environmental Research* 38 (1985): 46–53.

7. A.F., "The Chemistry of Wood Finish" (letter), *Nontoxic and Natural News*, March/April 1986, 8–9.

8. "Product Information," *The Human Ecologist* #31 (Winter 1985–86): 11.

9. Ruth Dabes, "Particle Board" (letter), *The Human Ecologist* #4 (August 1979): 14.

10. Dadd, *Nontoxic and Natural*, 148.

11. Richard C. Barnes, President of Negley Paint Co., personal correspondence, February 26, 1987.

12. Ralph Mayer, *The Artist's Handbook of Materials and Techniques* 3rd ed. (New York: Viking Press, 1970).

13. Dadd, *Nontoxic and Natural*, 149–150.

14. *2000 Down Home Skills & Secret Formulas for Practically Anything* (Laguna Beach, CA: Gala Books, 1971 reprint), 223.

15. Bruce A. Tichenor, "Measurement of Organic Emissions from Indoor Materials—Small Chamber Studies," Paper presented at EPA/APCA Symposium on Measurement of Toxic Air Pollutants, Raleigh, NC on April 28, 1986.

Chapter 20. Kitchens and Bathroom

1. Debra Lynn Dadd and Alan S. Levin, *A Consumer Guide for the Chemically Sensitive* (San Francisco: Nontoxic Lifestyles, Inc., 1982): 133.

2. Dadd, *Nontoxic and Natural*.

3. Golos, *Coping*.

Chapter 21. Mechanical Components

1. Theron G. Randolph, *Human Ecology and Susceptibility to the Chemical Environment* (Springfield, IL: Charles C. Thomas, 1962): 106.

2. Casimir M. Nikel, "Residential Space Heating," *The Human Ecologist* #15/16 (March 1982): 6–8.

3. John D. Spengler and Martin A. Cohen, *Emissions from Indoor Combustion Sources*, in *Indoor Air and Human Health*, by Richard B. Gammage and Stephen V. Kaye (Chelsea, MI: Lewis Publishers, 1985): 267–268.

4. "Ban Ordered on Wood Fires in Smoggy Reno," *Nontoxic and Natural News*, January/February 1986, 1.

5. Richard E. Honicky, Scott Osborne III, and C. Amechi Akpom, "Symptoms of Respiratory Illness in Young Children and the Use of Wood-Burning Stoves in Indoor Heating,"*Pediatrics* 75 (March 1985): 587–593.

6. Gregory W. Traynor, "Selected Organic Pollutant Emissions from Unvented Kerosene Heaters," Paper #86-52.5, presented to the 79th Annual meeting of the Air Pollution Control Association in Minneapolis, MN on June 22–27, 1986.

7. Isaac Turiel, *Indoor Air and Human Health* (Stanford, CA: Stanford University Press, 1985): 66.

8. D. Moschandreas and others, "Emission Rates from Unvented Gas Appliances," *Environment International* 12 (1986):247–253.

9. "Natural Gas Appliance," *Everything Natural*, March/April 1987, 3.

10. Randolph, *An Alternative Approach*, 56.

11. Ibid., 53.

12. Nikel, "Residential Space Heating."

13. Pfeiffer, *Household Environment*, 69.

14. Sidney J. Heiman, "Petrochemicals and Plastic Synthetic Gases," in *Clinical Ecology*, ed. Lawrence Dickey (Springfield, IL: Charles C. Thomas, 1976): 273–274.

15. "Keeping Cool Without Air Conditioning," *Home*, July 1982, 62–67.

16. Harold W. Newball and Sami A. Brahim, "Respiratory Response to Domestic Fibrous Glass Exposure," *Environmental Research* 12 (1976): 201–207.

17. CPSC, *Asbestos in the Home*, 8.

18. Nikel, "Residential Space Heating."

19. Don L. Jewett, "Product Information, Heaters," *The Human Ecologist* #15/16 (March 1982): 17.

20. Eva Lydahl, *Infrared Radiation and Cataract* (Stockholm, Sweden: Department of Ophthalmology and Medical Biophysics, 1984).

21. Forrest Wilson, "Doctors for Building," *Technology Review*, May/June 1986, 49–58.

22. John Ott, *Health and Light* (New York: Pocket Books, 1973).

23. Richard J. Wurtman, "The Effects of Light on the Human Body," *Scientific American* 233 (1975): 68–77.

24. John Ott, "Effects of Unnatural Light," *New Scientist* 429 (February 4, 1965): 294–296.

25. Zee Randegger, "Focus on Light, Part I: Full Spectrum Health Benefits," *Environ* #3 (Winter 1985/1986): 14–16.

26. National Indoor Environmental Institute, *Indoor Air Pollution: A Serious Health Hazard* (Plymouth Meeting, PA: NIEI, 1983).

27. Ellen Greenfield, *House Dangerous* (New York: Vintage Books, 1987): 65.

28. Norman E. Rosenthal and others, "Seasonal Affective Disorder," *Archives of General Psychology* 41 (January 1984): 72–80.

29. Thomas A. Wehr, "Phototherapy of Seasonal Affective Disorder," *Archives of General Psychology* 43 (September 1986): 870–875.

30. Environmental Protection Agency, *Lead in Drinking Water* (Washington, DC: EPA, April 1987), #OPA-87-006.

31. Zamm, *Why Your House*, 131.

32. Golos, *Coping*, 196.

33. Linda S. Sheldon and Kent W. Thomas, "Volatile Organic Emissions From Building Materials," Paper #86-52.3 presented to the 79th Annual Meeting of the Air Pollution Control Association in Minneapolis, MN on June 22–27, 1986.

Chapter 22. Filters and Purifiers

1. "Air Cleaners," *Consumer Reports*, January 1985, 7–11.

2. C.J. Weschler and others, "The Effect of Building Fan Operation on Indoor-Outdoor Dust Relationships," *Air Pollution Control Association Journal* 33 (January 1983): 624.

3. Harold Hopkins, "The Cans and Can'ts of Air Purifiers," *FDA Consumer*, October 1982, 5–7.

4. J. Gordon King, "Air for Living," *Respiratory Care* 18 (March/April 1973): 160–164.

5. Ibid.

6. "What You Should Know About Air Filtration," *The Human Ecologist* #23/24 (Fall/Winter 1983/84): 6–7.

7. Alayne Yates and others, "Air Ions: Past Problems and Future Directions," *Environment International* 12 (1986): 99–108.

8. Albert Paul Krueger and Eddie James Reed, "Biological Impact of Small Ions," *Science* 193 (September 1986): 1209–1213.

9. B.C. Wolverton, Rebecca C. McDonald, and E.A. Watkins, Jr., "Foliage Plants for Removing Indoor Air Pollutants from Energy Efficient Homes," *Economic Botany* 38 (1984): 224–228.

10. B.C. Wolverton, Rebecca C. McDonald, and Hayne H. Mesick, "Foliage Plants for Indoor Removal of the Primary Combustion Gases Carbon Monoxide and Nitrogen Dioxide," *Journal of the Mississippi Academy of Sciences* 30 (1985).

11. Godish, *Indoor Air Notes #2*.

12. Roul Tunley, "Time Bomb in Our Tap Water," *Reader's Digest*, January 1985, 90–96.

13. Randolph, *An Alternative Approach*, 226.

14. Halina Szejnwald Brown, Donna R. Bishop and Carol A. Rowan, "The Role of Skin Absorption as a Route of Exposure for Volatile Organic Compounds (VOCs in Drinking Water)," *American Journal of Public Health* 74 (May 1984): 479–484.

15. "Water Filters," *Consumer Reports*, February 1983, 68.

16. Debra Lynn Dadd, "Special Report: Water Filters," *Nontoxic & Natural Newsletter*, 1985, 1.

17. Pfeiffer, *Household Environment*, 114.

18. Sherman Hasbrouck and Linda Breece, *Removing Radon From Water Using Activated Carbon Adsorption* (Augusta, ME: University of Maine, April 1987), Information bulletin.

19. "Water Filters," *Consumer Reports*.

20. Leon Kim, "Catalytic Water Conditioning," *Water Conditioning and Purification*, February 1987, 72–79.

Appendix II Testing Materials

1. Small, *Susceptibility Report*, 30.
2. Levin, *Type 1/Type 2*, 44–45.
3. Sherry A.Rogers, "Diagnosing the Tight Building Syndrome," (Atlanta, GA: Proceedings of Indoor Air Quality '86, American Society of Heating, Refrigeration, and Air Conditioning Engineers, 1986): 772–776.

Selected Bibliography

BOOKS

Anachem, Inc. and Sandia National Laboratories. *Indoor Air Quality Handbook*. Albuquerque, NM: Sandia National Laboratories, September 1982. #SAND82-1773, UC-11.

Dadd, Debra Lynn. *Nontoxic, Natural and Earthwise*. Los Angeles: P. Tarcher, 1990.

Golos, Natalie, Frances Golos Golbitz and Frances Spatz Leighton. *Coping With Your Allergies*. New York: Simon and Schuster, 1979.

Good, Clint. *Healthful Houses*. Bethesda, MD: Guaranty Press, 1988.

Pfeiffer, Guy O. and Casimir M. Nikel. *The Household Environment and Chronic Illness*. Springfield, IL: Charles C. Thomas, 1980.

Randolph, Theron G. and Ralph W. Morris. *An Alternative Approach to Allergies*. New York: Harper and Row, 1980; New York; Bantam Books, 1982.

Rousseau, David, W.J. Rea and Jean Enwright. *Your Home, Your Health, and Well-Being*. Berkeley, CA: Tom Speed Press, 1988.

Small, Bruce M. and Associates Limited. *Indoor Air Pollution and Housing Technology*. Ottawa, Ontario: The Canadian Housing Information Center, Canada Mortgage and Housing Corporation, 1983. Cat No. NH 17-23/1983E.

Turiel, Isaac. *Indoor Air Quality and Human Health*. Stanford, CA: Stanford University Press, 1985.

Zamm, Alfred V. and Robert Gannon. *Why Your House May Endanger Your Health*. New York: Simon and Schuster, 1980.

PERIODICALS

Environ, P.O. Box 2204, Ft. Collins, CO 80522, Quarterly, $15 per year.

Safe Home Digest, 24 East Ave., Suite 1300, New Caanan, CT 06840, Monthly, $27.96 per year.

Index

Absorption, 69
Acoustical ceiling tiles, 257–258
Acid rain, 50
Activated carbon air filters, 76–77, 91, 290, 320–323
  sensitivities to, 321
  illus. 322
Activated carbon water filters, 332, 344
  illus. 331
Addiction and sensitivity, 27
Admixtures, concrete, 114–116
Adsorption, 69, 320
Aerial photographs, 46
Agricultural chemicals, 42, 49
Air barriers, 83–87, 220–222, 246, 341, see also Wind barriers
  illus. 85
Air conditioners, 73, 79, 291–292
  illus. 298
Air filters, 288, 290, 292, 311–326
  illus. 325
Air-Krete insulation, 217, 219
Air silencer, 97
  illus. 98
Air testing, 357–358
Airtight Drywall Approach, 66, 83–84, 106–107, 304, 338, 343
Airtightness, 7–8, 89–92, 102–107, 338–339
Air to air heat exchanger, see Heat recovery ventilator
Allergies, 22, 23, 27, 51–52, 56, 72–73, 146, 268
Aluminum foil tape, 107, 193, 221, 293
Ammonia fumigation, 17
Apartments, 36–37
Appliances, 6, 8, 56, 69, 76, 79, 101, 128, 280–281, 344
Arsenic treated lumber, 124, 148, 154–155
Asbestos, 11, 14–15, 65
  in ductwork, 293
  in flooring, 64, 232
  health effects, 14

  in insulation, 208, 217
  in joint compound, 255
  on piping, 294
  in roofing, 172–173
  sealing, 14
  siding, 65, 178, 188
Asphalt shingles, see Composition shingles
Asthma, 25, 39, 217
Author's home, 337–346
  illus. 340, 342

Baseboard heaters, 296–297
Basements, 131–135
  illus. 133
Bathroom, 77, 273–282
Bathtub, 278–279
Beeswax, 241
Board insulations, 211–214
Books, 57, 75, 134
Breathing of houses, 89–90, see also Airtightness
Bricks, see Masonry
Building codes, 59, 200
Building materials, 58–59, see also specific type
Building-related illness, 21–30, 32
  symptoms, 21–23
Built-up roofing, 174

Cabinets, 65–66, 78, 101, 273–276, 343
  reducing outgassing, 275
  illus. 274
Calcium chloride, 49, 80
Canaries, 25, 65
Carbon, see Activated carbon
Carbon dioxide, 12–14
Carbon monoxide, 12, 97
Carpeting, 31, 64, 75, 227–231
Carusorb, 320
Caulking, 75, 271–272
Cedar trees, 52

387